KT-568-611

Theory and research in promoting public health

Promoting public health: skills, perspectives and practice

This book forms part of an innovative series of structured teaching texts from The Open University, aiming to improve readers' understanding of modern multidisciplinary public health. The series consists of three books, *Theory and research in promoting public health* edited by Sarah Earle, Cathy E. Lloyd, Moyra Sidell and Sue Spurr, *Policy and practice in promoting public health*, edited by Cathy E. Lloyd, Stephen Handsley, Jenny Douglas, Sarah Earle and Sue Spurr, and *A Reader in promoting public health: challenge and controversy*, edited by Jenny Douglas, Sarah Earle, Stephen Handsley, Cathy E. Lloyd and Sue Spurr. These books form the core texts for The Open University's third-level undergraduate course, K311 *Promoting public health: skills, perspectives and practice*.

The books have four core themes:

- **power** and control and the ways these influence public health
- **change** in policy and practice and challenges to inequalities in health
- **diversity** of views, experiences and values about health and wellbeing
- **values and evidence** and how these inform public health theory and practice.

Theory and research in promoting public health

Edited by Sarah Earle, Cathy E. Lloyd, Moyra Sidell and Sue Spurr

The Open University

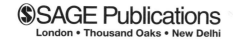

SAGE Publications
London • Thousand Oaks • New Delhi

Published by

Sage Publications
1 Oliver's Yard
55 City Road
London EC1Y 1SP

in association with

The Open University
Walton Hall
Milton Keynes MK7 6AA

First published 2007

Copyright © 2007 The Open University

All rights reserved. No part of this publication may be reproduced, stored in a retrieval system, transmitted or utilised in any form or by any means, electronic, mechanical, photocopying, recording or otherwise, without written permission from the publisher or a licence from the Copyright Licensing Agency Ltd. Details of such licences (for reprographic reproduction) may be obtained from the Copyright Licensing Agency Ltd, Saffron House, 6–10 Kirby Street, London EC1N 8TS; website http://www.cla.co.uk/

Open University course materials may also be made available in electronic formats for use by students of the University. All rights, including copyright and related rights and database rights, in electronic course materials and their contents are owned by or licensed to The Open University, or otherwise used by The Open University as permitted by applicable law.

In using electronic course materials and their contents you agree that your use will be solely for the purposes of following an Open University course of study or otherwise as licensed by The Open University or its assigns.

Except as permitted above you undertake not to copy, store in any medium (including electronic storage or use in a website), distribute, transmit or retransmit, broadcast, modify or show in public such electronic materials in whole or in part without the prior written consent of The Open University or in accordance with the Copyright, Designs and Patents Act 1988.

Edited and designed by The Open University.

Typeset in India by Alden Prepress Services, Chennai.

Printed and bound in Malta by Gutenberg Press.

This book forms part of an Open University course K311 *Promoting public health: skills, perspectives and practice*. Details of this and other Open University courses can be obtained from the Student Registration and Enquiry Service, The Open University, PO Box 197, Milton Keynes MK7 6BJ, United Kingdom: tel. +44 (0)870 333 4340, email general-enquiries@open.ac.uk

http://www.open.ac.uk

A catalogue record for this book is available from the British Library.

Library of Congress Control Number: 2006925363.

ISBN 978-1-4129-3070-3 (hardback)

ISBN 978-1-4129-3071-0 (paperback)

1.1

Mixed Sources
Product group from well-managed forests, and other controlled sources
www.fsc.org Cert no. TT-CoC-002424
FSC © 1996 Forest Stewardship Council

The paper used for this book is FSC-certified and totally chlorine-free. FSC (the Forest Stewardship Council) is an international network to promote responsible management of the world's forests.

Contents

Introduction *Sarah Earle*

Part I   Promoting public health

Introduction *Sarah Earle*

Chapter 1   Promoting public health: exploring the issues
Sarah Earle   1

Chapter 2   Exploring health *Sarah Earle*   37

Chapter 3   The factors that influence health *Sarah Earle and
Terry O'Donnell*   67

Chapter 4   Who promotes public health? *Jennie Naidoo and
Sarah Earle*   101

Chapter 5   Theoretical perspectives on promoting public health
Jane Wills and Sarah Earle   129

Chapter 6   Focusing on the health of children and young people
Sarah Earle   163

Part II   Researching health

Introduction *Sarah Earle*

Chapter 7   Researching health *Clive Pearson, Judy Thomas
and Cathy E. Lloyd*   199

Chapter 8   Studying the population's health *Moyra Sidell and
Cathy E. Lloyd, incorporating previously published material
from Jeanne Katz (2000)*   231

Chapter 9   Qualitative research towards public health
Linda Finlay   273

Chapter 10 Using research to plan multidisciplinary public
health interventions *Revised by Jenny Douglas, Cathy E. Lloyd
and Moyra Sidell, from an original chapter by Jones, Katz
and Sidell (2000)*   297

TMA 01

Chapter 11 Evaluating public health interventions *Revised
by Jenny Douglas, Moyra Sidell, Cathy E. Lloyd and Sarah Earle
from original chapters by Alyson Peberdy (2000)*   327

Chapter 12 Understanding obesity *Sarah Earle*   355

Index   393

About the authors

Sarah Earle is a Lecturer in Health and Social Care at the Open University and has been teaching in higher education for nearly fifteen years. She is a medical sociologist with an interest in reproductive health, sexuality and healthcare education and practice. She convenes the British Sociological Association's Human Reproduction Study Group and chairs the Birth and Death Research Group at the Open University. She is the co-author of *Sex in Cyberspace: men who pay for sex* (Ashgate, 2007) and co-editor of *The Sociology of Healthcare: A Reader for Health Professionals* (Palgrave, 2007), *Sociology for Nurses* (Palgrave, 2005) and *Gender, Identity and Reproduction: social perspectives* (Palgrave, 2003) as well as many other book chapters, papers and articles.

Cathy E. Lloyd is a Senior Lecturer in Health and Social Care at the Open University. She has worked in public health and epidemiology for more than twenty years both in the UK and USA. Her research interests include psycho-social aspects of chronic conditions, mental health, and minority ethnic health issues. She is Honorary Secretary of the Psycho-social Aspects of Diabetes Study Group and has a range of publications in national and international journals. She is currently principal investigator of a study examining alternative modes of data collection in South Asian communities in the UK. Before coming to the Open University nin years ago she was a Research Fellow at the University of Birmingham, Department of Epidemiology & Public Health.

Moyra Sidell was a Senior Lecturer in the Faculty of Health and Social Care at The Open University until 2003. She has published in the fields of women's health and the health of older people and has carried out research commissioned by the Department of Health on end of life care in care homes for older people.

Jenny Douglas is a Senior Lecturer in Health Promotion at the Open University. She has worked in health promotion and public health for more than twenty years. Her current research interests include 'race', ethnicity, gender and health; the organisational positioning of health promotion specialists; and cigarette smoking in African-Caribbean young women. Jenny has undertaken research and written widely about the health experiences of minority groups. Jenny chairs the Public Health and Health Promotion Research Group at the Open University. She is co-editor of *Promoting Health: Knowledge and Practice* (Palgrave/ Open University, 2000), *The Challenge of Promoting Health: Exploration and Action* (Palgrave/ Open University 2002) and *Debates and Dilemmas in Promoting Health* (Palgrave/ Open University 2003).

Judy Thomas is the Learning and Teaching Librarian Team Leader for the Faculties of Health and Social Care and Science at the Open University. She has led a number of initiatives in both faculties to ensure that students have the opportunity, when studying Open University courses, to develop their information literacy skills. Before joining the Open University she worked in nursing and medical libraries for more than ten years.

Sue Spurr is a Course Manager in the Faculty of Health and Social Care. She has contributed and edited a range of co-published Open University core texts and has a particular interest in complementary and alternative medicine.

Linda Finlay is a freelance Academic Consultant offering training and mentorship on how to apply qualitative research in health care. She also teaches and writes with the Open University in the Social Science and Health and Social Care faculties. Qualifying originally as an occupational therapist, she practised in the mental health field. She then pursued a more academic path after obtaining a psychology degree and PhD. She has published widely, being best known for her textbooks on psycho-social occupational therapy and groupwork. In the qualitative research area she has co-edited *Qualitative Research for Allied Health Professionals: challenging choices* (Wiley, 2006) with Claire Ballinger and *Reflexivity: A Practical Guide for Researchers in Health and Social Sciences* (Blackwell Publishing, 2003) with Brendan Gough.

Terry O'Donnell is a Health Sociologist who works in the Carnegie Faculty of Sport and Education at Leeds Metropolitan University. She has worked in post-registration health promotion education and training within further education and managed The Health Promoting College action research project in that sector. Current work is concerned with the sociology of the body, especially in relation to physical activity, and with critical perspectives on public health promotion.

Jennie Naidoo is Principal Lecturer in Health Promotion and Public Health at the University of the West of England. She has a background in sociology, health promotion, research and education. Jennie worked in health promotion and research for several years prior to taking up her post at UWE. Her research interests include gender and health, ethnicity and health and health in primary care and voluntary sector settings. She has written extensively on health promotion practice and theory, including the popular text *Health Promotion: Foundations for Practice*, which she co-authored with Jane Wills.

Jane Wills is a Reader in Public Health and Health Promotion at London South Bank University. Jane has taught health promotion for many years and published several textbooks. She has a particular interest in the development of the health promotion profession and has acted as a consultant to many NHS public health departments as they have developed their health improvement function. Jane is also visiting Professor of Health Promotion at the University of Witwatersrand, Johannesburg where she is developing a training programme for health promoters and involved in the evaluation of several community-based initiatives.

Clive Pearson is a sociologist. He has lectured at the University of Bradford and the University of Luton and held management positions at the University of Aberdeen and the Open University. He has tutored for the Open University since 1985. His most recent work has been with the Centre for Widening Participation at the Open University and he is co-author of Y157 *Understanding Society*, and Y158 *Understanding Health*. He is currently Development Officer for the Scottish Executive community development programme 'Initiative at the Edge', and a freelance educational consultant.

Other contributors

This book has grown out of debates and discussions in the K311 course team at The Open University. Besides the named authors, other team members who have contributed to the development of the book include Diane Charlesworth (Regional Academic (South West Region) in the Faculty of Health and Social Care), Philip Greaney (editor), Liz Rabone (editor), Gill Gowans (Copublishing), Cherryl Lewis (Course Team Assistant) and Liliana Torero-De-Clements (Course Team Assistant). The Open University course team would like to thank critical readers and developmental testers for their valuable comments on earlier draft chapters, and especially Professor Jackie Green, Leeds Metropolitan University, who, in her capacity as External Assessor, provided insightful and valuable comments.

Introduction

Sarah Earle

Promoting public health is everybody's business in that, directly or indirectly, everyone is involved in promoting the health of others, and everyone is affected by the health-promoting – and health-harming – actions of other people. This raises the question of whether it is possible to promote public health successfully without an understanding of some of the theoretical, conceptual or research issues that underpin public health practice. In this book, it is argued that effective modern multidisciplinary public health practice should be underpinned by relevant theoretical, conceptual and methodological knowledge, as well as the appropriate skills to enable individuals, families, communities, organisations and others to promote their own and other people's health.

Modern multidisciplinary public health in the twenty-first century includes a diverse range of practice, from the health education and health promotion activities carried out by public health practitioners working with individuals, groups and communities, to the actions of public health agencies involved in prevention, and the protection and surveillance of the public's health. It also includes the public health actions performed daily by lay people in promoting their own and other people's health, and the actions of the media and private commercial organisations, as well as those of civil society organisations such as faith groups and trade unions. As this book demonstrates, public health can be promoted both formally and informally within a wide variety of settings, including homes, hospitals, schools, nightclubs, and both on and off the street.

This book challenges everyone to promote public health in a way that recognises issues of power and diversity, acknowledges opportunities for change, and questions the values and evidence that can underpin public health practice and action. These issues – or themes – are developed throughout the book. 'Thinking points' – short, sometimes provocative questions – have been included and are designed to encourage the reader to reflect on the ever-changing debates and issues in the complex field of public health promotion.

The book is organised into two parts. Part I, 'Promoting public health', focuses on theoretical and conceptual concerns, while Part II, 'Researching multidisciplinary public health', focuses on issues of research, planning and evaluation. Each part contains six chapters and the final chapter within each part focuses on a substantive public health issue; this should encourage the reader to consider further the material presented in each part, and to reflect on and consolidate what they have read.

In Part I, some of the key issues and debates within public health are introduced, enabling the reader to develop a critical awareness of the concepts, models and values that underpin public health practice and action. Part I also introduces some of the key theoretical perspectives which help to shape knowledge, understanding and practice of public health. In addition, it provides a historical overview of modern multidisciplinary public health and introduces some of the key individuals who, and agencies and organisations which, are involved in, or influence, public health. In Chapter 6, the final chapter in Part I, these issues are brought together through an exploration of the health of children and young people.

Part II focuses on researching public health, as well as on planning and evaluating public health interventions. It seeks to make explicit the links between research and knowledge about health, to show that research influences how health issues are defined, how health policy is made and how public health initiatives are planned, carried out and evaluated. It contains discussion of both methodology and methods and critically analyses a variety of research methods in terms of their use and usefulness in public health promotion. This part of the book also aims to provide an analysis of the planning and evaluation of public health promotion initiatives. At the end of Part II, Chapter 12 brings these issues together in an exploration of obesity.

This book is part of the third level Open University course *Promoting public health: skills, perspectives and practice* (K311) and is published together with the companion volumes *Policy and Practice in Promoting Public Health* and *A Reader in Promoting Public Health: Challenge and Controversy*. All books are designed to engage the reader in a systematic review and critical assessment of current ways of working to promote public health, and seek to provide the skills, knowledge and understanding for the development, implementation and evaluation of new forms of practice. Each book aims to inform and empower everyone involved in promoting public health by exploring issues, innovations and dilemmas in modern multidisciplinary public health, with the two texts using a range of topical case studies, examples and thinking points.

In writing this book, the authors made use of text and illustrations from *Promoting Health: Knowledge and Practice* (edited by Jeanne Katz, Alyson Peberdy and Jenny Douglas) and *The Challenge of Promoting Health: Exploration and Action* (edited by Linda Jones, Moyra Sidell and Jenny Douglas), both published by Palgrave Macmillan for the preceding Open University course *Promoting health: skills, perspectives and practice* (K301). Any substantial use of these previous materials has been indicated in the list of authors of a particular chapter, but special thanks go to Linda Jones, Alyson Peberdy and Jeanne Katz.

Part 1
Promoting public health

Promoting public health begins from the premise that improving public health is a worthwhile activity, and Part I of this book encourages the reader to consider their responses to some of the many questions to which this inevitably gives rise. What is health-promoting activity? How should public health be promoted? Whose values are most important? Is one health promotion model more appropriate than another? Which theories can help inform public health practice? Part I provides a critical introduction to the theoretical and conceptual issues that underpin public health practice and action, and aims to engage the reader in relevant and contemporary debates.

Modern multidisciplinary public health is complex, diverse and continuously changing. Chapter 1, 'Promoting public health: exploring the issues', begins by analysing why public health promotion is fundamentally worthwhile and provides a brief historical overview of the field. This chapter also reflects on the importance of values and ethics in public health practice. However, just as the definition and history of modern multidisciplinary public health is complex and diverse, so, too, is the concept of health itself. Chapter 2, 'Understanding health', encourages critical reflection on health and considers the relationship between health and diversity. The chapter explores and contrasts several models and approaches to health, including the biomedical and social models, and holistic and salutogenic approaches. Concepts of health, as well as experiences of health, illness and disease, are socially stratified; inequalities in health and illness are long standing and well documented. Chapter 3, 'The factors that influence health', critically maps competing theoretical explanations for inequalities in health, exploring a range of factors that influence health, illness and disease, including, for example: sex and genetics; lifestyle and behaviour; community; living and working conditions; and social and environmental issues.

Given the very wide range of factors that influence health, promoting public health encompasses a broad range of activities that take place in a variety of settings. Chapter 4, 'Who promotes public health?', focuses on who is involved in promoting public health in both lay and professional capacities at local, regional, national and international levels. It introduces the reader to some of the people, settings, agencies and organisations that work – either directly or indirectly – to promote public health.

Chapter 5, 'Theoretical perspectives on promoting public health', discusses theories and models of health promotion, encouraging reflection on, and understanding of, the relationships between theory and practice. Theory can be used to analyse, predict or explain phenomena and, thus, can be helpful when deciding how best to promote public health. This chapter examines theories which explain behaviour at both individual and community levels, as well as focusing on theories of communication. It also examines models of health promotion which identify and map discrete approaches to public health practice.

The final chapter in Part I – Chapter 6, 'Focusing on the health of children and young people' – brings together some of these theoretical and conceptual issues. This chapter begins by looking briefly at the social construction of childhood and considers the politics and diversity of children's health, showing how childhood and children's health are both contested concepts which continue to change over time. It also draws on the views of children and young people to critically explore their concepts of health, focusing specifically on injury prevention, promoting positive mental health in schools, and promoting children's and young people's sexual health.

Chapter 1

TMA 01

Promoting public health: exploring the issues

Sarah Earle

Introduction

Promoting public health in the twenty-first century is a multidisciplinary endeavour ranging from the surveillance of health and disease in populations, through to the provision of health advice and information. It occurs at all levels, from the actions taken by individuals through to those taken by national and international agencies. It also takes place in many different settings: for example, in homes, workplaces, schools, hospitals, youth centres, nightclubs, and on the street.

There is widespread agreement on the significance of health, and improving the health of populations continues to be a major concern at local, national and international levels. National surveys in the UK (for example, see *British Social Attitudes Survey*, 2005) and more globally (for example, see Mossialos, 1997) have demonstrated that people are willing to spend more money on health services and that they rate good health as centrally important in living a full and satisfying life. There is now a heightened awareness of the need to promote public health.

But why promote health? To answer this question, this chapter begins by exploring the fundamental premise that every individual has the right to a healthy life. It then moves on in Section 1.2 to consider the historical origins of modern multidisciplinary public health, and in Sections 1.3 and 1.4, the role of values and ethics in promoting public health are considered.

1.1 Why promote public health?

In accordance with the UN Universal Declaration of Human Rights (1948), it is widely acknowledged that the right to health is inextricably linked to the ideal of freedom from fear and want. Rights can, therefore, be articulated positively (as the 'right to') and negatively (as 'freedom from'). This is further supported by Article 12 of The UN International Covenant on Economic, Social and Cultural Rights (1966) which recognises the right of everyone to the enjoyment of the highest attainable standard of physical and mental health. Of course, this does beg the question: what is health? This is discussed at length in the following chapter but, for the time being, one of the most commonly cited definitions of health is given below:

> Health is a state of complete physical, mental and social well-being and not merely the absence of disease or infirmity.
>
> (WHO, 1946, preamble)

It appears obvious that the absence of disease might be an achievable human right, but is a complete state of wellbeing achievable? In 1977 it was decided that the main social goal of governments and the World Health Organization (WHO) in the coming decades should be the attainment of a level of health that would permit all people to lead a socially and economically productive life; this goal is commonly known as *Health for All by the Year 2000* (HFA) (WHO, 1977). In the 1990s, HFA was developed to become *Health 21* (WHO, 1998), a new strategy for the twenty-first century which is thought to represent a more rigorous approach to health (see Box 1.1).

Box 1.1 *Health 21*: strategy for action

- Multisectoral strategies to tackle the determinants of health, taking into account physical, economic, social, cultural and gender perspectives, and using health impact assessment.

- Health-outcome-driven programmes and investments for health development and clinical care.

- Integrated family and community-oriented primary health care, supported by a flexible and responsive hospital system.

- A participatory health development process that involves relevant partners for health at home, school and work and at local community and country levels, and that promotes joint decision-making, implementation and accountability.

(WHO, 1998, p. 9)

According to this view, the matter of rights can be linked with the idea of citizenship and social justice. Both of these concepts are useful in understanding why public health should be promoted. According to Plant (1998), citizenship confers a right to central resources which provide health, education and economic security; the right to which exists irrespective of a person's standing in their society. The concept of social justice is based on a belief in the intrinsic worth of all human beings. The four principles of social justice are outlined below:

1 The foundation of a free society is the equal worth of all citizens.

2 Everyone is entitled, as a right of citizenship, to be able to meet their basic needs.

3 The right to self-respect and personal autonomy demands the widest possible spread of opportunities.

4 Not all inequalities are unjust, but unjust inequalities should be reduced and where possible eliminated.

(The Commission on Social Justice, 1998, p. 48)

Thinking point   do you believe that every individual has the right to health?

You may or may not agree with the view that every individual has the right to health: indeed, this right is the subject of social and political struggles throughout the world. But the concept of health as a right is not a modern phenomenon and can be traced back for many thousands of years (Adams et al., 2002). As such, the concept has become firmly entrenched in contemporary thinking about public health.

However, the relationships between health, social justice and citizenship are not without their critics. First, the idea of social justice is considered vague and the principles outlined above have been contested. Second, it raises difficult questions about the (re)distribution of resources and the question of equity. Although health may well be a fundamental social right, it may be difficult to enforce such a right when resources are scarce. For example, imagine that a local authority was allocating funding to promote physical activity in the community. Initiatives could be developed to support particular groups: younger people, older people, men, women, or people from minority ethnic groups. In an ideal world, the local authority would be able to support initiatives targeting all of these groups. However, in practice, and when resources are finite, this cannot be the case. While practitioners may wish to distribute resources fairly, hard decisions need to be made when such resources are scarce. The allocation of resources is therefore not simply a question of rights, but is also a moral, political, economic and social issue. As Reidpath et al. (2005) note, in any society, goods and resources are finite and it is social forces that heavily pattern their distribution.

1.1.1 The question of rights and responsibilities

Any discussion of rights also entails the question of responsibilities. Thus it follows that if health is a right, then 'who is responsible for health?' A survey of attitudes to public health (King's Fund, 2004) found that 89 per cent of people surveyed believed that individuals are responsible for their own health. At the same time, more than 40 per cent believed that there are too many factors outside of individual control to hold people entirely responsible for their health. Consider the issue of healthy eating: is the individual responsible for what he or she eats, or are the governments and policy makers responsible for their role in the politics of food production; and what of the role of manufacturers and marketing companies? Equal consideration should also be given to the way that choices are constrained by factors such as income and the cost of food, as well as the availability of 'healthy choices' in cafés, restaurants and shops.

Thinking point   who is responsible for your health?

To a certain extent it could be argued that everyone is individually responsible for their own health. But this is often mediated by other people, and influenced by factors that are often outside individuals' immediate control. Adams, Amos and Munro argue that health is: 'not primarily the result of individual choices or genetic lottery, but of the social structures and economic interests which surround us' (Adams et al. 2002, p. 1). Thus, health is fundamentally about the organisation of power and power relations.

Questions of freedom also enter into this debate: for example, consider how freedom may be restricted when the social right to health is enforced. Many travellers will experience long waiting times at airports while searches are conducted in the interests of security. It could be argued that, although inconvenient, this is a small price to pay for the protection of the wider public good. Box 1.2 illustrates how the banning of smoking in public places may be construed within a context of protecting the public from passive smoking. However, it also restricts the individual freedom of those who wish to continue smoking.

Box 1.2 The right to smoke

A man who was told by doctors he lost both his legs because of cigarettes is against plans to make Coventry a smoke-free city.

Wheelchair-bound Ron Morgan, who runs the city centre's toy museum in Much Park Street, had his right leg amputated below the knee in 1972. He lost his left leg two years later. The amputations were necessary because of blood clots – one of the health risks of smoking. Six months ago, Mr Morgan – who had packed in the fags for 10 years – started puffing again. The 79-year-old said he was against the city council-backed plans, adding: 'I'm dead against it. It's an infringement of freedom. I think it is way over the top. Smokers are normal intelligent people. They have weighed up the possible consequences and decided that the pleasures of smoking are worth taking a risk for. They say it shortens your life by three years but three years at the end of your life does not make any difference. And my life is as rich and as good as ever.'

> The city council and health chiefs in Coventry are looking at banning smoking in public places after a survey showed most people in the city backed the idea. This is not just to discourage habitual smokers but to protect vulnerable people, like bar staff, from the effects of passive smoking.
>
> (McCarthy, 2004)

The example above illustrates how difficult it can be to balance freedom **to** act (i.e. smoke) against freedom **from** other people's actions (i.e. passive smoking). However, in spite of the difficulties of putting this concept into practice, the right to health appears fundamental to the promotion of public health and seems to be widely accepted.

1.1.2 Health: the means to an end or an end in itself?

In the UK, patterns of health and disease have changed considerably over the last 150 years. Whereas life expectancy has increased worldwide, in the developed world the burden of disease has moved away from infectious, toxic and traumatic causes of death towards the challenges of managing the longer-term conditions associated with longevity and industrialisation (Wanless, 2002). In developing countries, many societies are also experiencing this transition. However, patterns of illness and disease have become increasingly complex with new infectious diseases such as HIV/AIDS and avian influenza (bird flu) affecting both the developed and developing worlds.

No doubt these shifts have influenced our overall sense of 'health consciousness', which Crawford defines as: 'a general heightened awareness and interest in health' (Crawford, 1980, p. 368). This heightened interest in health can be expressed in one of two ways: health can be seen as a means to an end or as an end in itself. Regardless of either position adopted, it is also important to consider health in relation to individuals, societies and the role of those who seek to promote good public health. Each of these positions is explored in turn.

If health is perceived as the means to an end, then good health is the vehicle to achieve other rewards in life. Seedhouse (1986) describes health as the 'foundations for achievement'. This implies that, without good health, the life chances – that is, individuals' ability to work, enjoy education, and establish and maintain social and personal relationships – are considerably reduced.

One way of thinking about this issue is to consider the effects of poor health. At the level of the individual, poor health is thought to considerably affect a person's life chances. In general, poor health is thought to prevent full participation in society. For example, consider the issue of employment.

Many studies have suggested that poor health can make it more difficult for individuals to move in and out of, and remain in, employment (for example, see Van de Mheen et al., 1999 and Elstad and Krokstad, 2003). Similar patterns can be found when comparing the effects of poor health on education. While not suggesting that poor health leads directly to all forms of inequality, it is clear that poor health can prevent individuals from enjoying their lives and participating fully in society. For example, in discussing the introduction of a Comprehensive Peace Agreement in Sudan following decades of war, David Nabarr, the WHO Representative of the Director-General states:

> the people of Sudan are not yet healthy enough to benefit fully from this opportunity. To reap the benefits of peace, Sudan's people must survive threats of disease ... Health must be given priority as experience from elsewhere indicates that sound investments in health are central to creating peace and promoting prosperity through consolidated public systems.

(WHO, 2005a)

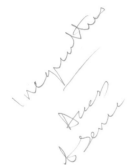

An alternative view is to see health as an end in itself. In other words, good health is seen as something that should be enjoyed for its own sake and other factors, such as poverty, are seen to influence the likelihood of being able to achieve good health. For example, a study of the Family Support Service in the multiracial area of Tower Hamlets, East London (Gray, 2003) describes how factors such as poverty, racism and overcrowding can exacerbate inequalities in health and prevent access to appropriate services. (Box 1.3 describes the account of an elderly Bangladeshi woman and her experiences of social isolation.) Gender, too, is another important factor. A gendered analysis of health shows how understandings of health, access to services and the policy agenda are gendered concerns – an issue that will be considered in later chapters (for example, see Cameron and Bernardes, 1998).

Box 1.3 Social isolation, crime and harassment

Both young and older people from the Bangladeshi community in Tower Hamlets said they felt vulnerable to theft and harassment:

'I had a mugger who took my money. The mugger was a boy from the flats. The mugger hit me as well, so I reported it to the police ... I lost so much blood and was in a very bad way ... Now I'm afraid to go outside myself and I'm afraid for my son to go outside alone.'

(Gray, 2003, p. 370)

The idea of health as an end in itself is not without its critics. Crawford, for example, suggests that health has become synonymous with good living, arguing that:

> In short, health has become not only a preoccupation; it has also become a pan-value or standard by which an expanding number of behaviors and social phenomena are judged. Less a means towards the achievement of other fundamental values, health takes on the quality of an end in itself. Good living is reduced to a health problem, just as health is expanded to include all that is good in life.
>
> (Crawford, 1980, pp. 380–1)

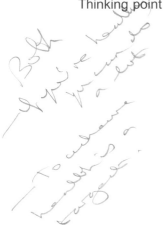

Thinking point   do you consider health to be a means to an end or an end in itself?

Although health can be seen as either a means to an end or an end in itself, in practice, health is often both a means and an end. Whatever your point of view, the relationship between health and achievement can be complicated further still. In relation to developing countries, Manderson states:

> Economic development, in general, in the long term will usually result in improved health for the population, but the ability of a country to invest in economic development is impeded where the health status of the population is poor, and certain development strategies and projects may compromise rather than improve people's health.
>
> (Manderson, 1998, 109–10)

For example, the International Financial Institutions (IFI) – the International Monetary Fund (IMF) and the World Bank (WB) – have been heavily criticised for their policies of structural adjustment. (These include currency devaluation, managed balance of payments, cuts in social spending, and business deregulation.) While the IMF claims that such a policy will reduce poverty, others argue that it has increased poverty and reduced spending on health, education and development in favour of debt repayment and economic restructuring. Chapter 4 considers the important role of international organisations in health. The next section provides a brief historical overview of the origins of modern multidisciplinary public health.

1.2 The origins of modern multidisciplinary public health

This chapter began with a statement describing the promotion of public health in the twenty-first century as a multidisciplinary endeavour. In outline, it consists of a range of activities, performed by different people in a variety of settings and levels, and is thus both complex and diverse. It includes people working within different paradigms, or worldviews, and (as you will see in Section 1.3) with different yet overlapping sets of values. It also embraces a range of multidisciplinary approaches to health research, planning, evaluation, policy making and action, all of which will be addressed in subsequent chapters. Modern multidisciplinary public health is referred to as 'public health' throughout this book.

1.2.1 What is modern multidisciplinary public health?

Public health may be improved by treating disease, by minimising or preventing the onset of sickness and enhancing the health of those who are already reasonably healthy. In addition, health maintenance for those who are sick – those who have become known as 'healthy ill people' – has become widely accepted within the remit of health and social care for those with long-term conditions. Reducing inequalities in health by improving the health of individuals and communities in a sustained manner also falls within the remit of promoting public health. In short, modern multidisciplinary public health includes a wide range of activities, reflecting the diversity of its historical origins, and because of this, many terms and definitions are used to describe the actions that promote public health. These terms are outlined in Figure 1.1, which provides a brief definition of each and an illustrative example. Of course, whilst attempts at definitions can be useful, it is worth bearing in mind that the meaning and significance of these terms has changed over time and will continue to do so. In practice (and within the literature on the subject) these terms are often used interchangeably and, sometimes, without proper consideration. For example, Tilford, Green and Tones (2003) have suggested that the terms 'health development' and 'health promotion' could be used interchangeably without serious difficulty. Likewise, MacDonald has argued: 'That it would not be reasonable to assume that ... those with a "health promotion" label do anything very different from those with either the "public health", "health improvement", or "health development" labels' (MacDonald, 2001, p. 38). As the Chief Medical Officer for England has stated: 'All these definitions reflect the fact that health and wellbeing is dependent on a range of social, economic, environmental, biological and service factors ... Different words are used to describe similar goals by those in organisations that contribute to better health and wellbeing.' (DoH, 2001. p. 6).

Figure 1.1 Promoting public health: scope of activity

Health education	A process that includes: giving of information and advice; the development of knowledge, attitudes, values and skills to enable individuals to take control of their own health; and empowering people to make informed choices about their health (e.g. breastfeeding support)
Health development	First used in 1997 by the WHO to describe a process of continuous, progressive improvement of the health status of individuals and groups in a population with an emphasis on sustainability (e.g. Healthy Cities Programme)
Health improvement	This tends to be used in connection with the health aspect of community planning, in particular focusing on the tackling of health inequalities at a local level (e.g. food co-operatives)
Health policy	The actions of governments, and others, aimed at maintaining and improving the population's health by 'adding years to life' and 'adding life to years' (e.g. the National Service Framework for Diabetes)
Healthy public policy	This focuses on structural change and is based on the 1986 Ottawa Charter for Health Promotion (WHO, 1986) and the Adelaide Charter (WHO, 1988) (e.g. fiscal measures)
Health promotion	The process of enabling people to increase control over, and to improve their health (WHO, 1986) (e.g. Healthy Living Centres)
Health protection	The protection of populations from: communicable diseases (e.g. tuberculosis); non-communicable environmental hazards (e.g. chemical fires); and to deliver emergency responses (e.g. to bioterrorist attack)
Modern multidisciplinary public health	The science and art of preventing disease, prolonging life and promoting health through organised efforts of society (see Acheson, 1998)
'New' public health	The 'new' public health movement began in the 1970s and is ideologically linked to the health reforms of the nineteenth century. It recognises the limitations of healthcare in improving public health and looks beyond this to the social, economic and environmental factors that influence health (e.g. the recommendations made by the Acheson Report, 1998).
Prevention of ill-health	Three levels of prevention can be identified: • Primary prevention, which aims to prevent the onset of disease (e.g. immunisation) • Secondary prevention, which aims to detect and cure disease at an early stage (e.g. cervical cancer screening) • Tertiary prevention, which aims to minimise the effects or reduce progression of an already established disease (e.g. hip-replacement surgery)
'Old' public health	In the nineteenth and early twentieth centuries, the public health movement aimed predominantly to control filth, odour and contagion (e.g. National Public Health Act, 1848). The rise of social medicine as a medical specialism in the twentieth century also led to the establishment of surveillance systems for disease.

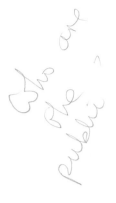

In any discussion of promoting public health it is also necessary to ask the question: **who is the 'public'**? Heller, Heller and Pattison (2003) suggest that there are four different ways of conceptualising the 'public' in public health, namely as:

1   merely decorative, a label used to make interventions more acceptable to the public
2   legitimising population-level interventions as sanctioned by the 'public'
3   a way of denoting the all-encompassing scope of a profession
4   a political endeavour, hence accountable to the public.

Thinking point   what do you understand by the 'public' in public health?

The concept of the 'public' is sometimes used in place of 'community' (Handsley, 2007). However, when thinking about promoting public health it is important to remember the issue of diversity and the fact that there is likely to be more than one public, comprising of a collection of groups with different interests, as well as more than one way of relating to these 'publics'.

Public interest in health is also becoming increasingly commonplace. Sang (2004) suggests four reasons for this increase in public involvement:

1   We are all fellow citizens with rights and responsibilities in relation to health.
2   We need to learn to facilitate dialogue at every level in every process.
3   We need to learn to manage our own lives and health journeys to enable us to challenge dominant cultures.
4   We need to be aware that co-operation between service users, across service boundaries can make a positive difference.

(Adapted from Sang, 2004)

Distinction needs to be made, however, between public consultation, defined as an attempt to seek the views of a broad constituency of persons, and user involvement, defined as a local attempt to include organised groups of service users in the planning, management and evaluation of services (Harrison and Mort, 1998). It is also important to ask whether increasing public participation in health should serve to increase consumer choice or simply to give a voice to the public.

These are all important issues, but to better understand modern multidisciplinary public health it is essential to consider its history (for example, see Sram and Ashton, 2007). While this is often neglected, a historical overview can enhance understanding of both public health action and research (Perdiguero et al., 2001).

There are numerous descriptions which trace the roots of modern public health and the adversarial tension between prevention and treatment back into antiquity. Of particular importance are the Greek mythological characters Hygeia and Panakeia, both daughters of the god of healing, Asclepius. Hygeia, the goddess of health (and from where we take the term 'hygiene') represented the preservation of health by living healthily. Her worshippers emphasised prevention rather than cure, and the importance of living in harmony with the environment. In contrast, goddess Panakeia (meaning 'cure-all') represented the restoration of health by the cure and treatment of disease. This adversarial tension is reflected in the diverse history of what is now described as modern multidisciplinary public health. This section now turns to a discussion of public health's more recent history, beginning with a discussion of public health in the nineteenth century.

1.2.2 Nineteenth-century public health

In the nineteenth century rapid industrialisation and urbanisation, coupled with a doubling of the population from an estimated nine million to eighteen million, led to a crisis in public health which had never known such urgency (Hodgkinson, 1973). Most histories of public health begin with a discussion of what is known as the 'sanitation phase' in the mid-nineteenth century, a period characterised by concentration on environmental issues such as housing, working conditions, the supply of clean water and the safe disposal of waste, also known as 'old' public health. Explanations for this vary but the motivating force of this public health movement is thought to be a concern with economic efficiency and better social cohesion between the working poor and other sectors of society (Webster and French, 2002). However, philanthropic concern and notions of social justice were also influential at this time.

There has also been a significant investment in many countries in creating infrastructures and services to protect health and to prevent ill-health. In most industrialising countries over the last 150 years, public health regulations and health and safety legislation have been enacted to provide safeguards for the industrial workforce, to control pollution levels in rivers, and to ensure proper sewerage and drainage, even if they have not always been enforced (see Figure 1.2). In nineteenth-century England, sanitary reformers and radical politicians argued, on economic grounds, for ill-health prevention through public policy interventions. In 1847 William Henry Duncan was appointed the first Medical Officer of Health (MOH). This was followed by the appointment of John Simon as MOH for the City of London in 1848. In that same year, the first Public Health Act introduced a Central Board of Health and, after that, MOHs were appointed in other areas, and took the lead in supervising improvements in health. Joseph Chamberlain, mayor of Birmingham, pushed through an ambitious improvement programme in 1875 by claiming that: 'We may hope to see disease and crime removed' and: 'The cost of the gaol, the hospital and the workhouse is infinitely greater than that of any sanitary improvement which the most extravagantly-minded man can devise' (Jones, 1995).

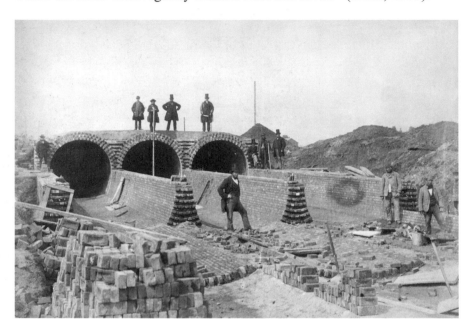

Figure 1.2   Sanitary improvements in nineteenth century England

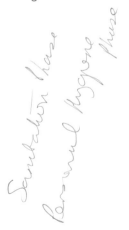

At around this time voluntary visiting of the poor began to gain popularity. Volunteer visitors were usually well-meaning middle-class women who were appalled by the dreadful living conditions of the urban poor. It is thought that the health visiting role emerged from this, supported by the MOHs, in 1867 the Manchester and Salford Ladies Sanitary Reform Association employed a 'respectable' working woman to assist the 'lady volunteers' in their sanitary inspection work (Dingwall, 1977).

Slum clearance, the paving of city streets and other similar measures were seen as paying long-term dividends in creating healthy and orderly communities run on hygienic principles (Jones, 1995). The sanitation phase of the public health movement emphasised environmental change. This sanitation phase, which led to a considerable and measurable reduction in infectious diseases – especially diphtheria, tuberculosis and cholera – was followed by the second phase, known as the personal hygiene era of the early twentieth century.

1.2.3 The rise of health education in the early twentieth century

The focus on environmental health was eclipsed by a more individualistic approach to health. During the personal hygiene era, the assertion that 'prevention was cheaper than cure' helped to persuade local authorities to extend health services beyond prevention of disease towards a notion of improving health through health education. For example, schoolchildren were taught hygienic principles (see Figure 1.3) and parents (particularly mothers) were instructed in hygiene, nutrition and childcare through home visiting (Lewis, 1980).

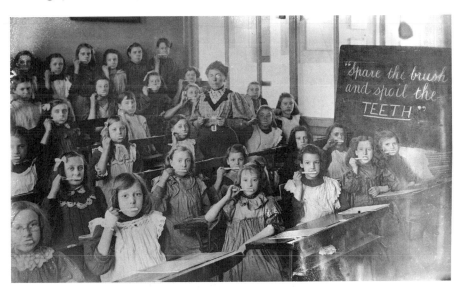

Figure 1.3   Teeth brushing. 'Spare the brush and spoil the teeth'. Schoolgirls in a dental hygiene class

This phase focused on the vulnerable in society and is typified by a focus on education and hygiene, locating the responsibility for improvements in health firmly with the individual. Children's health was seen as vital for ensuring adult health – a view that perpetuates (see Chapter 6). However, the Newsholme Report (1936), whilst identifying the importance of poverty, maintained that 'motherhood ignorance' was largely to blame for poor child health. Continuing with the role of the 'mothers' friend', health visiting by the 1920s had become a part of the expanding local authorities' services, and were accountable to the MOHs.

The initial focus of health provision in the UK was on health education, and for many health professionals providing information, advice, personal skills and support remains a key concern. The Central Council for Health Education was first established in 1927, financed by local authority public health departments. Its main tasks were to provide information which would persuade the public to change to healthier habits, in particular to safer sexual practices. The Health Education Council (HEC) was created in England in 1968 as a non-governmental organisation with an objective to create: 'A climate of opinion generally favourable to health education, develop blanket programmes of education and (target) selected priority subjects' (HEC, 1968). Similar health education agencies were set up in

Northern Ireland, Wales and Scotland. In addition to mass publicity campaigns, the HEC launched national programmes such as 'Look After Yourself' (LAY), which emphasised the links between personal behavioural changes and better health.

Fierce lobbying and political manoeuvring characterised the HEC's history (Sutherland, 1987; Pattison and Player, 1991). Above all, the links between smoking and lung cancer and between poor diet and illhealth, which had been well researched and were increasingly hard to ignore, pointed to the need to confront tobacco companies and even to try and influence food producers through the body responsible, the Ministry of Agriculture, Fisheries and Food. Yet pressure was exerted to ensure that the health messages targeted individual behaviour (see Figure 1.4). *Prevention and Health: Everybody's Business* (Department of Health and Social Security (DHSS), 1976), commenting on smoking-related diseases, alcohol misuse and other drug dependencies, obesity and its consequences, and sexually transmitted diseases, saw all these as 'preventable problems' about which 'the individual must decide for himself [sic]' (DHSS, 1976). At this time, the huge expenditure on advertising the risks of health damaging products was at this stage not seen as a central health issue.

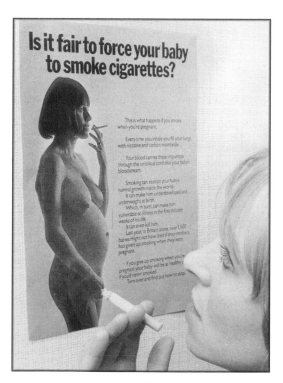

Figure 1.4   Health warning

1.2.4 The 'new' public health movement

The Lalonde Report, *A New Perspective on the Health of Canadians* (Lalonde, 1974), represents an important milestone in thinking about health, and it provided the first real framework for action. (This influential report is explored in more detail in Chapter 3.) The Lalonde Report was timely in that it reflected the current concerns of many governments with the high levels of spending on health services without the subsequent high returns in health improvement. The Health Field Model developed by Lalonde, which focused on environment, lifestyles, healthcare organisations and human biology, sought to show how health could be improved by focusing on all four aspects of health. Here began what is known as the 'new' public health movement, which recognised the importance of environment as well as individual behaviour and eventually re-established the importance of the wider social and economic factors in influencing health – moving the focus away from healthcare services.

During the 1980s, a flurry of reports indicated the need to take broader action on health. The HEC and the Scottish Health Education Group increasingly tangled with government departments over the extent to which both should attempt to influence and change public policy. The National Advisory Committee on Nutritional Education (NACNE, 1983) reported that the British diet was too high in saturated fats, sugar and salt, and too low in fibre; and that this was adding to the burden of cardiovascular and digestive tract diseases. The British Medical Association (BMA) strongly backed a campaign against smoking (Action on Smoking and Health, or ASH) which called for a ban on tobacco advertising and stricter regulation of sales.

The links between poverty, unemployment and poor health, which had been highlighted in many parts of Europe at the end of the nineteenth century, began to be 'rediscovered'. In many ways this was a response to the more individualistic and, some would say, victim-blaming approach of health education. In the UK, for example, a major study of poverty (Townsend, 1979) and a government-sponsored report on health (*The Black Report on Inequalities in Health*, DHSS, 1980) both pointed to the close relationship between health and poverty. Social-class gradients in health were identified: in other words, semi- and unskilled groups had much lower life expectancy and experienced more illhealth than those in the non-manual and professional groups. A follow-up report sponsored by the HEC indicated that in some areas the health gap had widened (Whitehead, 1987). The official launch of this report was cancelled and an alternative press conference hastily convened. This was soon followed by the demise of the HEC, considered an undesirable QUANGO (Quasi-Autonomous Non-Governmental Organisation) and its replacement by the Health Education Authority (HEA) which was less independent from government. Whitehead's report indirectly fuelled the call for a broader view of health and health services, which acknowledged how agencies outside the health

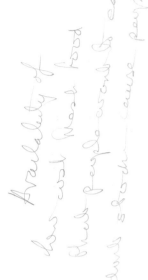

sector might enhance or damage health, and a shift of resources towards prevention, health protective legislation and health promotion (Rodmell and Watt, 1986).

1.2.5 The health promotion movement

By the mid-1980s it became more widely acknowledged that effective health education involved making healthier choices easier by modifying the circumstances, environment and policy frameworks within which people led their lives so that they had more opportunities to choose a healthier lifestyle. This required health to be prioritised on the public policy agenda so that policy making in every sector became newly 'health promoting'. *Health For All by the Year 2000* (WHO, 1977, 1985), while endorsing health education, proposed a wider agenda which involved socio-economic change. There were calls to change health sector priorities and invest in health promotion and prevention rather than clinical and curative services. Health promotion embraced the community development approach which involved supporting local residents in actions to improve their health. The health promotion movement recognised that people's capacity to take action was limited by environmental circumstances.

The *Ottawa Charter for Health Promotion* (WHO, 1986) provided a further impetus to an emerging modern health promotion movement, also focusing on the significance of empowerment. It identified five key themes, helping to define and shape the promotion of health (see Box 1.4).

Box 1.4 The Ottawa Charter

- **Build healthy public policy**: putting health on the agenda of policy makers in all sectors and at all levels, directing them to be aware of the health consequences of their decisions and to accept their responsibilities for health.

- **Create supportive environments**: systematic assessment of the health impact of a rapidly changing environment... is essential. The protection of the natural and built environment and the conservation of natural resources must be addressed in any health promotion strategy.

- **Strengthen community action**: health promotion works through concrete and effective community action in setting priorities, making decisions, planning strategies and implementing them to achieve better health. At the heart of this process is the empowerment of communities.

- **Develop personal skills**: health promotion supports personal and social development through providing information, education for health and enhancing life skills.

> • **Reorientation of health services**: the role of the health sector must move increasingly in a health promotion direction, beyond its responsibility for providing clinical and curative services.
>
> (Adapted from WHO, 1986)

In relation to promoting public health, empowerment refers to: 'A process through which people gain greater control over decisions and actions affecting their health' (Nutbeam, 1998, p. 6). The concept stems from the work of Freire (1970), a Brazilian philosopher and educator, who was concerned with the powerlessness of the lowest social classes and the relationship between power and knowledge. However, empowerment is not just a process, but can also be a goal in that it is also defined as the possession of power (Tones, 1994). Nutbeam (1998) also makes the distinction between individual and community empowerment. Individual empowerment (or self-empowerment) refers to the ability of the individual to have power over his or her own life. In health terms, community empowerment refers to the way in which individuals can act collectively to influence the determinants of health and the quality of life in their community. Although the concept of empowerment is not without criticism, it has become the cornerstone of practice for many individuals and groups engaged in public health action.

Over the last twenty years the Ottawa Charter has been highly influential and a constant point of reference for all those involved in promoting public health. However, despite its role as a significant landmark in the field, it has been criticised for creating a catch-all framework for promoting health in which priorities are unclear. Empowering communities, for example, means attending to their agendas for change, but which may be in tension with demands to build healthy public policy and supportive environments. Developing personal skills, which relates to the fourth aspect of the Ottawa Charter, implies that, once in place, people will opt for healthier lifestyles. Yet people are often sceptical about health information and offering them more may not alter this.

Some critics maintain that health and illhealth are determined by socio-economic and political structures and power relationships, and that attempts to change personal behaviour through empowerment are essentially misconceived (Tesh, 1988). For others, such as Kelly and Charlton (1995), the concern lies in the requirement that health should be prioritised by agencies, governments and individuals, who may have other valid priorities. The broad, all-encompassing agenda in the Ottawa Charter also extends health and the promotion of health into yet more parts of social life - global governance, communities, relationships, self-care - a trend that Armstrong (1993, 1995) has termed 'the rise of surveillance medicine'.

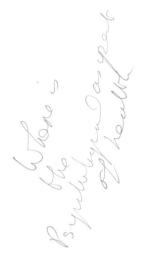

Surveillance critics, building on a long-standing critique of the medicalisation of everyday life (Zola, 1972, Crawford, 1980) claim that health promotion acts as a form of social regulation by shaping people's thinking about their bodies, relationships and lifestyles (Nettleton and Bunton, 1995); more is said about this in the next chapter.

Of course, not everyone would agree with these criticisms. The Ottawa Charter drew attention to the wide range of factors that influence health. Indeed, creating environments that enable people to live healthier lives has now become a central concern of health promotion. Successive WHO conferences over the last twenty years have emphasised healthy public policy as a central part of promoting health, and there has been a call to build on older public health traditions which improved people's health by tackling housing, sanitary and environmental causes of illhealth. Contemporary health promotion puts great emphasis on improving health through changing people's environments and living conditions (Ashton and Seymour, 1988) and focuses on public policy change rather than individual behaviour.

The roots of modern health promotion, therefore, lie in a concern with both the environment and collective measures in health improvement, health education and the individual. The influence of the WHO in mobilising modern health promotion cannot be underestimated.

The Bangkok Charter for Health Promotion in a Globalized World (WHO, 2005b) which was developed, amid some controversy, at the 6th Global Conference on Health Promotion, builds upon the principles of the Ottawa Charter. Here it was argued that the global context of health has changed considerably since the development of the Ottawa Charter, and that changing patterns of consumption and communication, increased urbanisation and commercialisation, and increasing inequalities within and between countries require a charter that addresses the determinants of health in a globalised world. An outline of the Bangkok Charter is given below in Box 1.5.

Box 1.5 The Bangkok Charter

Effective interventions

- Progress towards a healthier world requires strong political action, broad participation and sustained advocacy.
- Health promotion has an established repertoire of proven effective strategies which need to be fully utilized.

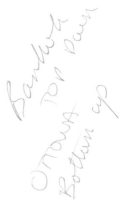

Required actions

To make further advances in implementing these strategies, all sectors and settings must act to:

- **advocate** for health based on human rights and solidarity.

- **invest** in sustainable policies, actions and infrastructure to address the determinants of health.

- **build capacity** for policy development, leadership, health promotion practice, knowledge transfer and research, and health literacy.

- **regulate and legislate** to ensure a high level of protection from harm and enable equal opportunity for health and well-being for all people.

- **partner and build alliances** with public, private, nongovernmental and international organizations and civil society to create sustainable actions.

A commitment that required actions will be to make promotion of health

- central to the global development agenda

- a core responsibility for all of government

- a key focus of communities and civil society

- a requirement for good corporate practice.

(Adapted from WHO, 2005b)

Thinking point   how does the Bangkok Charter relate to the themes set out in the Ottawa Charter?

The Bangkok Charter focuses on the first three themes of the Ottawa Charter, probably because these have been the most neglected within health promotion. However, that is not to say that personal health skills and reorienting health services are unimportant. Arguably, if all five strands of the Ottawa Charter were pursued in parallel then this would have a huge impact on health (IUHPE, 2001).

1.2.6 Promoting public health in the twenty-first century and beyond

To date, the promotion of public health in the twenty-first century has been characterised by considerable change and, some would say, has come full circle, returning to 'old' public health. The uneasy relationship between health promotion and new public health, and their respective haggling for territories, has not been resolved. Of late, their histories have been characterised by a concern with the so-called demise of health promotion and (for most people) its incorporation under the banner of modern multidisciplinary public health (see Tilford et al., 2003; Douglas, 2007). A concern with clarifying the nature of the public health function, the restructuring of the public health workforce and the ongoing development of competency frameworks are also characteristic of this field in the twenty-first century and beyond.

In *The Report of the Chief Medical Officer's Project to Strengthen the Public Health Function* (DoH, 2001), the public health workforce was organised into three key categories:

1   **Public health specialists**: those working at a strategic or senior level to promote the public's health (e.g. Directors of Public Health; Consultants in Public Health Medicine)

2   **Public health practitioners**: those who spend all or most of their time working in public health practice (e.g. health visitors; specialist community public health nurses; environmental health officers)

3   **The wider public health workforce**: those who promote public health through their work (e.g. nurses, transport engineers and social workers).

Drawing on this, Wanless carried out an independent review of the long-term resource requirements for the NHS published in two main reports. *Securing our Future Health: Taking a Long-term View* (Wanless, 2002) set out the challenge of full engagement in health. This 'fully engaged scenario' is described as:

> levels of public engagement in relation to their health are high: life expectancy increases go beyond current forecasts, health status improves dramatically and people are confident in the health system and demand high quality care. The health service is responsive with high rates of technology uptake, particularly in relation to disease prevention. Use of resources is more efficient.
>
> (Wanless, 2002, p. 35)

The White Paper *Choosing Health: Making Healthier Choices Easier* (DoH, 2004) endorsed the idea that individuals need more information and support to help them make healthier choices and sought to encourage healthier lifestyles.

In the second report, Wanless (2004) highlighted the importance of the wider public health workforce, and the need to strengthen the role of public health practitioners and the specialist workforce in realising this fully engaged scenario. As part of this, the Royal Institute of Public Health and Hygiene, the Faculty of Public Health, and the Multidisciplinary Public Health Forum (under the banner of the Tripartite Group) have developed ten standards for public health specialists (see Box 1.6). These ten standards map onto the broad areas developed as the national occupational standards for the practice of public health by *Skills for Health* (2004) which currently has sixty-eight competencies. *Read*

Box 1.6 Ten standards for public health specialists

1 Surveillance and assessment of the population's health and wellbeing

2 Promoting and protecting the population's health and wellbeing

3 Developing quality and risk management within an evaluative culture

4 Collaborative working for health

5 Developing health programmes and services and reducing inequalities

6 Policy and strategy development and implementation

7 Working with and for communities

8 Strategic leadership for health

9 Research and development

10 Ethically managing self, people and resources

(Skills for Health, 2004, p. 6)

The Tripartite Group has also set up the UK Voluntary Register for Public Health for those who meet the standards. The voluntary register was opened in 2003 for 'generalist specialists' – those working at consultant, specialist or director level. The UK Voluntary Register Board is also expected to outline registration for 'defined specialists', such as health promotion practitioners, in 2006.

These changes have also coincided with changes to the role of Director of Public Health and their appointment within primary care. However, unlike the Directors of Public Health, who had to be medically qualified in the former health authorities, this is not the case for Primary Care Trust (PCT) Directors of Public Health. Arguably, this change will bridge the gap between clinical and non-clinical leadership in public health and provide equality of professional status between the two. However, not everybody agrees with this: 'The idea that harmonised public health ... will somehow bridge the competency gap between those with extensive clinical experience and those without, is a fallacy' (Patterson, 2001, pp. 1593–6). Other changes have also taken place. For example, in 2004 the Nursing and

Midwifery Council opened a three-part register which includes the specialist community public health nurse – formerly a health visitor – with a remit for preventing illhealth and protecting and promoting health. Some see this as an opportunity for health visitors to engage in more radical health promotion activities within a wider public health role (Smith, 2004; Weeks et al., 2005), whereas others are more sceptical.

Now that the historical origins and more contemporary history of modern multidisciplinary public health have been considered, this chapter considers the role of values in promoting public health.

1.3 Exploring values in multidisciplinary public health

Values are important to the way that we think and act. The definition of promoting public health that we feel comfortable with, and the values underpinning it, will reflect our education and professional training (if any) and will be influenced by our work and life experiences. Some people may feel comfortable with a definition that emphasises medical treatment: that is, they may value secondary and tertiary prevention with a strong emphasis on the individual. On the other hand, others may well question this approach and see the central thrust of promoting health as influencing healthy public policy, valuing health development and improvement. Some may be less concerned with health at the level of the individual than with influencing groups and populations through media campaigns, community action or legislative change, thus valuing justice and equality. Yet for others, key values may be promoting client autonomy and anti-discriminatory practice.

To some extent the distinction between these different occupational groups is artificial and there are as many overlaps as there are differences. In a study of values amongst the public health workforce, Tilford et al. (2003) found that the values of those who identified themselves as working in 'health promotion' were slightly different from those working in 'public health', although there were considerable overlaps (see Box 1.7).

Box 1.7 Core values in the public health workforce

Health Promotion workers value	Public Health workers value
Equity	Equity
Equality	Equality
Justice/fairness	Justice/fairness

Autonomy/self determination	Autonomy
Empowerment	Empowerment
Health	Prevention
	Protection

(Adapted from Tilford et al., 2003, p. 77)

[handwritten annotations: "Difference" (circling Autonomy/self determination), "Difference", "Only Differences", "Difference"]

Thinking point   what are your own values in relation to public health?

[handwritten margin notes: "Cause of Population as a whole Communities", "Vaccination Programmes", "Health + Safety policy", "personal access to Health", "Individual"]

Writing about the role of values in promoting public health, Tilford et al. argue that:

> Values influence the ways that health issues are understood, the ways that knowledge and theoretical bases are developed and the nature of strategies identified for health improvement ... the selection of activities that are undertaken to promote health and the priorities accorded to actions, the balance between activities at individual and population levels, the relationships with individuals and communities who participate in initiatives, the goals which are being sought, and decisions about means and ends in achieving the goals.
>
> (Tilford et al., 2003, p. 120)

However, Seedhouse (2004), writing specifically about health promotion, argues that many people continue to avoid asking one of the most fundamental questions of all: **what is it that drives health promotion?** (See Box 1.8). St Leger (2001) also argues that although many practitioners and specialists are developing and employing high levels of technical competency, concerns with benchmarking and best practice are dominating our thinking about promoting public health. Like Seedhouse, he argues that there is a need to focus on what drives the promotion of public health. Exploring the underlying values adopted within this diverse field is fundamental to understanding activities that are designed to promote public health.

[handwritten margin note: "? Swine Flu"]

Box 1.8 Promoting public health: what drives health promotion?

Is public health promotion driven by evidence?

1   There is evidence of preventable health problems (this evidence is either factual or highly probable – and it is health promotion's main drive).

2   There are strategies designed to deal with the preventable problems (there is usually a choice of strategy, and values may be one of the factors influencing the choice).

Driven by values?

1   Health promoters hold particular values and political philosophies.

2   There is evidence of preventable health problems (this evidence is selected according to values and political philosophy – even the decision to call something a health problem or not is thus inspired though this is not to say that the evidence is entirely shaped by prejudice – there can be better and worse reasons to intervene).

3   Strategies designed to deal with preventable health problems are selected according to values, political philosophy and evidence – the key questions are: do we think this ought to be done and will it work?

(Adapted from Seedhouse, 2004, p.90, Figures 7 and 9)

A value implies a positive ethical ideal: many social scientists believe that the way in which the social world is understood is not neutral in that it is shaped by values. It is important to recognise that actions are shaped by values even when individuals believe themselves to be behaving objectively or independently. Although objectivity is not possible, and often not desirable, recognising the influence of values or 'prejudices' (Seedhouse, 2004) on practice is important.

The status of knowledge and 'evidence' will be discussed in more detail in later chapters, but first it is important to make good the claim that promoting public health involves values. The judgements people make about health grow out of their life experiences and influence their attitudes and the actions they take. There is a strong connection between thinking and doing and this is the case in public health promotion as well. Values are integral to promoting public health even though they are sometimes implicit rather than explicit. The next section draws on ethics to further explore the role of values.

1.4 Ethical issues in promoting public health

Ethics is a branch of philosophy concerned with the basis of moral judgements, principles and values. At its most abstract, ethics is concerned with questions such as the meaning of 'right' and 'wrong', but it is also concerned with the practical application of ethics, such as those that affect health and social care. An awareness of ethical issues is fundamental to an understanding of public health promotion since ethical dilemmas arise at almost every turn in the practice of promoting health. Wikler and Cash suggest that the following dilemmas are particularly salient:

> Those who would save lives through public health measures must prioritise and, thus, decide which lives to save.
>
> Interventions usually protect health, but because they sometimes carry risks, the claims of those who might be harmed must be heard.
>
> Public health programmes sometimes require compromises with values such as privacy and liberty.
>
> The pursuit of global public health takes place in an unjust world, demanding its practitioners judge when and to what extent to compromise their ideals and standards in order to remain effective.
>
> Practitioners of public health must sometimes choose between the objectives and interests of the communities they serve, the donors and sponsors and themselves.
>
> (Wikler and Cash, 2003, p. 226)

Working within multidisciplinary public health inevitably involves values because judgements are being made about what is 'good health' and how this could be achieved. The ethical principles most favoured within the promotion of public health are: beneficence (doing good), non-maleficence (doing no harm), respect for autonomy, and justice (for example, see Beauchamp and Childress, 2001). This section explores these ethical principles and considers some of the problems they raise.

1.4.1 Beneficence and non-maleficence

Two central tenets in promoting public health are to do good and to avoid doing harm. Both of these are aspects of Utilitarianism, which states that people should secure the greatest good for the greatest number of people. However, it is not always possible to simultaneously do good and to avoid harm. For example, by making individuals aware of the threat of terrorism and encouraging vigilance, one is potentially doing good by reducing the likelihood of successful terrorist attack. However, one may also be doing harm by inadvertently encouraging public fear and insecurity.

Thinking point   think of another example in which promoting public health may breach the principle of non-maleficence.

Screening, which is now firmly embedded in public health practice, has also come under increasing public scrutiny. Although it may improve public health outcomes, it raises many ethical, legal and social concerns at both the level of the individual and society (Hodge, 2004, p.66). A qualitative study of genetic testing for prostate cancer risk involving twelve focus groups with ninety men illustrated exactly this (Doukas et al., 2000). Box 1.9 highlights some of the main concerns raised by men when asked for their views on genetic screening for prostate cancer risk.

Box 1.9 Men's views on genetic testing for prostate cancer risk

Beliefs about consequences

Men expressed concern with maintaining or obtaining health and life insurance.

Expectations

Pragmatic concerns arose as to how useful the test would be when there is no definitive cure or conclusive results.

Beliefs about barriers

Men expressed a belief that, if they tested positive, treatment for cancer would hurt their sex life and could result in unnecessary surgery. These consequences could then cause decreased quality of life whether through an adverse treatment outcome, or from the anxiety of a possible cancer outbreak. Some thought that the creation of worry, anxiety and stress might make testing not worth the effort of combating cancer.

(Adapted from Doukas et al., 2000)

Consider, also, the case of a play worker at a nursery who is involved in dealing with a young child exhibiting antisocial behaviour towards other children, for example, by biting them. If the play worker refuses to accept the biting child within the play setting, then the other children are protected from this harm. However, the play worker must also consider the harm being done to the biting child and his or her family, who will be left without childcare. In any decision made, the play worker is simultaneously doing good and doing harm. Can utilitarian principles solve this dilemma by securing the greatest good for the greatest number? In making a decision the play worker would need to consider the needs of the biting child and his/her family, as well as the needs of all the children and their families.

This highlights a central problem with utilitarianism. It is open to many interpretations, according to what is understood by benefit or harm and how they are weighed against one another. Of course, utilitarianism is not the only way to do good and avoid harm but it is one of the most commonly used ethical principles.

1.4.2 Respect for autonomy

The ethical principle of autonomy is also key to promoting public health. The notion of autonomy is central to western societies and is bound up with notions of the sovereign individual who has the ability to reason, understand and therefore make rational choices within his or her environment. In other societies, and among some minority ethnic groups in the UK, the sovereign individual has not been of such importance, and the family, the group, or the community are more highly valued. Some critics have pointed out that, traditionally, the principle of autonomy has been reserved for men, and has trampled over the rights of women and children. The particular symbols of autonomy in contemporary society, such as the right to vote or own property, were granted to women only relatively recently. Some critics argue that women are not always perceived as rational, nor seen as having the ability to understand, reason and make choices. For example, a study of childfree women who chose to be sterilised (Campbell, 1999) showed how such women were often ignored, pathologised or not taken seriously by their doctors when requesting this operation. Box 1.10 gives an excerpt from the diary of Emma, a twenty-three year old woman who 'always knew' that she did not want to have children, which recounts her experience of a medical consultation.

> ## Box 1.10 Emma's diary: thoughts on a medical consultation
>
> What a waste of fucking time. He had the response all worked out and didn't even ask me how I felt. The 'statistics' show that it is not advisable to sterilize me as 'we' changed our minds ... and 'although he realizes I'm an individual...' Well, no, – didn't realize I'm an individual because he didn't ask me any questions, just made assumptions about my body and my reasons ... But I was so angry, so fucking angry that he has the power to sit in judgement over me, make decisions on my behalf. He didn't want to hear the same reasons he'd heard before from some pathetic little girl who would inevitably change her mind – that's if he even 'allowed' me the luxury of having a mind.
>
> (Campbell, 1999)

Thinking point   which groups in society might be seen as incapable of autonomy?

You might have commented that until recently people with learning disabilities were seen as non-autonomous, and this is still a contested area. Children and prisoners are also treated as dependent, but for different

Children

I keep worrying about a point of public health ???

reasons: prisoners may be seen as having forfeited their rights through acting irresponsibly towards others; children may not yet be seen as responsible, independent or fully rational. However, perceptions of children and their rights are constantly changing, and this is discussed further in Chapter 6.

Respecting autonomy raises dilemmas for all those involved in promoting public health. If an individual makes a choice that you consider harmful, you may be torn between respecting that person's autonomy, doing good, and avoiding harm. This issue revolves around the question: **by what right am I intervening and how do I justify the action I am taking?** The answer to this question may, of course, be influenced by whether the individual is harming her/himself or others. Decisions about the right to intervene involve ethical judgements about the rules and principles that should apply in this area of human conduct. Although dramatic interventions involving life or death decisions immediately come to mind (e.g. decisions about withholding medical treatment, abortion, sectioning and care orders), there are also dilemmas in more everyday decision making and action. The most frequently cited conflict is over health protection: some groups argue that the government ought to intervene to protect public health, whereas others claim that legislation and regulation infringe people's freedom of choice. For example, there is considerable debate concerning the fluoridation of water, with some researchers arguing that fluoridation prevents tooth decay (Medical Research Council, 2002), and anti-fluoridation campaigners, such as the Fluoride Action Network, arguing that it is unhelpful, unethical, harmful and ineffective.

1.4.3 Justice

The principle of distributive justice is bound up with the principles of avoiding harm and doing good. Promoting public health by necessity involves the dividing of time and resources between individuals and communities; between high-risk groups and whole populations. Activities such as setting up a youth centre for young people excluded from school, putting more police officers on the streets, or regenerating play areas are underpinned by assumptions about the value that should be placed on individuals or communities in promoting public health.

The principle of justice involves considerations about the degree to which promoting public health should be influenced by need, merit and equality. The Ottawa Charter (WHO, 1986) places equity at the forefront of promoting health, emphasising the importance of both individual empowerment, as well as healthier public policies as a means of improving health. This means that other objectives, such as unbridled economic growth or policies that undermine people's rights or fail to offer them protection against disease, are seen as unacceptable – and, indeed, as unethical in terms of promoting public health. It is on the grounds of justice that the structural adjustment policies of the IFI, discussed earlier, have been criticised.

1.4.4 Making 'ethical' decisions

One of the first questions that springs to mind when faced with a discussion of ethical issues is: **how do I know when I am doing good, avoiding harm, respecting autonomy and being just?** Moral codes exist in religious teachings, for example, in ideas concerning respecting the value of (all) life, or in the notion of treating others as you yourself would wish to be treated. Occupational groups in health and social care also have codes of ethics which set guidelines for action. One of the most well known is probably that of medicine – the Hippocratic Oath – which requires doctors, as a first principle, to avoid doing harm. Although the original Hippocratic Oath is no longer in use, at least half of all UK medical schools require doctors entering the profession to swear an oath of some kind. Social workers also follow a specific set of guidelines which help shape their practice. According to the British Association of Social Workers (BASW), social work is committed to five basic values:

> human dignity and worth
>
> social justice
>
> service to humanity
>
> integrity
>
> competence.

(BASW, 2005)

Although professional, moral and religious codes can guide action, individuals have to take responsibility for accepting, interpreting and applying ethical principles to their own health promoting activities. Seedhouse (1988) developed an ethical grid to enable systematic and critical reflection on ethical decisions (see Figure 1.5). Developed initially for healthcare professionals, it is meant to assist rather than to replace personal reflection and individual responsibility. Starting from the premise that individuals will answer honestly, the grid offers an opportunity to work through decisions in terms of key principles and potential consequences. It is not, however, morally neutral and Seedhouse signals his values by stating that individuals should approach the grid with the intention of finding opportunities to promote health.

Seedhouse suggests that practitioners should interrogate a proposed action in four main ways. Working from the centre outwards, in the centre quadrants (Layer 1) he asks: does it safeguard equity, respect and further the creation of autonomy? In Layer 2 he focuses on duties and reflects the moral code of health promoting work: what those working for health 'ought' to do; is it doing good and avoiding harm? Layer 3 deals with the consequences of action: will the consequences of the action be good and for whom? In Layer 4, Seedhouse asks: how does a proposed course of action measure up against external considerations, such as weight of evidence, legal responsibilities or risks? You can find these issues set out systematically within the four quadrants of the grid. The questions it raises about health promotion are further explained elsewhere (Seedhouse, 1996).

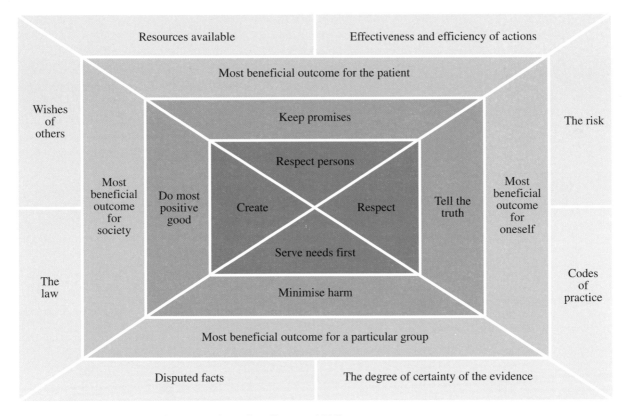

Figure 1.5 The ethical grid (Adapted from Seedhouse, 1988)

1.5 Conclusion

This chapter has covered a good deal of ground. It has encouraged you to reflect on the importance of health and on the relationships between health, rights and social justice. By now it should also be clear that multidisciplinary public health includes a complex and controversial range of activities. It is a difficult area of practice to define and will continue to be a contested and widely debated concept. The question has also been posed: **what drives the promotion of public health?** You have considered the important role of values in promoting public health and reflected on the ethical principles that underpin these value judgements. From relatively narrow and discrete origins, multidisciplinary public health – defined in the widest sense – has a broad, some would say, all-encompassing remit, which aims to work at the level of individuals, communities, public and private organisations, governments and through international agencies. The following chapters explore some of the main concepts, models and theories which underpin public health promotion.

References

Acheson, D. (1998) *Independent Inquiry into Inequalities in Health: Report*, London, The Stationery Office.

Adams, L., Amos, M. and Munro, J. (eds) (2002) *Promoting Health: Politics and Practice*, London, Sage.

Armstrong, D. (1993) 'From clinical gaze to regime of total health' in Beattie, A. et al. (eds) *Health and Wellbeing: A Reader*, Basingstoke, Macmillan/Milton Keynes, The Open University.

Armstrong, D. (1995) 'The rise of surveillance medicine', *Sociology of Health and Illness*, vol. 17, no. 3, pp. 393–404.

Ashton, J. and Seymour, H. (1988) *The New Public Health*, Milton Keynes, Open University Press.

Beauchamp, T.L. and Childress, J.F. (2001) *Principles of Biomedical Ethics*, Oxford, Oxford University Press.

British Association of Social Workers (BASW) (2005) *Code of Ethics for Social Work*, BASW, Birmingham [online], http:www.basw.co.uk/articles.php?articleId=2 (Accessed 4 April 2006).

Bunton, R., Nettleton, S. and Burrows, R. (eds) (1995) *The Sociology of Health Promotion*, London, Routledge.

Cameron, E. and Bernardes, J. (1998) 'Gender and disadvantage in health: men's health for a change', *Sociology of Health and Illness*, vol. 20, no. 5, pp. 673–93.

Campbell, A. (1999) *Childfree and Sterilized: Women's Decisions and Medical Responses*, London, Cassell.

Crawford, R. (1980) 'Healthism and the medicalisation of everyday life', *International Journal of Health Services*, vol. 10, no. 3, pp. 365–88.

Cribb, A. and Duncan, P. (2002) *Health Promotion and Professional Ethics*, Oxford, Blackwell.

Department of Health (DoH) (2001) *The Report of the Chief Medical Officer's Project to Strengthen the Public Health Function*, London, HMSO [online], http://www.dh.gov.uk/assetRoot/04/06/23/59/04062359.pdf (Accessed 4 April 2006).

Department of Health (DoH) (2004) *Choosing Health: Making Healthy Choices Easier*, London, Department of Health.

Department of Health and Social Security (DHSS) (1976) *Prevention and Health: Everybody's Business*, London, HMSO.

Department of Health and Social Security (DHSS) (1980) *The Black Report on Inequalities in Health*, London, HMSO.

Dingwall, R. (1977) 'Collectivism, regionalism and feminism: health visiting and British social policy 1850–1975', *Journal of Social Policy*, vol. 6, no. 3, pp. 291–315.

Douglas, J. (2007) 'Promoting the public health: continuity and change over two centuries' in Douglas, J., Earle, S., Handsley, S., Lloyd, C.E. and Spurr, S. (eds) (2007) *A Reader in Promoting Public Health: Challenge and Controversy*, London, Sage/Milton Keynes, The Open University.

Doukas, D.J., Fetters, M.D., Coyne, J.C. and McCullough, L.B. (2000) 'How men view genetic testing for prostate cancer risk: findings from focus groups', *Clinical Genetics*, vol. 58, pp. 169–76.

Elstad, J.I. and Krokstad, S. (2003) 'Social causation, health-selective mobility, and the reproduction of socio-economic health inequalities over time: panel study of adult men', *Social Science and Medicine*, vol. 57, no. 8, pp. 1475–90.

Freire, P. (1970) *Pedagogy of the Oppressed*, New York, Seabury Press.

Gray, B. (2003) 'Social exclusion, poverty, health and social care in Tower Hamlets: the perspectives of families on the impact of the Family Support Service', *British Journal of Social Work*, vol. 33, no. 3, pp. 361–80.

Handsley, S. (2007) 'Community involvement and civic engagement in public health promotion' in Lloyd, C.E., Handsley, S., Douglas, J., Earle, S. and Spurr, S. (eds) *Policy and Practice in Promoting Public Health*, London, Sage/Milton Keynes, The Open University.

Harrison, S. and Mort, M. (1998) 'Which champions, which people? Public and user involvement in health care as a technology of legitimation', *Social Policy and Administration*, vol. 32, no. 1, pp. 60–70.

Health Education Council (HEC) (1968) *Annual Report*, London, HEC.

Heller, R.F., Heller, T.D. and Pattison, S. (2003) 'Putting the public back into public health. Part I. A redefinition of public health', *Public Health*, vol. 117, no. 1, pp.62–5.

Hodge, J.G. (2004) 'Ethical issues concerning genetic testing and screening in public health', *American Journal of Medical Genetics,* vol. 125, no. 1, pp.66–70.

Hodgkinson, R. (1973) Public Health in the Victorian Age: Debates on the Issue from 19th Century Critical Journals, Farnborough, Gregg.

International Union for Health Promotion and Education (IUPHE) (2001) *The Evidence of Health Promotion Effectiveness: Shaping Public Health in New Europe*, IUPHE, France.

Jones, L.J. (1995) 'Business interests and public policy making' in Jones, H. and Lansley, J. (eds) *Social Policy and the City*, London, Avebury.

Kelly, M. and Charlton, B. (1995) 'The modern and the post-modern in health promotion' in Bunton et al. (eds) (1995), pp. 78–90.

King's Fund (2004) *Public Attitudes to Public Health Policy*, London, King's Fund.

Lalonde, M. (1974) *A New Perspective on the Health of Canadianss – A Working Document, Ministry of Supply and Services*, Ottawa, Ministry of Supply and Services [online], http://www.hc-sc.gc.ca/hcs-sss/alt_formats/hpb-dgps/pdf/pubs/1974-lalonde/lalonde_e.pdf (Accessed 4 April 2006).

Lewis, J. (1980) *The Politics of Motherhood*, London, Croom Helm.

McCarthy, J. (2004) 'My right to smoke', *Coventry Evening Telegraph*, 18 September 2004. http://iccoverty.icnetwork.co.uk/0100news/0100localnews/tm_method=full%26objectid=14656843%26siteid=50003_name_page.html (Accessed 7 December 2006).

MacDonald, G. (2001) *Making the Shift: A Report of Two Research Projects carried out for the Health Development Agency and the Society for Health Education and Promotion Specialists*, Birmingham/London, SHEPS/HDA.

Manderson, L. (1998) 'Health matters in developing economies' in Petersen, A. and Waddell, C. (eds) *Health Matters: A Sociology of Illness, Prevention and Care*, Buckingham, Open University Press, pp. 97–113.

Medical Research Council (2002) *Water Flouridation and Health*, London, Medical Research Council Working Group Report.

Mossialos, E. (1997) 'Citizens' views on health care systems in the 15 member states of the European Union', *Health Economics*, vol. 6, no. 2, pp. 109–16.

MORI (2002) 'Tax and Spend' [online], www.mori.com/mrr/2002/c020510.shtml (Accessed 4 April 2006).

National Advisory Committee on Nutrition Education (NACNE) (1983) *Nutritional Guidelines for Health Education in Britain*, London, Health Education Council.

National Centre for Social Research (2005) *British Social Attitudes: 22nd Report*, London, Sage.

Nettleton, S. and Bunton, R. (1995) 'Sociological critiques of health promotion' in Bunton et al. (eds) (1995), pp. 41–59.

Newsholme, A. (1936) *The Last Thirty Years of Public Health: Critical Analyses of Consumption, Lifestyle, and Risk*, London, Allen & Unwin.

Nutbeam, D. (1998) *Health Promotion Glossary*, Geneva, World Health Organization.

Patterson, F. (2001) 'Competencies, equivalence and the non-medical public health specialist', *British Medical Journal*, vol. 322, pp. 1593–6 [online], [bmj.bmjjournals.com/cgi/eletters/322/7302/1593 (Accessed 4 April 2006).

Pattison S. and Player, D. (1991) 'Health education: the political tensions' in Doxiadis, S. (ed.) *Ethical Issues in Health Education*, Chichester, Wiley.

Perdiguero, E., Bernabeu, J., Huertas, R. and Rodriguez-Ocana, E. (2001) 'History of health, a valuable tool in public health', *Journal of Epidemiology and Community Health*, vol. 55, pp. 667–73.

Plant, R. (1998) 'Citizenship, rights, welfare' in Franklin, J. (ed.) *Social Policy and Social Justice: The IPPR Reader*, Cambridge, Polity, pp. 57–72.

Reidpath, D.D., Chan, K.Y., Gifford, S.M. and Allotey, P. (2005) '"He hath the French pox": stigma, social value and social exclusion', *Sociology of Health and Illness*, vol. 27, no. 4, pp. 468–90.

Rodmell, S. and Watt, A. (eds) (1986) *The Politics of Health Education*, London, Routledge and Kegan Paul.

Sang, B. (2004) 'Choice, participation and accountability: assessing the potential impact of legislation promoting patient and public involvement in health in the UK', *Health Expectations*, vol. 7, pp. 187–90.

Seedhouse, D. (1986) *Health: The Foundations for Achievement*, Chichester, Wiley.

Seedhouse, D. (1988) *Ethics: The Heart of Health Care*, Chichester, Wiley.

Seedhouse, D. (1996) *Health Promotion: Theory and Practice*, Chichester, Wiley.

Seedhouse D. (2004) *Health Promotion: Philosophy, Prejudice and Practice* (2nd edn), Chichester, Wiley.

Sidell, M. (2007) 'Older people's health: applying Antonovsky's Salutogenic Paradigm', in Douglas et al. (eds) (2007).

Sindall, C. (2002) 'Does health promotion need a code of ethics?', *Health Promotion International*, vol. 17, no. 3, pp. 201–3.

Skills for Health (2004) *National Occupational Standards for the Practice of Public Health Guide*, Bristol, Skills for Health.

Smith, M.A. (2004) 'Health visiting: the public health role', *Journal of Advanced Nursing*, vol. 45, no. 1, pp. 17–25.

Sram, I. and Ashton, J. (2007) 'Millennium Report to Sir Edwin Chadwick' in Douglas et al. (eds) (2007).

St Leger, L. (2001) 'Building and finding the new leaders in health promotion: where is the next wave of health promotion leaders and thinkers? Are they emerging from particular regions, and are they less than 40 years old?', *Health Promotion International*, vol. 16, no. 4, pp. 301–3.

Sutherland, I. (1987) *Health Education: Half a Policy*, London, Allen & Unwin.

Tesh, S.N. (1988) *Hidden Arguments: Political Ideology and Disease Prevention Policy*, New Jersey, Rutgers University Press.

The Commission on Social Justice (1998) 'What is social justice?' in Franklin, J. (ed.) *Social Policy and Social Justice: The IPPR Reader*, Cambridge, Polity, pp. 37–49.

Tilford, S., Green, J. and Tones, B.K. (2003) *Values, Health Promotion and Public Health*, Leeds, Centre for Health Promotion Research, Leeds Metropolitan University.

Tones, B.K. (1994) 'Health promotion, empowerment, and action competence' in Jensen, B. and Schnack, K. (eds) *Action and Action Competences*, Copenhagen, Royal Danish School of Educational Studies.

Tones, B.K. and Tilford, S. (1994) *Health Education: Effectiveness, Efficiency and Equity*, London, Chapman Hall.

Townsend, P. (1979) *Poverty in the United Kingdom*, Harmondsworth, Penguin.

United Nations (1948) 'Universal Declaration of Human Rights. General Assembly Resolution 217A (III)' [online], www.unhcr.ch/udhr/lang/eng.html (Accessed 20 July 2005).

United Nations (1966) 'The UN International Covenant on Economic, Social and Cultural Rights' [online], www.hrweb.org/legal/escr.html (Accessed 20 July 2005).

Van de Mheen, H., Stronks, K., Schrijvers, C.T.M. and Mackenbach, J.P. (1999) 'The influence of adult ill health on occupational class mobility and mobility out of and into employment in the Netherlands', *Social Science and Medicine*, vol. 49, no. 4, pp. 509–18.

Wanless, D. (2002) *Securing our Future Health: Taking a Long-term View*, London, HMSO.

Wanless, D. (2004) *Securing Good Health for the Whole Population: Final Report*, London, HMSO.

Webster, C. and French, J. (2002) 'The cycle of conflict: the history of the public health and health promotion movements' in Adams, L., Munro M. and Munro, J. (eds) *Promoting Health: Politics and Practice*, London, Sage, pp. 5–12.

Weeks, J., Scriven, A. and Sayer, L. (2005) 'The health promoting role of health visitors: adjunct or synergy?' in Scriven, A. (ed.) *Health Promoting Practice: The Contribution of Nurses and Allied Health Professionals*, Basingstoke, Palgrave.

Whitehead, M. (1987) *The Health Divide*, London, Health Education Council.

Wikler, D. and Cash, R. (2003) 'Ethical issues in global public health' in Beaglehole, R. (ed.) *Global Public Health: A New Era*, Oxford, Oxford University Press, pp. 226–42.

World Health Organization (WHO) (1946) *Preamble to the Constitution of the World Health Organization as adopted by the International Health Conference, New York, 19 June – 22 July 1946; signed on 22 July 1946 by the representatives of 61 States (Official Records of the World Health Organization, no. 2, p. 100) and entered into force on 7 April 1948*, Geneva, WHO.

World Health Organization (WHO) (1977) *Health for All by the Year 2000*, Geneva, WHO.

World Health Organization (WHO) (1985) *Health for All in Europe by the Year 2000*, Copenhagen, WHO.

World Health Organization (WHO) (1986) *Ottawa Charter for Health Promotion*, WHO, Geneva.

World Health Organization (WHO) (1997) *The Jakarta Declaration on Health Promotion into the 21st Century*, Geneva, WHO.

World Health Organization (WHO) (1988) *Adelaide Recommendations on Healthy Public Policy*, Adelaide, WHO.

World Health Organization (WHO) (1998) *Health 21: Health for All in the 21st Century*, Copenhagen, WHO.

World Health Organization (WHO (2005a) *Health is Key to Sustained Peace and Prosperity in Sudan*, 11 April [online], http://www.who.int/hac/crises/sdn/sudan_peace/en/index.html (Accessed 4th April 2006).

World Health Organization (WHO) (2005b) *The Bangkok Charter for Health Promotion in a Globalised World*, Bangkok, WHO [online], http://www.who.int/healthpromotion/conferences/6gchp/bangkok_charter/en/ (Accessed 4th April 2006).

Zola, I. (1972) 'Medicine as an institution of social control', *The Sociological Review*, vol. 20, no. 4, pp. 487–504.

Chapter 2

Exploring health

Sarah Earle

Introduction

Chapter 1 explored the significance of health as both a means to an end as well as an end in itself. But what, exactly, is meant by 'health'? Kelman (1975) has argued that perhaps the most perplexing and ambiguous issue in the study of health since its inception concerns how it should be defined. But how should health be defined? And why is defining it so important when promoting public health? Hughner and Kleine (2004) provide one answer to the last of these questions when they argue that the way in which people think about health and wellbeing influences their health behaviours. So if you are concerned with understanding, changing and influencing health, then it is important to understand what is meant when people talk about their 'health'. Also, if initiatives to promote public health are to be effectively designed, delivered and evaluated, then understanding health and interrogating its meaning form a necessary and fundamental starting point. As you shall also see in later chapters, understanding health is fundamental to health research – the basis of modern multidisciplinary public health.

This chapter examines concepts and definitions of health and explores some of the models and approaches that have been developed to enable you to make sense of health. Such definitions provide a useful starting point for thinking about the components and parameters of promoting public health. In focusing not just on absence of disease but on the attainment of a more positive and holistic state this chapter presents a challenge to think more seriously about what makes for good health within different contexts and in relation to diverse experiences and settings.

2.1 Understanding health

At different times and places and across different cultures, people have understood health in various ways. For example, in most traditional societies, fatness was regarded as healthy whereas now, in many modern societies, thin bodies are seen as ideal. In primitive societies, health and illness were thought to be influenced by magic and witchcraft, whereas in most contemporary societies this is no longer the case (Blaxter, 2004). Many studies have been conducted which explore the ways in which individuals understand health and illness. The majority of these have, however, explored understandings of illness, rather than health. The smaller, more focused body of research which examines how people think about health has been conducted predominantly in Europe, with the majority of studies having been carried out in the United Kingdom (Lawton, 2003).

Images of health are also built on media messages and prevalent ideas about health rights, awareness of health issues, access to services and levels of service provision. Health is an abstract concept which some people find difficult to define. Understanding and knowledge of health has, traditionally, been dominated by medicine, with its focus on treatment and disease, which may partly account for the emphasis on illness rather than health within research. Indeed, research suggests that individuals often find it difficult to talk about health without reference to illness (Dines, 1994), and this is explored later in this chapter. The published studies also show that good health tends to be something that people can take for granted (Hughner and Kleine, 2004). They also show that there can be a significant difference between people's knowledge and beliefs in comparison to their actual health behaviours (Lawton, 2003). For example, although many people may know that physical activity is good for their health, they may, nonetheless, lead sedentary lifestyles. It is important to bear this in mind when promoting public health at all levels.

In the *Health and Lifestyles Survey* – one of the most comprehensive surveys of what health means in the United Kingdom – Cox et al. (1987) interviewed over 9,000 individuals. This survey asked respondents to consider their own health as well as the health of other people. Two key issues were raised: (1) Think of someone you know who is very healthy. Who are you thinking of? How old are they? What makes you call them healthy? (2) At times people are healthier than at other times. What is it like when you are healthy? Analysis of responses to these questions revealed ten major lay concepts of health (see Box 2.1). The term 'lay' is used to describe people who are not experts or professionals. Concepts of health refer to the way in which individuals understand and think about their own health and those of others. These concepts can be fluid and interchangeable.

Box 2.1 Lay concepts of health

- Health as not ill
- Health as absence of disease/health despite disease
- Health as a reserve

- Health as behaviour

- Health as physical fitness

- Health as energy

- Health as a social relationship

- Health as function

- Health as psycho-social wellbeing

- Negative answers (i.e. not relevant, not interested in health)

(Adapted from Blaxter, 1990)

Analysis of the *Health and Lifestyles Survey* (Cox et al., 1987; Blaxter 1990) and other research studies found that although health is an individual experience, it is through influences such as culture, class and gender that these experiences are shaped. For example, young people are much more likely to define health in relation to physical fitness or health behaviours than older people, who are more likely to define health in relation to experiences of illness, disease and functionality (Williams, 1983; Calnan, 1987; McKague and Verhoef, 2003). People in the lowest socio-economic groups tend to consider themselves healthy if they do not need to take time off work (Calnan, 1987), whereas women are much more likely than men to focus on emotional health and the maintenance of social relationships (Blaxter, 1990).

Thinking point   do you think that an understanding of lay concepts of health is helpful in promoting public health?

Arguably, an understanding of the crucial differences in the way that diverse individuals and groups make sense of health should underpin all public health action. For example, there is little point in attempting to promote the health of people for whom health appears irrelevant. Similarly, caution should be taken when attempting to promote mental health among groups who value physical health above all else. Recognising diversity is a key feature of successful modern multidisciplinary public health.

In a recent and comprehensive review of the research on health, Hughner and Kleine (2004) identified eighteen concepts of health within the literature (see Figure 2.1) which they have classified into the following four areas:

- Definitions of health

- Explanations for health

- External and/or uncontrollable factors impinging on health

- The place health occupies in people's lives.

Figure 2.1 Eighteen key concepts of health

Eighteen key concepts of health

Theme		Example statement
1	Health is the absence of illness	If I am not sick (e.g. running a fever), I generally consider myself healthy
2	Health is functional ability	As long as I am able to carry out my daily functions (e.g. going to work, taking care of the household), I consider myself healthy
3	Health is equilibrium	The mind, body and spirit are all connected; all need to be in sync for good health
4	Health is freedom	Good health is freedom; with it comes the ability to do what I want to do, to live how I want to live
5	Health is constraint	Good health can be constraining; with it individuals have to conform to the demands of society
6	Health through meditation or prayer	Health and wellness can be maintained through meditation and/or prayer
7	Health is dependent upon mental attitude	The power of a positive outlook or attitude can prevent sickness
8	Health through working	As long as I keep going, I tend not to get sick – keeping busy doesn't allow one to have the time to get sick!
9	Religious and supernatural explanations	God works in mysterious ways; health and sickness are part of the divine plan
10	Health maintained through rituals	The use of certain rituals is helpful in the maintenance of health (e.g. reciting a prayer or psalm)
11	Health is a moral responsibility	I have a responsibility to my family to maintain my health
12	Health is maintained through internal monitoring	I believe visiting a medical doctor for regular check-ups is important to maintain good health
13	'Self-blame'	Many people suffer from illnesses caused by their own bad habits
14	Health as policy and institutions	I believe good health is, in part, the product of governmental institutions that ensure the health of citizens
15	Modern way of life	Many diseases of modern life result from the stressful and polluted environment in which people live
16	Health is genetics	Often, getting sick just happens and little can be done about it.
17	The value and priority placed on health	I have more important goals in my life than the pursuit of optimal health
18	Disparity between health beliefs and behaviours	I know a lot about how to keep healthy (e.g. which type of eating and activity behaviours are considered healthy); however, I often do not practise this health knowledge

(Adapted from Hughner and Kleine, 2004, p. 419)

Modern multidisciplinary public health is unlikely to improve health and to bring about change unless those involved develop an understanding of health concepts, focus on why and how people's ideas about health differ, and can adjust health priorities and actions to meet the expressed needs of different social groups. Building on this, you will now explore definitions of health.

2.2 Defining health

Definitions of health contain complex ideas about what it is to be healthy, whose responsibility it is to maintain health and how illness and disease should be interpreted. Definitions of health can be described as statements about health, although like concepts of health, these too can change and be reworked over time. Such definitions may project officially sanctioned ways of viewing health which have passed into 'common sense' understandings, and thus become part of popular thinking.

2.2.1 Disease, illness and sickness

The terms disease, illness and sickness are frequently used interchangeably, although they describe very different states.

Disease refers to a specific condition, or pathological state, in a person. From the viewpoint of modern scientific medicine this can usually be identified by an actual change (lesion or abnormality) on the surface of, or inside, some part of the body. Diseases are classified by being entered in the International Classification of Diseases (ICD) index. In theory, a specific disease should characterise every episode of reported sickness. In practice, health workers treat patients and sign them off work in some cases where no disease can be identified; some disease categories, such as repetitive strain injury or chronic fatigue syndrome (ME), are hotly contested. It is also possible for an individual to be diseased and yet not feel ill for example, a person with controlled diabetes or epilepsy.

Thinking point   how far do you think that the definition of disease can be applied to mental heath problems?

Defining mental health and mental health problems is complex, and an important task of mental health promotion. Definitions of disease often favour physical health rather than mental health (Handsley, 2007). However, as the Mental Health Foundation argues:

> we are all 'mental' beings – in the same way as we are all 'physical' beings. And mental health is just as important as physical health. If we are to grow and to flourish and if we are to contribute individually and collectively to society, we need to accept that we are 'mental' beings with emotional and spiritual needs, as well as physical ones.

> (Mental Health Foundation, 2005)

Mental health problems range from normal feelings of grief or worry that are experienced as part of everyday life, through to the most serious and potentially life-threatening conditions such as psychosis, self-harm and anorexia nervosa.

Illness, on the other hand, is the subjective state of feeling unwell; in other words, illness is based on an individual's own experience and feelings. This draws attention to the fact that illness is mediated through the individual: that is, illness is about how people feel – whether they feel 'healthy' or 'unhealthy'. For example, an individual may visit his or her general practitioner with a bad cough and be told that 'there is nothing wrong with you'. Although the individual may be reassured (or not), he or she may still feel very ill. Similarly, a person diagnosed with cancer may recognise the severity of their condition but may feel healthy and not at all ill.

Sickness refers to reported illness and describes the way in which an individual becomes a medical statistic. Hannay (1979) identified the concept of the 'clinical iceberg' to explain how only a proportion of individuals who feel ill will ever report their illness and thus officially become a medical statistic. Research suggests that most of the illness in society goes unreported.

However, Robinson (1971) suggests that a person's readiness to consider him or herself ill cannot always be explained by reference to the severity of symptoms. In other words, it seems that the pathology of the disease bears little relevance to the likelihood of someone becoming a medical statistic. As explored further in Chapter 8, sickness rates are calculated from the use of health services and absence from work records. Neither are very reliable indicators of illness because both are influenced by individual circumstances and different methods of recording and reporting sickness across the country (Whitehead, 1987). A classic study conducted by Mechanic (1968) revealed a wide range of factors that contribute to the likelihood of someone seeking medical assistance for their symptoms (see Box 2.2)

Box 2.2 Factors contributing to seeking medical assistance

The factors contributing to someone seeking medical assistance are:

- the extent to which symptoms are visible and recognisable
- their perceived seriousness
- the extent to which they impact on the sufferer's life
- their perceived frequency and persistence

- the degree to which an individual can tolerate them

- knowledge about what symptoms may mean

- anxiety about their perceived seriousness

- competing needs

- competing explanations for the symptoms

- availability of treatment and assistance.

(Adapted from Mechanic, 1968)

Zola (1973) has also suggested that there are particular triggers which lead individuals to seek medical attention:

- **The occurrence of an interpersonal crisis** An event which calls attention to a person's symptoms, forcing the individual to do something about them.

- **The *perceived* interference with social or personal relations** The extent to which symptoms interfere with everyday living.

- **Sanctioning** This refers to the involvement of another person who sanctions the decision to seek medical attention.

- **The *perceived* interference with vocational or physical activity** The extent to which symptoms interfere with occupational activity.

- **A kind of temporalising of symptomatology** The setting of a time period after which treatment will be sought.

(Zola, 1973, p. 683)

Thinking point   how would you define health?

Health can be variously defined; the next section in this chapter explores some of these definitions.

2.2.2 Health as absence of disease

Health has been most frequently defined as the 'absence of disease'. This definition has been one of the most pervasive definitions of health and is one that was commonly found in government reports and legislation, as well as in medical documents. Critics have labelled this the medical definition of health because it focuses not on health, but on disease: according to the medical view, health occurs when you are not classified as sick, or in need of medical attention. This can be regarded as a negative, rather than a positive, definition of health.

The definition of health as the absence of disease can be traced back as far as the ancient Greeks. However, René Descartes, seventeenth-century French philosopher and mathematician, has provided the best-known account of the difference between mind and body. This distinction, which is known as Cartesian dualism, has been a fundamental influence on medicine's largely reductionist focus on the body and disease, to the exclusion of other aspects of health and illness.

2.2.3 Health as wellbeing

In an attempt to move away from the characterisation of health defined solely as the absence of disease (and as highlighted in Chapter 1), in 1946 the World Health Organization defined health as: 'A state of complete physical, mental and social wellbeing and not merely the absence of disease or infirmity' (WHO, 1946, preamble). This marks a shift away from a definition of health that focuses solely on disease towards one that accepts some of the other factors that influence health. This statement conceptualises health as a positive state rather than a state of not being sick. People are viewed not only in physical terms, but also in psychological and social terms, and all-round health is seen as including the notion of 'wellbeing'. The Scottish Executive provides a useful definition of wellbeing: 'A person's sense of positive feeling about their life situation and their personal health, both physical and mental. You can have a physical illness, injury or mental health problem or illness and still have a sense of wellbeing' (Scottish Executive, 2002).

The concept of wellbeing is increasingly used in government strategy. For example, in their consultation document *Well Being in Wales*, the Welsh Assembly (2002) defined wellbeing in relation to community engagement, accessible health and social care, and a sense of happiness, safety and comfort.

Wellbeing is also being widely used within the academic literature on health, but it is used in different ways and seldom as explicitly defined as it is above. For example, Lee and McCormick (2004), writing about the wellbeing of people with spinal cord injuries, suggest that it is a concept that includes both the subjective experiences of individuals, as well as the functional and more objective measures of quality of life. Subjective wellbeing, Diener (1994) argues, refers to the individual judgement of the pleasantness of one's life.

In a study of older people and the end of life (Lloyd, 2000), five key outcomes were identified in relation to the promotion of wellbeing:

- promoting non-institutionalised services
- encouraging openness about illness and dying

- enabling older people to exercise choice and control over caring interventions

- minimising the fear of death

- maintaining family and other social networks.

(Lloyd, 2000, p. 179)

A recent review of the term 'wellbeing' within health research and health promotion (Cronin de Chavez et al., 2005) revealed an even wider variety of uses and definitions. For example, within medical research the term was often used unreflectively and interchangeably with physical health, whereas those promoting public health tended to use the term in relation to health outcomes. Social science approaches were informed by their different disciplinary traditions. For example, psychologists focused on aspects of wellbeing related to subjectivity and a sense of self, whereas economists focused on the realisation of wellbeing within the context of achievable opportunities.

However, moving the definitional boundaries in this way raises difficult questions about what being healthy really involves and takes us back to some of the issues discussed in Chapter 1. It begs the question of whether anyone can ever hope to attain a state of complete health, or wellbeing, and whether this can ever be a realisable human right. The 1946 WHO definition of health puts forward health as a goal – an end in itself rather than a means to an end. Some commentators have argued that this definition is both unrealistic and unattainable (Lupton, 1995), thus serving to cause inevitable failure within multidisciplinary public health. Crawford has argued that health has simply become synonymous with 'good living' – or a metaphor for 'all that is good in life' an idea he describes as 'healthism' (Crawford, 1980, p. 365). Drawing on this, and on the work of Illich (1976), Fitzpatrick (2000) is also critical of what he terms the contemporary 'tyranny of health', arguing that governments exaggerate risks to health and seek to intervene further and further into the lives of people who are not sick. This, he argues, is having an unhealthy effect on the population.

Thinking point   identify one example of how promoting public health might be considered unhealthy.

It could be argued that making health the sole ambition is an unhealthy state. As already outlined in Chapter 1, some would also suggest that health screening programmes (e.g. cervical screening) can cause fear and anxiety, thus promoting illhealth. Next, you turn to an alternative approach to health, which positions health as a resource, rather than the objective of living.

2.2.4 Health as a resource

The Ottawa Charter for Health Promotion (WHO, 1986) reinforced the concept of wellbeing but defined health more cautiously:

> To reach a state of complete physical mental and social wellbeing, an individual or group must be able to identify and to realize aspirations, to satisfy needs, and to change or cope with the environment. Health is, therefore, seen as a resource for everyday life, not the objective of living. Health is a positive concept emphasizing social and personal resources, as well as physical capacities.

(WHO, 1986)

This definition emphasises the way that health is embedded in the processes and actions of people's everyday lives. It relates health to the ability to cope and adapt within a particular environment. Unlike the earlier WHO definition from 1946, it deliberately avoids viewing health as an object – or a goal – seeing it instead as a 'resource' for living. It signals that health might be understood in different ways, and emphasises the dynamic interaction between individuals and their environment.

Initiatives such as Sure Start are based on the principle that good health is a resource for living and the cornerstone of tackling inequality, deprivation and social exclusion in both rural and urban areas (see Box 2.3).

Box 2.3 Sure Start: the Travelling Tutor scheme in Deeside, Scotland

A local Community Learning Worker identified the need for support for rurally isolated parent and toddlers groups in Deeside. After piloting, the Travelling Tutor scheme was established to provide physical play, messy play, storytelling and music during term times and the summer holidays. Skilled tutors travelled to many of the smaller villages and ran sessions for an hour and a half. Sessions were well received and eagerly participated in by parents and toddlers.

(Adapted from Sure Start Scotland, 2003, p. 5)

2.3 Approaches, models and accounts of health

This final section of Chapter 2 explores models and approaches to health, as well as lay accounts. These models and approaches provide accounts of health and illness which not only create stories about beliefs but also about practices. The models are a representation of how health operates in the real world and can also become a blueprint for action. Such models and approaches can be understood within the wider context of discourses (Foucault, 1973): that is, comprehensive frameworks of conceptualising ('knowing') and practising ('doing') health work. Discourses of health are explored in more detail in Chapter 7.

2.3.1 A medical model

The medical model, which draws on the definition of health as an absence of disease, informs the most powerful and influential discourse about health and, as you have already seen, one that defines health quite narrowly. The medical model is the most dominant system of medical knowledge within the modern western world. Its central activity is the treatment of disease in individuals. This is underpinned by an explanation of the causes of illhealth that privileges the physical body (see Box 2.4).

Box 2.4 The medical model of health

In this model:

- health is viewed as the 'absence of disease'

- illness can be reduced to disordered bodily functions within the individual

- health services treat sick and disabled people largely within specialisms (e.g. paediatrics; obstetrics; podiatry etc.)

- health services are predominantly remedial and curative

- each disease is thought to be caused by a specific (potentially identifiable) pathogen or genetic marker

- the production of medical knowledge via the use of 'scientific' research methods is valued over the use of qualitative research methodologies

- health professionals are the 'experts' with the power to diagnose disease and decide on treatment, and supervise the withdrawal of patients from their everyday lives.

(Adapted from Earle, 2005, p. 53)

This view of disease has dominated western thinking for the past two centuries. It is linked to the rise of clinical pathology and the scientific investigation of disease by a growing body of specialist doctors and researchers, and to the emergence of health work as a formal, professionalised area of expertise (Friedson, 1970). Conventionally, this is underpinned by a set of power relationships between doctors and patients and between other health and social care workers and their clients, in which the patient or client is conceptualised as the inactive recipient of 'expert' knowledge and intervention.

Medicine and public health

If multidisciplinary public health views health positively as a resource for living, it sees people being in an active and dynamic interaction with their social, economic and physical environments. It focuses both on individuals and on entire populations or groups and one of its functions is to enhance health by preventing disease before it strikes. This is difficult to reconcile with a medical model of health (Box 2.4), which focuses mainly on treatment and cure. A significant part of multidisciplinary public health deals with prevention and risk reduction strategies and the contribution these can make towards the improvement of health. Public health has often focused on medical risk factors as a basis for developing campaigns and projects aimed specifically at groups 'at risk' in the population. The publication of the UK health strategies and the focus on health targets and prevention make such an approach more justifiable, even though health promotion specialists, and others, continue to broaden their approach by developing programmes and community-based approaches that incorporate a range of settings.

Medicine has traditionally placed a high value on scientific knowledge and using quantitative and experimental methods of research, while tending to give a lower status to qualitative evidence. (The areas of qualitative and quantitative research are defined and discussed in Chapters 7, 8 and 9.) Many epidemiological studies of the state of a person's health have been produced over the years, whereas most qualitative research has been produced outside the field by social scientists. However, as you shall see later on in this book, this is beginning to change; social epidemiology, in particular, is beginning to embrace a wider range of methodological approaches, and those researching in public health are using a wide range of mixed methodologies, reflecting the broad range of activities that take place, their position in relation to values and evidence, as well as its multidisciplinary nature.

The shortcomings of the medical model are more generally apparent as public health gradually becomes recognised as a broader activity being undertaken by professionals and lay people, within the health and social care sector, within voluntary organisations, and in schools and at home. Social workers, for example, have found it difficult to work within a medical framework. Other professional groups in the field of health have also been critical, such as occupational therapists who aim to work within a more positive model of occupational performance. Drawing on this broad public health remit, general practitioners have also called for a reorientation of health services and a redistribution of resources towards public health and primary care. Nurses, too, aim to work within a model which is not exclusively focused on the treatment of disease.

2.3.2 A salutogenic approach to health

The medical model of health is pathogenic, focusing on treatment and on why people become sick and die. The work of Antonovsky (1987; 1993) adopted the opposite approach, focusing on what it is that keeps people healthy. He argued that working within this salutogenic (or health producing) framework focused attention for almost the first time on why some people remained healthy. He emphasised that stressors and disruption were unavoidable aspects of life rather than the demons they are portrayed to be within pathogenic models. This salutogenic framework suggests that the normal state of affairs is one of entropy (or disorder) and of disruption of homeostasis, so that most people are neither diseased nor healthy but somewhere along a 'health–ease–disease' continuum.

The central focus within Antonovsky's work is on 'behavioural immunology': that is, the successful coping with adverse conditions in life. One group studied by Antonovsky was concentration camp survivors from the Second World War. These studies of survivors suggested that people were enabled to cope by having developed by early adulthood a feeling of confidence that the world had meaning and was predictable, that they had the resources to cope with the challenges they faced, and that these challenges were worth responding to. Antonovsky suggested that these three components – comprehensibility, manageability and meaningfulness – together created 'a sense of coherence' which he defined as:

> a global orientation that expresses the extent to which one has a pervasive, enduring though dynamic feeling of confidence that: i) the stimuli deriving from one's internal and external environments in the course of living are structured, predictable and explicable; ii) the resources are available to one to meet the demands passed by these stimuli; and iii) these demands are challenges worthy of investment and engagement.

(Antonovsky, 1987, p. 19)

Salutogenic research explores, in any given setting, how changes can be made so that the sense of coherence is strengthened, rather than blaming the victims who fall sick. In the workplace, for example, people's sense of coherence will be enhanced if they have work that is meaningful, not over-stressful, and if a sense of autonomy and participation is fostered (Antonovsky, 1987; Cooper and Clarke, 2003; Sidell, 2007). In relation to chronic illness, salutogenesis can offer people a positive way forward: public health can assist them in moving along the health–ease–disease continuum towards better health, expressed in terms of relief from symptoms, increased mobility and greater independence by ensuring that the factors contributing to their sense of coherence are strengthened. Within midwifery and the maternity services, the concept of salutogenesis is also being used to support the Royal College of Midwives' *Campaign for Normal Birth* by focusing on the factors that encourage 'normal' birth rather than the risk factors associated with complicated deliveries (RCM, 2005).

Antonovsky criticises the pathogenic paradigm because it not only focuses our attention on disease, illness and medical treatment as abnormal, but also on contributing factors, such as stressors and disruption, as abnormal too. He proposes a salutogenic approach that would emphasise stress and change as being essential aspects of life, able to be dealt with providing people have the resources to do so. Then the essential research question is to ask why some people are successful at coping and others are not. Those who have enough in their lives that is manageable and meaningful, and for whom life is sufficiently predictable to be understood, are more likely to cope and remain healthy. The investigation of how people cope and remain healthy further demonstrates the dynamic relationship between people and their environment. Good management of stressors depends not just on personal resources, but on relationships, social support and supportive environments.

Thinking point   what factors would increase your own sense of coherence?

Some of the factors that increase a sense of coherence might include: good relationships with family, friends and wider networks; supportive working environments and peer support; financial security; and leisure interests. However, the concept of salutogenesis, underpinned by the theory of coherence, can be criticised for focusing too much on the individual and on the way in which he or she responds to external stimuli. It could be argued that just as pathogenesis locates the problem within the individual so, too, does salutogenesis, although this was not Antonovsky's intention. You will now turn to an alternative model of health.

2.3.3 A social model of health

The concept of salutogenesis, while not without its critics, is a useful bridge from the medical approach to health to an approach that sees health as influenced by political, economic, social, psychological, cultural and environmental as well as biological factors. This is not to say that the social model of health dispenses with modern medicine; far from it. But there is a fundamental assumption that the medical model is only part of the answer.

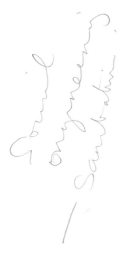

In response to the limitations of the medical model, a social model of health is now well established within the canon of literature on health, illness and disease (Annandale, 1998). A social model of health posits that the concept of health (and illness) is socially constructed, and can be socially caused. Social construction, which has had a profound influence on the way in which health is understood, refers to the way that reality is constructed through human interaction, rather than it being independently real (Blaxter, 2004). Social scientists have also argued that health cannot be fully understood without first understanding subjective experiences of health, illness and disease. Indeed, Turner argues that health is 'fundamentally a social state of affairs' (Turner, 1995, p. 37), rather than a biological one.

2.3.4 The social causation of health and illness

One of the most significant contributions made by social scientists has been to show how health and illness are influenced by a wide range of social factors (these factors are explored in more depth in Chapter 3). Fitzpatrick (1986) has shown how patterns of disease have changed over time, arguing that modern societies have passed through three distinct disease patterns:

1   **Disease in pre-agricultural societies**

    Before 10,000 B.C. evidence suggests that most people died from environmental or safety hazards, such as exposure. Deaths arising from infectious diseases are thought to have been uncommon.

2   **Disease in agricultural and early industrial societies**

    A range of infectious diseases, such as tuberculosis and cholera, were the most common forms of death in these societies.

3   **Disease in the modern industrial era**

    By the mid-twentieth century, infectious diseases were no longer a primary cause of death. Chronic and degenerative diseases, such as cancer, diabetes and cardiovascular disease have become more common.

Even more recently, modern industrialised societies have seen a return of infectious diseases such as tuberculosis. Changes in the prevalence of disease illustrate the relationship between disease and society. It could be argued that advances in medicine and health and social care provision have had a significant impact on the prevalence of certain types of disease. This may be true in a limited number of cases, but social scientists would argue that if you examine the changing patterns of disease within any given society, you can see a strong relationship between health, and social and economic factors.

2.3.5 The medicalisation of everyday life

Social scientists have been instrumental in outlining the ways in which the very concepts of health and disease are dependent upon the nature of the society and cultures in which people live. Sociologists, in particular, have argued that what comes to be defined as a disease is dependent upon a range of political and economic factors. For example, Hunt (1994) and Lee (1998) have pointed out that the construction of the menopause as an oestrogen deficiency disease developed in the 1960s and was strongly associated with the development and availability of hormone replacement therapies.

Just as some processes, experiences or behaviours become medicalised, others become demedicalised. A good example of this is the demedicalisation of homosexuality which, until 1973, appeared in the Diagnostic and Statistical Manual of Mental Disorders as a pathological psychiatric disorder. This highlights how the labelling of any process or behaviour as a medical problem is only tangentially related to a distinct physiological or psychological occurrence.

Medicalisation has been widely criticised. For example, Illich (1976) developed the theory of iatrogenesis to highlight the harmful effects of medicine on society. He identified three specific types of iatrogenic effect:

- **Clinical iatrogenesis** refers to the harm done by medicine through treatment, ineffectiveness of treatment, or medical uncertainty.
- **Social iatrogenesis** refers to the way that individuals become dependent upon medicine and become consumers of healthcare.
- **Structural iatrogenesis** refers to the way in which society can become dependent on medical attention and on the medical model of health.

Thinking point   can you think of other examples of the medicalisation of everyday life?

Sociologists have also shown how other healthy physical processes, such as menstruation, pregnancy and childbirth, have come to be seen as medical problems requiring surveillance and intervention. Some would also argue that other experiences, such as sadness and worry, have also become medicalised and are now defined as depression and stress. In discussing the problem of such medicalisation, Zola argued that: 'If anything can be shown in some way to affect the workings of the body and to a lesser extent the mind, then it can be labelled ... "a medical problem"' (Zola, 1973, p. 261).

2.3.6 Taking into account lay experiences

The social model is concerned with both the 'upstream' and the 'downstream' determinants of health; in other words, with the wider, structural factors that contribute to health and illness, as well as the actions of individuals and communities. This draws on an idea developed by McKinlay (1975), in which he used the analogy of a river to represent illness, in response to his frustration with the medical model of health. McKinlay argued that doctors were so caught up in rescuing people from the river that they had no time to look upstream to see who was pushing them into the water. He argued that doctors should stop focusing on downstream efforts, or individual interventions, and should refocus upstream, where the real problems – and solutions – lie. Since people themselves often have the greatest insight into the impact of these upstream determinants, a central concern within the social model of health is to start where people are in terms of the stream: that is, to understand and value the views of lay people and to recognise that their ideas and concerns about health and illness may not necessarily coincide with professional views and priorities. A good example of this relates to housing. In strictly scientific terms it has taken years to prove the adverse impact of damp housing on health because of the intervening variables which make precise measurement very difficult. But people living in poor housing have had a very clear and detailed understanding of the impact of housing on their families' health, for example, in the case of childhood asthma (Hunt et al., 1986). For them, better housing is a central priority whereas smoking is of less importance.

It is only since the 1980s that experts at an international level have systematically developed strategies to involve and listen to the views of lay people through community action and development, healthy cities projects and healthy partnerships. Such initiatives have been underway for some time, but it remains difficult to ensure that lay people's voices and their expressed needs are heard. Intervention based on a social model would be more likely to respond to people's priorities rather than professional-led priorities for change, and would recognise how people's behaviour is shaped by structural factors. Good examples of such an initiative are the many Healthy Cities projects around the world, including some in the UK (e.g. in Belfast, Sheffield, Glasgow and Stirling), which are all part of the WHO's Healthy Cities Programme. Box 2.5 outlines a Healthy City project in Australia which was based on the needs of local residents.

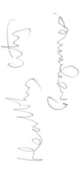

Box 2.5 Healthy Cities Illawarra, Australia

Bellambi suburb is a large public housing area. The coordinator of the neighbourhood centre was concerned about the bad press the suburb had been receiving. Healthy Cities Illawarra (HCI) held a vision workshop with residents who were asked to give their dreams for their neighbourhood. Many of the visions were simple, such as playground equipment, more trees, no sewerage leakage into the ocean, a swimming pool. An interagency committee was formed and further progress has been made on neighbourhood improvements.

A breakfast programme was started, a community food garden was set up and a major redevelopment of the suburb is underway. One important change is that the local community has developed the skills, networks and organisation to undertake change.

(Adapted from: www.healthycitiesill.org.au/)

At first glance, the social model seems to provide a much more accommodating framework for promoting public health. Its underlying philosophy is that the health of individuals and social groups is the result of complex and interacting material-structural and behavioural-cultural factors. For example, the most frequently stated guiding principles of health promotion – which draw on a social model of health – are a commitment to empowerment, to local participation, to equity in health, to accountability, and to co-operation and partnership with other agencies and sectors. This in turn creates distinctive objectives: to work to improve adverse features of the environment, such as pollution, bad housing or poor working conditions; to reduce health inequalities; and to work with groups such as refugees, older people, or homeless people, whose health needs may be overlooked. However, both the social and medical models are located within a pathogenic approach to health (with the focus on disease). For example, many programmes that claim to work within a social model of health (with some exceptions) will use WHO targets and UK targets for disease reduction.

2.3.7 A dissenting view

Some people involved in promoting health, however, have found some difficulty in pinning down what types of actions and interventions would be indicated by working within a social model of health. The social model is so broad that it can include different, and potentially competing, sets of priorities, including large-scale statutory interventions, small-scale self-help, lay power and shared lay and professional leadership. Health promotion projects, public health programmes, local health projects and campaigning groups have all used the rhetoric of the social model in a variety of ways, for example:

- as a set of underlying values – a philosophical approach to health
- as a set of guiding principles to orientate health work in a specific way
- as a set of practice objectives.

As the philosophy is turned into principles and then action, so the social model becomes characterised differently by groups with varying priorities and interests. One assumption has been that the social model is focused on local 'communities' even though community is an ill-defined concept which projects a vision of social solidarity and mutual interest that rarely exists in the twenty-first century. Large-scale health projects, such as those aimed at influencing change within a whole city, have also embraced the social model, but the types of changes planned have been ambitious and structural, sometimes making it difficult to respond to lay views or needs and evaluate their outcomes.

There have been criticisms of the social model, beyond and within multidisciplinary public health, particularly by sociologists. One criticism has focused on the perceived failure of this new approach to replace the epistemology (ways of knowing about knowledge) of the medical model. At the heart of the social model, it is argued, is an expert discourse about social causes of disease and social system breakdown that is analogous to the medical model's focus on biological cause and malfunction. This means that the social model links social structures to disease (in the same way that the medical model blames germs); although what epidemiological evidence actually demonstrates is that there is only a correlation (not a causal relationship) between social inequalities and health. Kelly and Charlton argue:

> In the medical model the pathogens are microbes, viruses or malfunctioning cellular reproduction. In the social model they are poor housing, poverty, unemployment and powerlessness. The discourse may be different but the epistemology is the same. The social model is not, in our view, an alternative to the discredited medical model. It is a partner in crime.
>
> (Kelly and Charlton, 1995, p. 82)

Another criticism of the social model as a new model of health concerns its imperialism or its success in taking over the whole of life. The social model is particularly culpable, because its approach is so much broader than that of the medical model. In this view, health now encompasses all contexts, structures and cultural styles. It has now been 'dispersed into non-medical surveillance and maintenance systems that target behaviours and beliefs, norms and mores and blur the boundaries between public and private, individual and social life in the name of "wellness"' (O'Brien, 1995, p. 204). So, in this sense, the social model serves to increase the 'medicalisation' of everyday life.

The social model of health is one among several philosophical approaches to health. Like others, it sets down principles and priorities for action. Hence there is a danger that such a broad-brush approach will deliver an equally vague set of outcomes. Linking everything to health could simply mean that health loses its meaning – and that health messages are discarded and that promoting public health can become frustrating.

Unchallenged, the medical model may perpetuate risk factors, further narrowly define high-risk groups and notions of normality, and will marginalise the broader socio-economic influence on health. If public health workers are really going to listen to lay people's views about the causes of poor health, then they will have to find a way to reconcile 'expert' discourses with lay beliefs.

2.3.8 A holistic approach to health

A holistic approach to health can be equated with the biopsychosocial model first proposed by Engel in 1977. This approach, introduced as a way of leading healthcare professionals away from what Engel believed to be the reductionist and deficient approach of mainstream medicine, attempted to integrate biological, psychological and social factors for the aetiology (the study of the causes of disease, as well as for the treatment) of illness. Since then, holism has been defined in numerous ways. Wynne, Brand and Smith (1997) have argued that holism is underpinned by an acceptance that health is determined and defined by interrelated social, psychological and biological factors. Others have defined holism in relation to the whole person (Kolkaba, 1997) or have argued that the whole is greater than the sum of its parts. Patterson (1997) has argued that holism implies mind, body and spirit.

Holistic approaches to health bear some similarities to a social model. However, holism tends to focus on individuals, whereas a social model tends to focus on the social structures within which the individual finds him or herself. Holistic approaches to health are commonly found within the nursing profession and, to some extent, within general practice (Armstrong, 1987; Hassed, 2004), although this is disputed (Reilly, 2001). Holism is also influential within the allied health professions, such as occupational therapy, and within specific areas of healthcare, for example, within pain management where an holistic approach is increasingly applied (Marcus et al., 2000).

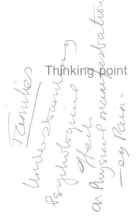

Thinking point   can you think of any examples where you have adopted a holistic approach?

Holistic approaches are applied to many areas of health and social care. For example, in palliative care, a holistic approach which includes the provision of spiritual care is dominant (Lloyd-Williams, 2003). Holism also commonly underpins many complementary and alternative approaches to health, such as acupuncture (Paterson, 2004). In social work, holism also provides a way of providing better care for clients in a way that crosses the boundaries between 'health' and 'social care' (see Box 2.6).

> ## Box 2.6 Holism, social care and older people
>
> The new role of a health-and social care-trained generic worker was developed to provide comprehensive care for older people living at home. The role is a cross between a nursing auxiliary, healthcare assistant and a community support worker. The evaluation of the one-year pilot project demonstrated that clients were very satisfied with the care they received, particularly the emotional aspects of care. A high proportion of the generic workers, time was spent listening and responding to their clients' mental health needs, and providing comfort and emotional support. Having been trained by local health professionals, the generic workers felt valued and respected, better able to communicate with their health colleagues, and therefore able to provide holistic care to their clients.
>
> (Hek et al., 2004, p. 237)

2.3.9 Concerns with holistic approaches

However holism is defined, concerns with a holistic approach to health have been widely expressed. As the blurring of 'health' and 'illness' increases, and health becomes defined more holistically, health can be considered as the totality of people's lives. Nettleton for example suggests that: 'A concern about this more 'holistic' approach to professional–patient interactions, one which takes the 'whole person' into account, is that medicine, or health care workers more generally, are legitimately able to encroach on more and more aspects of people's lives' (Nettleton, 1995, p. 157).

Foucault (1973) argues that individuals have become subject to surveillance and to 'the gaze' of the state. This is enacted through the professional and expert surveillance of social workers, public health specialists, police officers and others, but most importantly, through self-surveillance; that is, the responsibility everyone has to monitor their own health and those of their families. In other words, the power of the state and its agents is enacted through individuals themselves. Much attention has been given to the rise of surveillance medicine which has become an increasingly accepted part of everyday life in modern western societies. Writing about this, Armstrong (1986) argues that making this a normal process ensures that populations come under increased observation. Surveillance, such as cervical cancer screening or prenatal testing, is such that individuals are encouraged, and expected, to comply. Howson (1999) suggests that such expectations are not unproblematic but embedded within a moral framework of self-responsibility and social obligation. There is considerable evidence to show that surveillance medicine causes considerable tension and anxiety amongst the population (see Press,

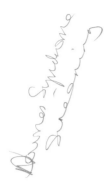

Fishman and Koenig, 2000). As Edwards et al. (2003) note, screening is designed to reduce morbidity in the population, but at an individual level other issues need to be considered. It is often a question of balancing harms – such as false positive results or unnecessary morbidity – against the benefits.

Williams, Cooke and May (1998) argue that it is important to recognise the difference between rhetoric and reality. Writing specifically about nursing (although their point is applicable to all), they suggest that there can be a big difference between how nurses say they practise and how they do practise. They argue that holism serves to reinforce an idealistic image of health workers which, in reality, does not hold true. Alonso (2004) also suggests that although the biopsychosocial model has found broad intellectual acceptance, in practice, a holistic approach to health is not pervasive in practical settings.

2.3.10 Lay accounts of health

Over the last thirty years, interest has grown in exploring the way that lay people understand health. Early accounts focused on classifying people's views. For example, an early classic study of the views of middle-class people in France (Herzlich, 1973), identified three different ideas about health:

1   health as existing in a vacuum

2   health as a reserve

3   health as equilibrium.

Elsewhere, this has been described as health in terms of having, doing and being (Blaxter, 2004). These findings have been echoed, in varying degrees, by other researchers (e.g. Blaxter and Patterson, 1982; Cornwell, 1984; Calnan, 1987). All of these early studies are characterised, however, by the idea that lay understandings of health and illness are separate from other ways of knowing about health, (e.g. the medical model), and that these understandings are best understood as lay **beliefs**, in that they differ from a more systematic way of conceptualising health.

However, later research on lay understandings of health pointed to the complexity of people's accounts. For example, Stainton Rogers (1991) shows that people draw on rich and varied experiences and insights, including medical ones, in order to make sense of health. (Box 2.7 shows different elements of lay knowledge of health.) This led researchers to endorse the idea of lay **knowledge** of health, rather than lay beliefs, thus, demonstrating the robustness of people's understandings of health and illness.

Box 2.7 Lay knowledge of health

1 The 'body as machine' account, in which illness is accepted as a matter of biological fact and modern biomedicine is seen as the only valid type of treatment.

2 The 'body under siege' account,, which sees the individual as under constant threat from germs, diseases, stresses and conflicts of modern life.

3 The 'inequality of access' account, which accepts modern biomedicine but is concerned about unequal access and treatment.

4 The 'cultural critique' of medicine account, which highlights how western biomedicine has oppressed women, minority groups and colonial peoples and which emphasises its 'social construction'.

5 The 'health promotion' account, which emphasises the importance of a healthy lifestyle and personal responsibility, although it also sees health as a collective responsibility.

6 The 'robust individualism' account, which emphasises the individual's right to live a satisfying life and their freedom of choice.

7 The 'God's power' account, which views health as righteous living and spiritual wholeness.

8 The 'will-power' account, which emphasises the moral responsibility of individuals to use their will to maintain good health.

(Stainton Rogers, 1991)

Drawing on this, others have even argued for a lay epidemiology of health, making a case for the way in which lay people theorise about health and illness. Supporting the idea of a lay epidemiology of health, Davison et al. (1991) argue that, in reality, most people carry out observations and create hypotheses to help them understand and explain their social worlds. Over time, richer and thicker descriptions of lay understandings of health have emerged, reflecting the changing lexicon, from 'lay beliefs' to 'lay knowledge' and 'lay epidemiology' (Popay et al., 2003).

Lay understandings of health do not exist in a vacuum in that they draw on other ways of knowing about health. Shaw (2002) problematises the concept of 'layness' further and argues that there are no lay understandings of health which are not informed by an expert conceptual framework of some kind. Given the increasingly blurring boundaries between lay and expert knowledge, Kangas (2002) argues that the boundaries between lay models of health and expert knowledge bases are vague. Indeed, the Expert Patients' Programme (DoH, 2001) is underpinned by a user-led service which draws on lay expertise. Similar local initiatives can be found in other countries within the UK: for example, the 'Braveheart Project' in Scotland and the 'Challenging Arthritis' course in Northern Ireland. What all of these programmes have in common is not just the desire to take into account lay experiences but to acknowledge lay expertise. However, Prior (2003) is highly critical of the concept 'lay expert' and, drawing on dictionary definitions of the words, 'layness' and 'expert', suggests that the 'lay expert' is an oxymoron:

> lay people – in the ordinary way of things – do have experiences of illness and disease. Nevertheless, they simply are not (as lay people) skilled and practised in the diagnosis and management of illness. Indeed, it is only by virtue of 'having experience' that we can even begin to think of such a creature as a lay expert. Lay people do, of course, have information and knowledge to impart ... And all in all, they are experts by virtue of 'having experience'. Yet, experience on its own is rarely sufficient to understand the technical complexities of disease causation, its consequences or its management. This is partly because experiential knowledge is invariably limited, and idiosyncratic.
>
> (Prior, 2003, p. 53)

Thinking point   how useful do you find the concept of the 'lay expert'?

Whether you agree or disagree with the concept of the lay expert, it does highlight the importance of people's own views of health and illness and the way that these might differ from those of professionals. It is also important to acknowledge the distinction between a lay expert and a lay person who has expertise in his or her own condition. Acknowledging these similarities and differences might be helpful for those involved in promoting health at different levels. Writing specifically about the role of lay knowledge in relation to public health research, Popay and Williams (1996) argue that it must use the insights offered by lay experts on the nature of health, illness and health behaviour.

2.4 Conclusion

Definitions of health are personal and individual, as well as social and cultural. Defining health is perplexing and ambiguous, but it is worthwhile since definitions and understandings of health influence the success of any activity designed to promote public health. It is also important to recognise that both explicitly and implicitly held concepts and models of health can influence the planning, delivery and evaluation of health promoting interventions.

Multidisciplinary public health adopts a broad view of health and illness. Although this is laudable, it is important to question the extent to which a person's 'health' can be distinguished from the totality of their lives. The impact of this idea on the likelihood of achieving a state of health and the consequences of this for promoting public health should also be reflected on.

References

Alonso, Y. (2004) 'The biopsychosocial model in medical research: the evolution of the health concept over the last two decades', *Patient Education and Counselling,* vol. 53, no. 2, pp. 239–44.

Annandale, E. (1998) *The Sociology of Health and Medicine: A Critical Introduction*, London, Polity.

Antonovsky, A. (1987) *Unravelling the Mystery of Health: How People Manage Others and Stay Well*, New York, Wiley.

Antonovsky, A. (1993) 'The sense of coherence as a determinant of health' in Beattie, A. et al. (eds) *Health and Wellbeing: A Reader*, Basingstoke, Macmillan/Milton Keynes, The Open University.

Armstrong, D. (1986) 'The problem of the whole-person in holistic medicine', *Holistic Medicine*, vol. 1, pp. 27–36.

Armstrong, D. (1987) 'Theoretical tensions in biopsychosocial medicine', *Social Science and Medicine*, vol. 25, no. 1, pp. 1213–18.

Blaxter, M. (1990) *Health and Lifestyles*, London, Routledge.

Blaxter, M. (2004) *Health*, Cambridge, Polity.

Blaxter, M. and Patterson, E. (1982) *Mothers and Daughters*, London, Heinemann.

Calnan, M. (1987) *Health and Illness: The Lay Perspective*, New York, Tavistock.

Cooper, C.L. and Clarke, S. (2003) *Managing the Safety Risk of Workplace Stress*, London, Routledge.

Cornwell, J. (1984) *Hard-earned Lives: Accounts of Health and Illness from East London*, London, Tavistock.

Cox, B.D., Blaxter, M., Buckle, A.L.J., Fenner, N.P., Golding, J.F., Gore, M., Huppert, F.A., Nickson, J., Roth, M., Stark, J., Wadsworth, M.E.J. and Whichelow, M.J. (1987) *The Health and Lifestyle Survey*, London, Health Promotion Research Trust.

Crawford, R. (1977) 'You are dangerous to your health: the politics and ideology of victim blaming', *International Journal of Health Services*, vol. 7, no. 4, pp. 663–80.

Crawford, R. (1980) 'Healthism and the medicalisation of everyday life', *International Journal of Health Services*, vol. 10, no. 3, pp. 365–88.

Cronin de Chavez, A., Backett-Milburn, K., Parry, O. and Platt, S. (2005) 'Understanding and researching well-being: its usage in different disciplines and potential for health research and health promotion', *Health Education Journal*, vol. 64, no. 1, pp. 70–87.

Davison, C., Davey Smith, G. and Frankel, S. (1991) 'Lay epidemiology and the prevention paradox: the implications of coronary candidacy for health education', *Sociology of Health and Illness*, vol. 13, no. 1, pp. 1–20.

Department of Health (DoH) (2001) *The Expert Patient: A New Approach to Chronic Disease Management for the 21st Century*, London, DoH.

Diener, E. (1994) 'Assessing subjective well-being: progress and opportunities', *Social Indicators Research*, vol. 31, pp. 103–57.

Dines, A. (1994) 'A review of lay health beliefs research: insights for nursing practice in health promotion', *Journal of Clinical Nursing*, vol. 3, no. 6, pp. 329–38.

Earle, S. (2005) 'What is health?' in Denny, E. and Earle, S. (eds) *Sociology for Nurses*, Oxford, Polity.

Edwards, A., Unigwe, S., Elwyn, G. and Hood, K. (2003) 'Effects of communicating individual risks in screening programmes: Cochrane systematic review', *British Medical Journal*, vol. 327, pp. 703–9.

Engel, G.L. (1977) 'The need for a new medical model: a challenge for medicine', *Science*, vol. 196, pp. 129–36.

Fitzpatrick, M. (2000) *The Tyranny of Health: Doctors and the Regulation of Lifestyle*, London, Routledge.

Fitzpatrick, R.M. (1986) 'Society and changing patterns of disease' in Patrick, D.L. and Scambler, G. (eds) *Sociology as Applied to Medicine* (2nd edn), London, Balliere Tindall, pp. 16–39.

Foucault, M. (1973) *The Birth of the Clinic: An Archaeology of Medical Perception*, London, Tavistock.

Friedson, E. (1970) *Profession of Medicine*, Chicago, University of Chicago Press.

Handsley, S. (2007) 'Mental health promotion' in Douglas, J., Handsley, S., Lloyd, C. and Spurr, S. (eds) *Policy and Practice in Promoting Public Health*, London, Sage/Milton Keynes, The Open University.

Hannay, D.R. (1979) *The Symptom Iceberg: A Study of Community Health*, London, Routledge and Kegan Paul.

Hassed, C.S. (2004) 'Bringing holism into mainstream medical education', *Journal of Alternative and Complementary Medicine*, vol. 10, no. 2, pp. 405–7.

Hek, G., Singer, L. and Taylor, P. (2004) 'Cross-boundary working: a generic worker for older people in the community', *British Journal of Community Nursing*, vol. 9, no. 6, pp. 237–44.

Herzlich, C. (1973) *Health and Illness: A Social Psychological Analysis*, London, Academic Press.

Howson, A. (1999) 'Cervical screening, compliance and moral obligation', *Sociology of Health and Illness*, vol. 21, no. 4, pp. 401–26.

Hughner, R.S. and Klein, S.S. (2004) 'Views of health in the lay sector: a complication and review of how individuals think about health', *Health: An Interdisciplinary Journal for the Social Study of Health, Illness and Medicine*, vol. 8, no. 4, pp. 395–422.

Hunt, K. (1994) 'A "Cure for All Ills?" Constructions of the menopause and the chequered fortunes of hormone replacement therapy' in Wilkinson, S. and Kitzinger, C. (eds) *Women and Health: Feminist Perspectives*, London, Taylor & Francis, pp. 141–65.

Hunt, S.M., McEwan, J. and McKenna, S.P. (1986) *Measuring Health Status*, London, Croom Helm.

Illich, I. (1976) *The Limits to Medicine*, Harmondsworth, Penguin.

Kangas, I. (2002) '"Lay" and "expert": illness knowledge constructions in the sociology of health and illness', *Health: An Interdisciplinary Journal for the Social Study of Health, Illness and Medicine*, vol. 6, no. 3, pp. 301–4.

Kelly, M. and Charlton, B. (1995) 'The modern and the post modern in health promotion' in Bunton, R., Nettleton, S. and Burrows, R. (eds) *The Sociology of Health Promotion*, London, Routledge, pp. 78–90.

Kelman, S. (1975) 'The social nature of the definition problem in health', *International Journal of Health Services*, vol. 5, no. 4, pp. 625–42.

Kolkaba, R. (1997) 'The primary holism in nursing', *Journal of Advanced Nursing*, vol. 25, no. 2, pp. 290–6.

Lawton, J. (2003) 'Lay experiences of health and illness: past research and future agendas', *Sociology of Health and Illness*, vol. 25, no. 3, pp. 32–40.

Lee, C. (1998) *Women's Health: Psychological and Social Perspectives*, London, Sage.

Lee, Y. and McCormick, B. (2004) 'Subjective well-being of people with spinal cord injury: does leisure contribute?' *Journal of Rehabilitation*, vol. 70, no. 3, pp. 5–12.

Lloyd, L. (2000) 'Dying in old age: promoting well-being at the end of life', *Mortality*, vol. 5, no. 2, pp. 171–88.

Lloyd-Williams, M. (ed.) (2003) *Psychosocial Issues in Palliative Care*, Oxford, Oxford University Press.

Lupton, D. (1995) *The Imperative of Health*, London, Sage.

McKague, M. and Verhoef, M. (2003) 'Understandings of health and its determinants among clients and providers at an urban community health center', *Qualitative Health Research*, vol. 13, no. 5, pp. 703–17.

McKinlay, J. (1975) 'A case for refocusing upstream: the political economy of sickness' in Enelow, A. et al. (eds) *Behavioral Aspects of Prevention*, Seattle, Washington, American Heart Association pp. 9–25.

Marcus, K.S., Kerns, R.D., Rosenfeld, B. and Breitbard, W. (2000) 'HIV/AIDS-related pain as chronic pain condition: implications of a biopsychosocial model for comprehensive assessment and effective management', *Pain Medicine*, vol. 1, no. 3, pp. 260–73.

Mechanic, D. (1968) *Medical Sociology*, New York, Free Press.

Mental Health Foundation (2005) *What is Mental Health?* [online], http://www.mentalhealth.org.uk/page.cfm?pagecode=PMWM (Accessed 4th April 2006).

Nettleton, S. (1995) *The Sociology of Health and Illness*, Oxford, Polity.

O'Brien, M. (1995) 'Health and lifestyles: a critical mess? Notes on the differentiation of health' in Bunton, R., Nettleton, S. and Burrows, R. (eds) *The Sociology of Health Promotion*, London, Routledge, pp. 191–205.

Paterson, C. (2004) 'Acupuncture as a complex intervention: a holistic model', *Journal of Alternative and Complementary Medicine*, vol. 10, no. 5, pp. 791–801.

Patterson, E.F. (1997) 'The philosophy and physics of holistic health care: spiritual healing and workable interpretation', *Journal of Advanced Nursing,* vol. 27, no. 2, pp. 287–93.

Popay, J., Bennett, S., Thomas, C., Williams, G., Gatrell, A. and Bostock, L. (2003) 'Beyond "beer, fags, egg and chips"? Exploring lay understandings of social inequalities in health', *Sociology of Health and Illness*, vol. 25, no. 1, pp. 1–23.

Popay, J. and Williams, G. (1996) 'Public health research and lay knowledge', *Social Science and Medicine*, vol. 42, no. 5, pp. 759–68.

Press, N., Fishman, J.R. and Koenig, B.A. (2000) 'Collective fear, individualised risk: the social and cultural context of genetic testing for breast cancer', *Nursing Ethics,* vol. 7, no. 3, pp. 237–49.

Prior, L. (2003) 'Belief, knowledge and expertise: the emergence of the lay expert in medical sociology', *Sociology of Health and Illness*, vol. 25 (Silver Anniversary Issue), pp. 41–57.

Reilly, C. (2001) 'Enhancing human healing', *British Medical Journal*, vol. 322, pp. 120–1.

Robinson, D. (1971) *The Process of Becoming Ill*, London, Routledge.

Royal College of Midwives (2005) *Campaign for Normal Birth: Salutogenesis in Support of Normality* [online], http://www.rcm.org.uk/data/info_centre/data/virtual_institute_salutogenesis.htm (Accessed 1 February 2006).

Scottish Executive (2002) *Well? Mental Health and Well-being in Scotland*, Scottish Executive [online], http://www.scotland.gov.uk/Publications/2002/09/15357/10707 (Accessed 4th April 2006).

Shaw, I. (2002) 'How lay are lay beliefs?' *Health: An Interdisciplinary Journal for the Social Study of Health, Illness and Medicine*, vol. 6, no. 3, pp. 287–99.

Sidell, M. (2007) 'Older people's health: applying Antonovsky's salutogenic paradigm' in Douglas, J., Earle, S. Handsley, S., Lloyd, C. and Spurr, S. (eds) *A Reader in Promoting Public Health: Challenge and Controversy*, London, Sage/Milton Keynes, The Open University.

Stainton Rogers, W. (1991) *Explaining Health and Illness: An Exploration of Diversity*, London, Harvester Wheatsheaf.

Sure Start Scotland (2003) *Bulletin 15*, Scotland, Sure Start.

Turner, B.S. (1995) *Medical Power and Social Knowledge* (2nd edn), London, Sage.

Welsh Assembly Government (2002) *Well Being in Wales*, Cardiff, Office of the Chief Medical Officer.

Whitehead, M. (1987) *The Health Divide: Inequalities in Health in the 1980s*, London, Health Education Council.

World Health Organization (WHO) (1946) *Preamble to the Constitution of the World Health Organization as adopted by the International Health Conference, New York, 19 June – 22 July 1946; signed on 22 July 1946 by the representatives of 61 States (Official Records of the World Health Organization, no. 2, p. 100) and entered into force on 7 April 1948*, Geneva, WHO.

Williams, R. (1983) 'Concepts of health: an analysis of lay logic', *Sociology*, vol. 17, pp. 185–204.

Williams, A., Cooke, H. and May, C. (1998) *Sociology, Nursing and Health*, Oxford, Butterworth Heinemann.

Williams, G. and Popay, J. (1994) 'Lay knowledge and the privilege of experience' in Gabe, J., Kelleher, D. and Williams, G. (eds) *Challenging Medicine*, London, Routledge, pp. 118–39.

World Health Organisation (WHO) (1958) *The First Ten Years of the World Health Organisation*, Geneva, WHO.

World Health Organization (WHO) (1986) *Ottawa Charter for Health Promotion*, Geneva, WHO.

Wynne, N., Brand, S. and Smith, R. (1997) 'Incomplete holism in pre-registration nurse education: the position of the biological sciences', *Journal of Advanced Nursing*, vol. 26, pp. 470–4.

Zola, I.K. (1973) 'Pathways to the doctor – from person to patient', *Social Science and Medicine*, vol. 7, no. 9, pp. 677–89.

Chapter 3

The factors that influence health

Sarah Earle and Terry O'Donnell

[handwritten margin note: What did Lalonde Report say?]

Introduction

This chapter begins by considering how changing understandings of health and illness can affect ways of thinking about multidisciplinary public health. It considers the influence of the Lalonde Report (1974) which, as you saw in Chapter 1, was an influential part of the 'new' public health and, some would say, represented an important shift in ways of thinking about health. In this chapter you also consider the issue of inequalities in health and some contemporary explanations for these. Building on these explanations, and drawing on the work of Dahlgren and Whitehead (1991), the remainder of this chapter focuses on the key factors that influence health: biology and genetics, lifestyle and behaviour, living and working conditions, social and community networks, and the wider social conditions in which individuals are located. Before reading on, consider the question in the thinking point.

[handwritten margin note: My mind My work My lifestyle — our eating / drinking / exercise My family Biology / genes]

Thinking point   what influences your health?

3.1 Changing understandings of health and illness

Changing understandings of health and illness can affect perceptions of the factors and the strategies that could be adopted to promote health. So, for example, a traditional medical model of health tends to focus predominantly on individual biology, whereas a more contemporary medical model widens this focus to pay attention to personal behaviours such as smoking or physical activity. A social model locates both individual biology and personal behaviours within wider social contexts and thus takes into account features such as income distribution, social deprivation, and the organisation of health and social care. This latter perspective is, furthermore, not just concerned with the incidence of illness and disease in particular points in time and space, but also recognises that experiences of health and disease are socially differentiated.

As described in Chapter 1, the origins of modern public health recognised the significance of poverty and environment on the population's health. However, individual responsibility for health was also recognised and sometimes individuals – especially the poor – were blamed for death and disease. In the early nineteenth century the high level of mortality – especially among the labouring masses – prompted an interest in the living and working environments of the poor. Nevertheless, within this overall focus on the environment, there were different perspectives. In his *Report on the Sanitary Conditions of the Labouring Population in Great Britain*, Chadwick (1842) showed that mortality rates were highest for the poorest and for urban dwellers. He also showed that the poorer classes lived in the most unsanitary areas. This led Chadwick to endorse the miasma theory – a belief that bad air caused infectious and respiratory diseases – and to argue for schemes to safely dispose of the filth he believed to be an inevitable consequence of industrialisation, and a danger to all.

Engels (1845), however, took a different stance. Using a variety of sources, including official reports from the Registrar-General, he also observed appalling living and working conditions among the poor. He argued that the propertied classes failed to deal with pollution and hazardous working conditions and charged workers high rents for bad housing. Engels argued that these actions, driven by profit, were directly responsible for the patterns of disease and early death in the working class and that they amounted to what he termed 'social murder'.

In the period between the First and Second World Wars, concerns with poverty and unemployment and their relationship to health remained on the agenda. At this time there was some academic interest in social medicine, and new thinking in public health emerged from experiments such as the Pioneer Peckham Health Centre in the 1930s (Webster and French, 2002). The Peckham Health Centre, which aimed to explore the impact of the environment on health, was housed in a building built by the renowned engineer, Sir William Owen, and designed to allow maximum air and sunlight to circulate, as well as allowing for observation of health centre members. Nine hundred and fifty families signed up for the Peckham experiment, and for one shilling per week they had access to a swimming pool, games and workshops, and an annual medical examination. In contrast to other forms of healthcare at that time, and the prevailing ethos of the newly formed NHS, the Peckham Health Centre emphasised the importance of preventative, rather than curative, healthcare, but in 1950, after several funding crises, the Centre closed down.

The introduction of the National Health Service (NHS) in 1948 revolutionised health care in the UK. The predominance of the medical model was a major driver of this health service (and other countries' healthcare systems). Subsequently, resources went into therapeutic medicine with the greatest emphasis being on the secondary care provided by hospitals, as opposed to the relatively low resourcing of the primary-care-based General Practitioner (GP). Despite widespread recognition of the way in which environment and living and working conditions could influence health, relatively fewer resources went to public health.

Concepts of health and their associated understandings of what influences health have been intimately connected to the continual shaping of healthcare systems and governmental policies on public health.

3.2 A paradigm shift: Lalonde's Health Field Concept

While the NHS and similar health systems in other countries have been described as revolutionary, rising costs and an ever increasing burden of disease prompted the necessity to think differently about health. The Lalonde Report (1974) represented an important milestone in changing understandings of health and illness. McKay (2000, p. 3) argues that it 'provided the conceptual framework to inspire a paradigm shift by officially announcing that health was more than health care'. Until this time health service provision was regarded as one of the most important ways of achieving better health, but Lalonde argued that 'The health care system ... is only one of many ways of maintaining and improving health. ... For these environmental and behavioural threats to health, the organized health care system can do little more than serve as a catchment net for the victims.' (Lalonde, 1974, p. 5).

This was supported by the ideas of McKeown (1976), who proposed that dramatic reductions in mortality were due to improved socio-economic conditions rather than attributable to medicine and healthcare.

The Lalonde Report identified four fields within which health could be improved, which it termed environment, biology/genetics, lifestyle and health services (see Figure 3.1). It suggested that while most attention had been paid to medical treatment provided by the health services, environment and lifestyle would offer the greatest opportunities for promoting public health in the future. Members of the Lalonde team also foresaw the increasing importance of genetic research for future health and believed that research should underpin policy and practice in all four health fields.

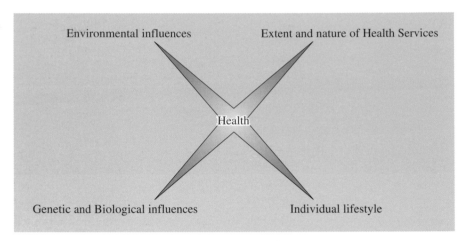

Figure 3.1 Lalonde's Health Field Concept (1974)

Thinking point   how far is it possible to focus on lifestyle and environmental issues at the same time?

In theory, it is possible to focus on both lifestyle and environmental issues at the same time and, as you saw in Chapter 1, the Ottawa Charter focused on both individuals and environments. However, although the Lalonde Report was undoubtedly important, it is not without its critics. For example, in its discussion of road traffic accidents, the report argued that behavioural changes to reduce speeding and careless driving and increase seatbelt use would result in the greatest benefits to health, with environmental changes to roads and car design being the second most important issue. Indeed, many commentators have suggested that the Lalonde Report placed greatest emphasis on individual lifestyle and behaviour modification and conceived the public solely as passive recipients of services (Raeburn and Rootman, 1989; McKay, 2000; Boyce, 2002). As you can see below, this legacy has been perpetuated.

3.3 Promoting public health: post Lalonde

3.3.1 Factors affecting health

After publication of the Lalonde Report, policy and strategy increasingly recognised the role of all four health fields. However, just as Lalonde was criticised for focusing mostly on lifestyle and behaviour so, too, were subsequent documents. For example, in the 1970s, *Prevention and Health: Everybody's Business* (DHSS, 1976) argued that the weight of responsibility for health lay on the shoulders of individuals themselves.

Amid concern with the efficacy and organisation of the NHS, increasing attention was paid to the problem of health inequalities, especially the difference in life expectancy between different socio-economic groups. Under the Chair of Sir Douglas Black, a report – which became known as the Black Report – was published which highlighted the considerable inequalities in health in Britain (DHSS, 1980). Indeed, the report was suppressed when it first came out. The Black Report offered four possible explanations for inequalities in health, as outlined in Box 3.1.

Box 3.1 Possible explanations for inequalities in health

Artefact: This proposes that the inequalities are an artefact of the way the statistics are produced, and that biases and changes in the composition of different social classes over time have made the evidence unreliable.

Social selection: This proposes that inequalities are a result of social mobility; that is, those in good health move up the social scale whereas those in poor health slip down.

Behaviour: Health inequalities are the result of people engaging in health-damaging behaviours and those in the lowest social classes are most likely to exhibit such behaviours.

Material circumstances: Poverty, poor environments and weak social networks, among other cultural and social factors, influence health and largely create health inequalities.

While multifactoral influences on health were recognised, in 1987 the British government published *Promoting Better Health* which, once again, emphasised the importance of behavioural change: 'Much distress and suffering could be avoided if more members of the public took greater responsibility for their own health ...' (DHSS, 1987, p. 3).

However, by the 1990s many researchers had highlighted the interconnections between the various factors that influence health, suggesting that action was required to combat inequalities at various levels: strengthening individuals, strengthening communities, improving access to essential facilities and services and encouraging macroeconomic and cultural change. So, in the early 1990s, the health strategy for England (DoH, 1992) aimed to ensure that health would be tackled at these different levels. However, it was widely criticised for not paying sufficient attention to broader economic and structural factors (such as the environment).

These wider factors are shown in Figure 3.2 (published in 1991), which offers a multifactoral illustration of the wider determinants of health.

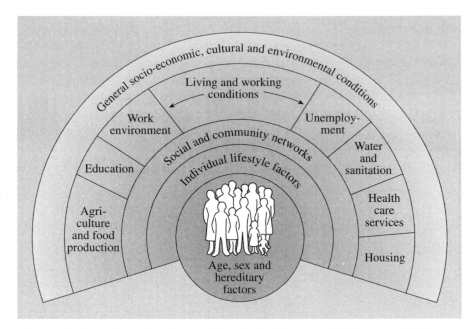

Figure 3.2 The main determinants of health (Dahlgren and Whitehead, 1991)

Thinking point   to what extent do you think that the factors identified by Dahlgren and Whitehead in Figure 3.2 influence your own health?

This multifactoral approach differentiates between individual and social factors, offering a diagram with layers which can be peeled away. The core of the diagram consists of inherited attributes relating to age, sex and hereditary factors. The inner layer suggests that health is partly determined by individual lifestyle factors, such as patterns of smoking, physical activity and diet. Moving outwards, the diagram draws attention to relationships with family, friends and significant others within the local community. As discussed in Chapter 2, these are the downstream determinants of health – the actions of individuals and communities. The next layer focuses on working and living conditions – housing, employment, access to healthcare services and so on. The outer layer highlights broader socio-economic, cultural and environmental forces such as economic development, shifts in welfare systems, political change, social forces and structures. These final two layers relate to the upstream determinants of health. Although it is not really shown in the diagram, there is potential for layer-to-layer interaction. For example, cutbacks in welfare services might adversely affect people's access to adequate housing and thus influence their health.

By the late 1990s the public health agenda across the UK gained prominence. New Labour, coming into power in 1997, adopted the concept of 'social exclusion' to show recognition of how social divisions (such as social class, ethnicity, gender and disability) resulted in unequal experience of, and access to, health and social care. An independent inquiry

Acheson Report 1998 /

into inequalities in health in England (known as the Acheson Report) was published in 1998. This influential report – which drew on the framework suggested by Dahlgren and Whitehead (1991) – made thirty-nine recommendations underpinned by a broad analysis of the social, economic and environmental determinants of health inequalities (Acheson, 1998). In England, the White Paper *Saving Lives: Our Healthier Nation* (DoH, 1999) and similar publications in Scotland, Northern Ireland and Wales also addressed social inequality and social exclusion.

The 1990s saw a multifactoral response to health become established within UK government policy and strategy. However, more recently, another shift has occurred. In England, for example, the government White Paper *Choosing Health: Making Healthier Choices Easier* (DoH, 2004) recognises the impact of social, environmental, economic and cultural trends, yet firmly locates the public health agenda within the context of individual behavioural change. The White Paper is based on three principles:

1   informed choice
2   personalisation
3   working together in partnership.

Each of these, in particular the first two principles, draws on notions of the responsible citizen and his/her 'choice' of health behaviours. A similar picture can be found in the Welsh Assembly initiative, 'Health Challenge Wales', which urges members of the public to improve their own health by taking up the professional advice, information and support available to them.

3.3.2 Contemporary explanations of inequalities in health

There is considerable research activity on the multifactoral causes of health inequalities which, as O'Donnell states: 'is developing our knowledge of the pathways that link the bodies of individuals to their life experiences, including their material resources, and how these are all shaped by the social structure' (O'Donnell, 2005, p. 150).

Bartley (2004) provides a useful account of contemporary explanations of health inequalities and suggests that there are three key explanations: psycho-social explanations, lifecourse explanations and neo-materialist explanations. These are examined in turn below.

Psycho-social explanations focus on the way in which the contemporary conditions of life produce social stresses that affect social groups unevenly, and on how members of these groups have uneven access to material and personal resources to manage these stresses. However, such stresses do not only affect mental wellbeing; they also affect the body through the cardiovascular, endocrine and immune systems. Siegrist et al.

(1990), for example, argue that occupational distress can occur when a high workload is matched with job insecurity, poor promotion prospects and low control over the work. They suggest that this effort/reward imbalance can lead to heart disease and its precursors, such as raised blood pressure. Outside of employment, hard-to-manage causes of stress (e.g. rising debt) can often lead to coping behaviours harmful to health, such as smoking, excessive alcohol consumption and an unhealthy diet. Figures in 2004 suggested that at least one third of all UK households had some sort of unsecured debt, such as a personal loan or credit card bill greater than they expected to pay off at the end of the month (ONS, 2004a). The ability to change these health-damaging behaviours is affected by restricted access to important resources of money, time and supportive outlets such as community networks and health clubs.

Lifecourse explanations consider how the health effects of adverse socio-economic circumstances accumulate throughout the lifecourse, from conception through to later life. Early work carried out by Barker (1989), for example, led to the concept of foetal programming, which suggests that maternal poverty can affect foetal development. Material and social disadvantage for adults can, thus, be reflected in the lower birth weight and poor health of their children. Childhood poverty has also been shown to have an independent effect on both adult health and socio-economic status. Indeed, the highest health risks have been found in those who both grow up, and remain, in disadvantaged material circumstances (van de Mheen et al., 1998). Whilst health problems in adult life do not necessarily result in downward social mobility, poor health in children and young adults, combined with poor socio-economic circumstances, can produce a negative downward effect. Theories of social selection have been virtually discounted, but it is important to consider the cumulative effect of socio-economic circumstance across the lifecourse.

Neo-materialist explanations focus on the way in which adverse socio-economic and psycho-social environments, and the health-damaging mechanisms associated with them, are products of material and social formations. According to these explanations, these social formations produce an unequal distribution of personal income and wealth which, in turn, shapes unequal access to food, transport, housing, healthcare and education, as well as unequal consumption of a healthy lifestyle. In the UK there is considerable inequality in income distribution. Inequalities in disposable income (the amount of income available for spending and saving) are also evident. Figure 3.3 shows that the top decile of earners account for 28 per cent of total disposable income. The bottom seven decile groups received nearly half of total income, with the other half going to the top three decile groups. Wealth is even less evenly distributed than income: most recent figures (ONS, 2005a) show that half the adult UK population own only 6 per cent of total wealth, whereas the wealthiest 1 per cent of the population own 23 per cent of all wealth.

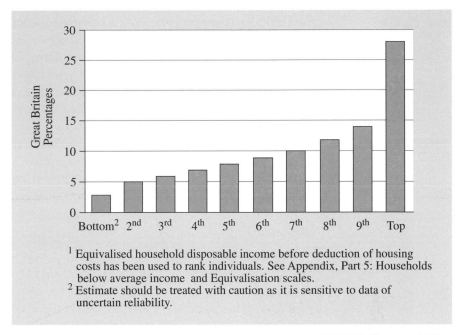

¹ Equivalised household disposable income before deduction of housing
  costs has been used to rank individuals. See Appendix, Part 5: Households
  below average income and Equivalisation scales.
² Estimate should be treated with caution as it is sensitive to data of
  uncertain reliability.

Figure 3.3 Shares of disposable income: by decile group 2002/03 (Source: ONS, 2005a, p. 73, Figure 5.14)

In 2002–03, 33 per cent of households in the United Kingdom reported having no savings at all. However, if the relationship between ethnicity and wealth is examined, further inequalities can be identified. Households headed by a Black/Black British or Asian/Asian British person are nearly twice as likely as households overall to have no savings. However, among Asian/Asian British households, those headed by someone of Indian origin are more likely to have savings than are those of Pakistani/Bangladeshi origin. Around half of all households headed by someone of Indian origin have no savings compared with three-quarters of households headed by someone of Pakistani/Bangladeshi origin.

So, there are inequalities both between, as well as within, groups, and it is these structured inequalities that produce social exclusion and low levels of social capital (these are discussed further below).

Thinking point   what are the difficulties of adopting a neo-materialist explanation?

Researchers working within a neo-materialist approach warn against putting too much emphasis on the consequences of inequality rather than on the need for structural change (Lynch et al., 2000). They suggest that by focusing on individuals and communities, rather than on unequal social structures, public health simply becomes another form of victim blaming. From a neo-materialist perspective, income inequality – together with the inequitable distribution of public resources (such as health services, schooling and social welfare provision) – produces inequalities in health. These wider inequalities are themselves produced by economic and political processes operating at a macro level and as such require major social interventions to create effective change (O'Donnell, 2005).

3.4 Exploring the factors that influence health

Using the framework provided by Dahlgren and Whitehead (1991), this chapter now moves on to explore the factors that influence health.

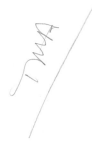

3.4.1 Age, sex and hereditary factors

In an attempt to move away from an exclusively biomedical approach to health towards one that does not equate health with healthcare, the significance of age, sex and hereditary factors have been somewhat overlooked in the last decade or so. However, more recently, and with considerable changes in science and technology, the importance of these factors in understanding inequalities and experiences of health and illness have, once again, come to the fore.

Genetics, health and the human genome

The Health Field Concept recognised the significance of human biology and genetics for health. Indeed, probably one of the most important endeavours undertaken in recent years has been the Human Genome Project (HGP), an internationally co-ordinated and funded undertaking which aims to map every gene in human DNA. As part of this project, and in what is widely described as the 'new genetics', the ability to identify gene mutations is making possible each of the following:

1   screening for carriers of recessively inherited disorders (e.g. cystic fibrosis)
2   identification of those who have the gene for a particular disorder (e.g. Huntingdon's Disease)
3   gene therapy for those affected with a disorder (e.g. cystic fibrosis).

Particular interest has been shown in the relationship between 'race', ethnicity and health. There has been much discussion and debate about whether genetic factors contribute to inequalities and differences in patterns of mortality and morbidity, particularly in relation to common chronic conditions such as diabetes, coronary heart disease and hypertension (DoH, 2000). However, while some researchers argue that the higher prevalence of these conditions among some ethnic groups is evidence of genetic differentiation between groups, other researchers have argued that environmental factors are most important. In a review of the epidemiological evidence on ethnic inequalities in health, Davey-Smith et al. (2000) argue that there is more genetic variation within ethnic groups than between ethnic groups, thus concluding that social and environmental factors are more significant than genetic ones.

Many commentators, including scientists, religious leaders, politicians, policy makers, academics and activists, have welcomed the potential outcomes of the HGP and see it as having enormous potential for promoting public health. However, others warn against the potential for abuse and discrimination (for example, see Albert, 2007) although this warning is by no means widespread (Earle and Sharp, 2007). Some of these concerns have been identified in Box 3.2.

Box 3.2 The human genome project: A dangerous future?

It has been predicted ... that insurance companies will insist on having detailed genetic profiles on all applicants for life or health insurance; that parents will try for perfect, designer babies, and select them (or abort them) on grounds such as intelligence, sex, or beauty; that traits not currently seen as being diseases, but as being part of normal human variation, will come to be seen as pathological conditions meriting treatment or eradication; and that the selection of marriage partners will be based on the exchange of genetic information. Further predictions are that we will become less sympathetic to and less able to cope with, or pay for, physical or mental disability, since it will be assumed that births of severely handicapped individuals can be avoided; that prospective parents will be under pressure to abort foetuses affected by genetic disorders, whether or not they personally approve of abortion; that ethnic groups with a tradition of marrying their cousins will be discriminated against in health-care provision and pressurized to change what for them may be socially valued practices; that employers will screen prospective employees for genetic conditions and that those likely to develop genetic disorders may not only be unemployable but also uninsurable; and that the health services will become overwhelmed by expensive programmes for genetic screening, diagnosis and therapy.

(Macintyre, 1995, p. 226)

Others have also been critical of the increasing emphasis on genetics and the human genome. Lippman, for example, refers to geneticisation, which she describes as: 'an ongoing process by which differences between individuals are reduced to their DNA codes, with most disorders, behaviors and physiological variations defined, at least in part, as genetic in origin' (Lippman, 1991, p. 19).

In a European study of the new genetics and of reproductive technologies, interviews with medical, legal and nursing professionals also show how geneticisation has become a 'public health story' (Ettorre, 2002, p. 56) in which health surveillance can claim competence in additional areas of personal and social life. Given these concerns, Wang et al. (2005) identify some of the opportunities for public health genetics in relation to health interventions, advocacy and promoting the public understanding (see Box 3.3).

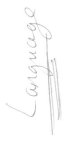

Box 3.3 Research and practice opportunities for public health genetics

Public understanding of genetics

- Methods to increase genetic literacy
- Genetic risk communication
- Informed consent and decision making
- Unintended outcomes of genetic information (e.g., fatalism, fear of discrimination)
- Media reporting of genetics

Interventions for health behavior change

- Impact of genetic information on screening and lifestyle behaviors
- Methods to incorporate genetic information into behavioral interventions
- Role of family history as a tool for public health prevention

Public health assurance and advocacy

- Advocacy against premature introduction of genetic services
- Methods to counter direct-to-consumer and direct-to-provider advertising
- Availability of comprehensive genetic services
- Equal access to genetic services
- Prevention of genetic discrimination (e.g. genetics and the workplace)

(Wang et al., 2005, p. 692, Table 1)

Whereas geneticisation places heredity at the fore of public health, the new genetics poses both problems and possibilities for improvement. It also creates a society in which individual characteristics are no longer fixed, but malleable and changeable by the manipulation of genes.

Sex, gender and health

It has long been assumed that sex (the **biological** differences between men and women), rather than gender (the **socially** defined differences between men and women), determines health. For example, in most countries, male life expectancy is lower than that of females and this is projected to continue (see Figure 3.4). However, in recent years this male disadvantage has become far less significant than before. For example, in England and Wales, between 1970 and 2003, male life expectancy increased by four years, but life expectancy for women increased by only three years, with the gap being 6.2 years in 1971 and 4.3 years in 2003 (ONS, 2005c). So while women were assumed to possess a biological advantage, given changes in patterns of life expectancy, this assumption is being challenged.

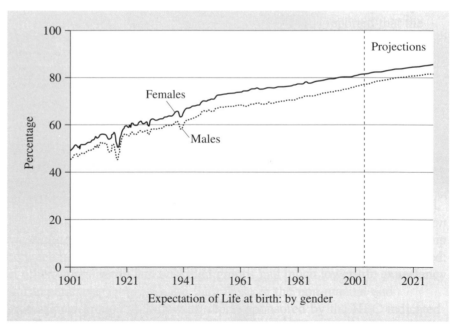

Figure 3.4 Life expectancy: 1901–2026 (Source: ONS, 2005c)

Thinking point   to what extent do you think that human biology is a major determinant of health?

Sex differences have also been drawn upon to explain patterns of mortality. For example, coronary heart disease (CHD), which is the leading cause of death in developed countries, was once thought to affect men more than women. Differences in CHD include a later age of onset for women, a greater prevalence of co-morbidity and differences in the initial manifestations of the disease (Bello and Mosca, 2004). However, psycho-social differences, and differences in lifestyle and in living and working conditions between men and women, are probably better indicators of susceptibility to CHD and associated co-morbidity than are biological factors (Fodor and Tzerovska, 2004) and, at least in relation to coronary heart disease, male anatomy is not destiny (Weidner and Cain, 2003, p. 769). So gender, rather than sex, is a better indicator of inequalities in health.

Age and the lifecourse: healthy ageing

Lifecourse perspectives draw on age, sex and hereditary factors to show how health effects accumulate throughout a person's life. Illness and ageing are seen to go hand-in-hand and old age is often portrayed as a period of decrepitude and decline. However, as Featherstone and Hepworth (1988) rightly note, there have been considerable attempts to deconstruct lifecourse explanations and to show how the 'mask of ageing' is socially constructed, rather than biologically determined. For example, a study of urinary incontinence (Mitteness and Barker, 1995) shows that whilst this condition is aggressively managed and treated in young people, in older people urinary incontinence is perceived as an inevitable and untreatable consequence of old age, in spite of the fact that it is often treatable and even reversible in some cases.

As a consequence of changes to the age structure of the population and a subsequent moral panic over welfare – which is discussed later in this chapter – the concept of positive, or healthy, ageing has been promoted as the way forward for older people. Whereas illness in old age was once seen as a consequence of chronology and biology, it is now recognised that behavioural, social and environmental factors all have a part to play (Sidell, 2007). Attention has been given to the relationships between ageing, activity and health. For example, particular emphasis has been given to the role of physical activity throughout the lifecourse and into later life (de Groot et al., 2004).

It is also important to recognise that later life and experiences of ageing are socially differentiated. For example, while many people believe that older people are now financially better off, what we have is a polarisation of the pensioner population with most of the wealth going to those who are already more wealthy. According to Age Concern (2005), in Scotland, one-quarter of households of older people have a low income (that is, below 60% of median disposable income), and many of these incomes are so low that the older people are entitled to claim other benefits.

This situation is most likely to affect older women, who are less likely to have paid into an occupational pension or state earnings related pension (SERPS).

Unusually high mortality in winter is also higher among the older population; however, this does not affect all older people equally. Although the exact numbers of people who die 'from the cold' are not known, older people are more likely to experience fuel poverty (generally defined as a household which needs to spend more than 10 per cent of its income on all fuel; slight variations in definition exist across the UK); this is largely caused by the cost of domestic fuel, the level of disposable income and the energy efficiency of the home. Older people are more likely to live on a low income, in poor quality housing and with expensive and inefficient heating systems.

3.4.2 Individual lifestyle factors

As you have seen above, emphasis on individual lifestyle as a determinant of health can be seen in most policies and strategies. In recent years the concept of a 'healthy lifestyle' has achieved considerable popular currency but, like many such concepts, the term can be widely used in many different contexts and can come to mean different things. Davison et al. provide a useful definition of 'lifestyle' which they describe as: 'the aspects of health-related behaviours and conditions which entail an element of personal action at the individual level ... strongly associated with the possibility of individual choice and the triumph of self control over self indulgence' (Davison et al., 1992, p. 675).

The main issues addressed usually include diet and physical activity, tobacco and alcohol use, drug intake and sexual activity, although, at various times, other issues have also fallen within this rubric, for example, exposure to the sun and use of seat belt or child car seat.

Many attempts to promote public health have focused on the individual and their lifestyle, and this seems to be a fairly common-sense approach. After all, it could be argued that if individuals ate a little less and took more exercise, then they would be less likely to become obese. If they smoked less and drank less alcohol they would be at a reduced risk of long-term conditions such as heart disease or cirrhosis, and if individuals engaged in safe sex, then they would be less likely to become infected with HIV or other sexually transmitted infections. Individual behaviour can play an important part in health and illness, so maintaining a healthy lifestyle could well be simply a matter of self-control. However, as outlined below, lifestyle accounts have been challenged on several counts.

Thinking point   how far is maintaining a healthy lifestyle simply a matter of self-control?

At a practical level, research has shown that it is very difficult to change individual behaviour. Although there have been some instances of success (e.g. the national HEA campaign to prevent cot deaths in the 1990s), there is still considerable debate about how far health can be improved through targeting individual behaviour. For example, although smoking has declined over time, a recent Omnibus Survey (Lader and Goddard, 2004) of smoking behaviour found that nearly 80 per cent of current smokers had tried (unsuccessfully) to give up smoking; and of these, 46 per cent had received advice on smoking cessation.

As explored later in Chapter 5, many theories and models have been developed to help explain individual health behaviours. However, one of the key problems facing those promoting public health is the failure of many individuals to follow healthy lifestyle advice. Two key explanations have been put forward to explain this. The first rests on the notion that the public are 'victims of their own ignorance' (Davison et al., 1992) and that with increased health education and advice, they will begin to embrace healthier lifestyles. This was the notion underpinning the government's HIV/AIDS prevention campaign in the late 1980s (see Figure 3.5).

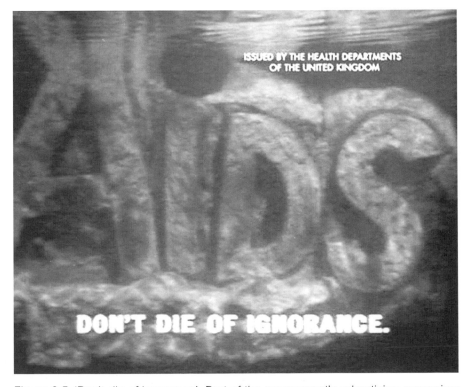

Figure 3.5 'Don't die of ignorance'. Part of the government's advertising campaign; this leaflet was distributed to all UK households. (See http://www.avert.org/his87_92.htm)

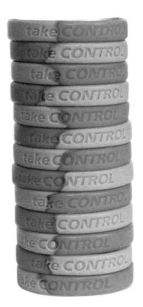

Figure 3.6 'Take Control' wrist band: part of Epilepsy Action's Take Control Campaign

The second explanation draws on the idea that individuals can believe that health is largely determined by external factors, therefore denying the relevance of individual behavioural change. Psychologists draw on the health 'locus of control' (Rotter, 1954) to describe the general expectancy that behaviour either is or is not directly related to health outcomes. An internal locus of control relates to the individual's feeling of control over health, whereas an external locus of control relates to factors outside of the individual's control. For example, a study of stress among mothers caring for children with intellectual impairments found an internal locus of control to be a protective factor (Hassall et al., 2005). A study of perceived risk for breast cancer also noted that women with an internal locus of control were more likely to engage in protective health behaviours such as attending screening (Rowe et al., 2005). The significance of this internal locus of control underpins the 'Take Control Campaign' launched by Epilepsy Action, which seeks to encourage all those with epilepsy to take control so as to achieve better management of their condition (see Figure 3.6).

The notion of taking control underpins many contemporary attempts within the public, private and voluntary sectors to promote public health. However, taking control is subject to the ability to take responsibility for health and to make choices, both of which are governed by power relations. In other words, not everyone is free to make decisions and choices, since individual choice and control can be constrained both by other people and by the factors that influence health.

While targeting individual behaviour might seem to be common sense, it is important to recognise that distinct patterns of behaviour can be found among different social groups. For example, Figure 3.7 shows that people in routine and manual occupations are more likely to smoke than people with non-manual occupations. Figure 3.8 shows changing patterns of excessive alcohol consumption, demonstrating that younger people are more likely to drink to excess and that women are now more likely to drink excessively in comparison to previous years.

Lifestyle accounts draw on notions of individual choice. However, if patterns of behaviour are considered – for example, those identified above – it is easy to see that 'choice' is not just an individual matter, but a social one. It is important to ask why young women are drinking to excess and why men in manual occupations are twice as likely to smoke as men in managerial or professional occupations. The rhetoric of choice and the 'right to choose' have become embedded in policy and practice. Writing specifically about reproductive choice, for example, Petchesky (1980) argues that, to be meaningful, the right to choose must carry with it the enabling conditions that will make that right concretely realisable and universally available:

> The 'right to choose' means very little when women are powerless ... women make their own reproductive choices, but they do not make them just as they please; they do not make them under conditions which they themselves create but under social conditions and constraints which they, as mere individuals, are powerless to change.

(Petchesky, 1980, pp. 674–750)

Figure 3.7   Prevalence of cigarette smoking, by sex and socio-economic classification, 2001–2004 (Source: ONS, 2005d, p. 9, Table 2.3)

All respondents

Socio-economic classification	2001	2002	2003	2004	2001	2002	2003	2004
	Percentage smoking cigarettes				Bases = 100%			
Men								
Managerial and professional occupations	17	17	16	16	586	647	625	637
Intermediate occupations	26	31	26	21	244	290	256	268
Routine and manual occupations	33	34	36	30	651	675	606	630
Never worked and long-term unemployed	26	22	30	29	68	135	142	114
Total	26	26	26	23	1549	1747	1628	1649
Women								
Managerial and professional occupations	20	16	15	18	544	574	564	527
Intermediate occupations	22	22	16	20	467	499	435	441
Routine and manual occupations	27	30	34	29	802	799	686	734
Never worked and long-term unemployed	14	24	20	20	131	203	207	197
Total	23	24	23	23	1944	2075	1891	1899
All								
Managerial and professional occupations	18	16	16	17	1132	1221	1189	1165
Intermediate occupations	24	25	19	21	711	790	690	711
Routine and manual occupations	30	32	34	29	1452	1474	1291	1365
Never worked and long-term unemployed	19	23	24	23	199	338	349	311
Total	24	25	24	23	3494	3823	3519	3552

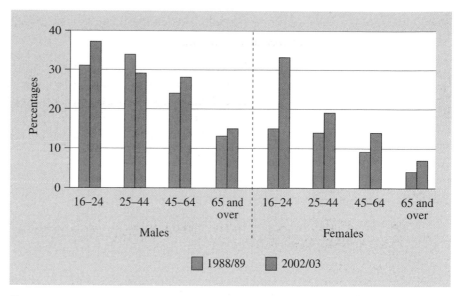

Figure 3.8 Adults exceeding weekly benchmarks of alcohol: by sex and age, 1988–89 and 2002–03, GB (Source: ONS, 2004b)

So, although lifestyle might be a factor that influences health, it is also important to focus on wider influences and the context within which individual 'choice' takes place.

3.4.3 Social and community influences

Here the role of social and community influences on health are considered. The concept of social capital has become very popular within public health in recent years, although, like many similar concepts, it been used in different ways by different people. Indeed, Wall et al. (1998) and Hawe and Shiell (2000) have argued that the concept is being used so widely and diversely that its explanatory power is being weakened.

The concept of social capital can be traced to one of several sources (Bourdieu, 1986; Coleman, 1988; Putnam, 1995); however, the work of Bourdieu is probably the most relevant here. He describes social capital as: 'the aggregate of the actual or potential resources which are linked to possession of a durable network of more or less institutionalized relationships of mutual acquaintance or recognition – or in other words to membership of a group' (Bourdieu, 1986, p. 248).

In a synthesis of the literature on social capital, Portes (1998, p. 1) describes it as 'the ability to secure benefits through membership in networks and other social structures' (see also Chapter 4 and Gibson, 2007). So social capital is both a resource enabling better access to goods and services as well as a network of relationships between individuals and between individuals and institutions.

A lifecourse approach would focus on how social capital is accrued throughout life and how it can be passed on from one generation to the next. Writing about education, Bourdieu (1999) discusses the way in which extra knowledge – or cultural capital – is passed on from parents to children and, drawing on this, Sullivan (2001) argues that this is one of the ways in which middle-class families ensure educational advantages for their children. Bagnall et al. (2003) carried out a study into involvement in parent / teacher associations (PTA) in the North West of England. Drawing on their analysis of 88 in-depth interviews they found that, while middle-class parents found PTA involvement a useful way of building social capital, working-class parents were more likely to generate social capital using their own family and other local social networks. For mobile middle-class people, the PTA enabled then to connect with 'like-minded' people as well as establishing institutional and relational links with the school as a means of 'getting ahead' (see Box 3.4).

Box 3.4 Social capital and 'getting ahead'

Interviewer: Why did you join the PTA?

Respondent (female, 40 years old):   Well, partly to meet people, partly to help fundraising for the school, and it's quite a good way of finding out what's going on as well.

(Bagnall et al., 2003)

For middle-class parents, PTA involvement is represented as the norm, but for working-class parents a lack of involvement is the norm. The latter are also much more likely to be dismissive of PTA involvement and more likely to describe themselves as being 'too busy'. Bagnall et al. suggest that working-class parents are more interested in 'getting by' rather than 'getting on', as illustrated by the following two quotes from this study in Box 3.5.

Box 3.5 Social capital and 'getting by'

Interviewer: [...] are you involved in any PTAs, or anything like that?

Respondent (male, 33 years old):   No, not at the moment, not involved at all ... I think the people who are attracted to it don't attract me, basically.

[...]

Interviewer: Did you get involved with the school – PTAs, things like that?

Respondent (female, 39 years old):   Not particularly PTAs, because having quite a lot on ourselves, because I do my husband's paperwork as well as doing the job myself, running the house, looking after the children, because he's so busy.

(Bagnall et al., 2003)

The relationship between social capital and health is disputed. Some writers have suggested that there is a direct relationship between inequalities in social capital and inequalities in health, whereas others (for example Kaplan et al., 1996) are less certain. Kawachi et al. (1997) argue that there is a clear relationship between increased morbidity and mortality and disinvestment in social capital. A study of physical activity and the social environment (i.e. culture, people and institutions with whom people interact) involving over 3,300 adults in six countries (Ståhl et al., 2001) also found that the social environment was the strongest predictor of physical activity. Those who perceived low levels of social support from their personal environment (i.e. family, friends, school and workplace) were twice as likely to be physically inactive compared to those who reported high levels of support. The study concluded that strategies to promote greater physical activity would need to focus more on social norms regarding active lifestyles, and on making activity more 'socially acceptable'. Thus, a settings approach, which is discussed further in the next chapter, seeks to enable different social environments – such as schools, workplaces, and so on – to maximise their health-promoting potential.

Social capital is, thus, linked to both social inclusion and social exclusion because, as you have already seen, it is not equally distributed. The Social Exclusion Unit (SEU) defines social exclusion as happening:

> when people or places suffer from a series of problems such as unemployment, discrimination, poor skills, low incomes, poor housing, high crime, ill health and family breakdown. When such problems combine they can create a vicious cycle.

> Social exclusion can happen as a result of problems that face one person in their life. But it can also start from birth. Being born into poverty or to parents with low skills still has a major influence on future life chances.

(Social Exclusion Unit, 2004)

Key groups who may suffer social exclusion include people with mental health problems, young runaways, teenage mothers and ex-prisoners, all of whom may lack membership of the networks and social structures that promote positive health and wellbeing. One of the goals of the SEU is the reintegration of people who, for one reason or another, have 'fallen through the net'.

Psycho-social approaches emphasise the importance of relational networks in promoting good health. For example, religiosity, or spirituality, has been found to increase a sense of belonging and, through various related activities, such as volunteering, promote good health (Yeung, 2004). Social and community influences can be important determinants of health, not just because of the material resources to which individuals may or may not have access, but also because of the relational networks within which individuals find, or locate, themselves. As Link and Phelan suggest: 'when a population develops the wherewithal to avoid disease and death, individuals' ability to benefit from that wherewithal is shaped by resources of knowledge, money, power, prestige, and beneficial social connections' (Link and Phelan, 2002, p. 730).

3.4.4 Living and working conditions

Social and community influences on health have been recognised for some time, but it is also important to consider the conditions in which people live and work. Graham's (1993) research on women and smoking, for example, showed that those who were poorest – low-income lone parents – were the most likely to smoke and that smoking was used as a strategy to cope with poverty and social exclusion. As one respondent in Graham's study stated: 'I smoke more if I've got bills coming in, I tend to get worried. Like Christmas is coming and I'm not able to afford the things I want' (Quoted in Graham, 1993).

Psycho-social explanations emphasise the way in which hard-to-manage stress, such as bringing up children alone and in poverty, can lead to health-damaging behaviours.

Other living conditions can also cause stress for people who are excluded or at risk of social exclusion. For example, whereas moving house can be a positive social and economic experience for some people, for people in transition such as those leaving hospital or care, and for traditionally mobile groups such as Gypsies, Travellers and seasonal workers, moving accommodation can compound the barriers they face. A report published by the Social Exclusion Unit (2004) found that instability in accommodation could:

- act as a barrier to securing work or training

- make accessing key services, such as health or social care, more difficult

- disrupt education
- and negatively affect physical and mental health.

Some of the findings of this report are outlined in Box 3.6 below.

Box 3.6 Accommodation instability, social exclusion and health

- One in three of the households who moved at least three times in the past year were not in work.

- Relationship breakdown is a major cause of homelessness: 13% of statutory cases involve domestic violence.

- 30% of young homeless people are estimated to have been in care.

- Shortage of site provision for Gypsies and Travellers is a major cause of frequent moving for these groups – between 1996 and 2003 there was a total net loss of 596 pitches for Gypsies and Travellers while the size of the Traveller population grew.

- There are significant gaps in achievement between mobile and non-mobile pupils.

- 9% of households accepted as homeless are in priority need because of a mental health problem.

- An estimated 40% of single homeless people have multiple needs, e.g. a mental health problem and one or more issues such as drug or alcohol misuse.

(SEU, 2004)

People living in poverty and social exclusion often have the greatest need for good healthcare, education, jobs, housing and transport. However, a report from the Joseph Rowntree Foundation (Wheeler et al., 2005) found evidence of the 'inverse care law' (Tudor Hart, 1971) – whereby those with the greatest need have least access to good quality services. Using data from the Millennial Census, the report compares the relationship between needs and supply across England, Wales, Northern Ireland and Scotland. Some of the key issues identified are detailed below:

- Areas with the highest levels of poor health have the lowest numbers of doctors, dentists and other health professionals living and working there.

- Areas with the greatest proportions of young people with no qualifications have the lowest availability of working teachers per head of population.

- The UK is divided between 'work rich' and 'work poor' areas. In areas with low unemployment, the people who have jobs are more likely to be working very long hours that may affect their health and wellbeing. In areas of higher unemployment those with jobs are less likely to work long hours, but unemployment itself is associated with physical and mental health problems.

As partly identified by the Joseph Rowntree Foundation report, harmful working conditions, such as poor ergonomic design and physical job demands, as well as work stresses related to effort / reward imbalance, can also lead to health-damaging behaviours and illness more generally. A survey analysis of working conditions conducted in Sweden (Hemström, 2005), for example, concluded that the work environment is an important means by which socio-economic class influences inequalities in health.

Interest in levels of sickness absence has been growing in recent years and absenteeism has been identified as an important public health issue, not just because such levels provide evidence of morbidity in the population but because absenteeism is costly for both the private and public sectors. According to a survey of over 1,000 employers by the Chartered Institute of Personnel and Development (CIPD, 2005), the most common cause of sickness absence for all workers was minor illness, followed by stress for non-manual employees, and back pain for manual staff. Box 3.7 outlines some of the key findings from a UK analysis of labour market trends and sickness absence (ONS, 2005b).

Box 3.7 Sickness absence

- In the three months from March to May 2004 some 1.7 million scheduled working days were lost to sickness absence among employees. Some 2.9 per cent of employees took at least one day off work because of sickness or injury.

- The days lost to sickness were fairly evenly spread across the weekdays. This is counter to the common perception that sickness absence is higher on Monday and Fridays as a result of non-genuine absence.

- Female employees and younger employees aged 16 to 34 were more likely than other groups to take at least one day off sick.

> • Lone mothers had the highest rate of sickness absence, followed
>   by women with no dependent children (4.4 per cent and 3.4
>   per cent respectively). Men without dependent children had the
>   lowest rate of absence.
>
> (ONS, 2005b, p. 149)

Recognising some of these issues, in a press release on 26 September 2005 the Government announced its plans to appoint a national director for occupational health (jointly appointed by the Departments of Health and of Work and Pensions) to oversee the implementation of the 'Health, Work and Wellbeing Strategy' (DfWP, 2005).

It is important to recognise, of course, that work stress should not just be tackled at the level of the individual but as noted in *Choosing Health*:

> The real task is to improve the quality of jobs by reducing monotony, increasing job control and applying appropriate HR practices and policies – organisations need to ensure that they adopt approaches that support the overall health and wellbeing of their employees.
>
> (DoH, 2004, p. 161)

More recently researchers have also begun to develop an interest in presenteeism, a concept describing how individuals work through illness and injury in spite of the need to be away from work. This, they argue, can lead to further morbidity and mortality which has encouraged some commentators to argue that more attention should be paid to presenteeism. However, a study of presenteeism in New Zealand (Dew et al., 2005) found that workers encounter very different organisations and relationships to management and other workers, and that this will influence the type of presenteeism that exists. For example, one of the respondents in their study – a nurse working in a public sector hospital – stated:

> 'I think nurses are a bit terrible like that. We actually go [to work when sick] and then can't even make it to lunchtime ... we are all determined to be here to not let anybody down.'
>
> (Quoted in Dew et al., 2005, p. 2279)

Dew et al. argue that presenteeism is expressed differently between social groups and operates in a distinct way according to social class and job market position.

Thinking point   reflect on your own work / life balance and consider the impact of this on your health.

Modern patterns of work tend to increasingly blur the boundaries between work and private space and time with employees often working longer and longer hours to the detriment of their health and lives. Whether your experience concurs with this or not, you may find that your work / life balance shifts over time and across your lifecourse. It will also relate to your own position with respect to factors such as age, gender, socio-economic status and whether or not you have caring responsibilities.

Concern with this 'work / life balance' is also evident in policy and strategy. For example, in 2000 the Department for Trade and Industry launched the 'Work–Life Balance Campaign' to help employers recognise the benefits of flexible working patterns, enabling staff to better balance their work with other aspects of their lives and, thus, be more productive. The *Long Hours Working Partnership Project*, administered by the Equal Opportunities Department, also has a remit for addressing work/life balance, focusing on issues such as high client demand (for example, 24-hour service provision), presenteeism and flexible working (DTI, 2005).

Living and working conditions are essential to the daily life experiences of individuals and groups. However, we will now move on to consider more general social conditions and their impact on health.

3.4.5 General social and environmental conditions

Neo-materialist explanations focus on the way in which adverse socio-economic and psycho-social environments, and the health-damaging mechanisms associated with them, are socially constructed. Concurring with this, Link and Phelan argue that social conditions remain fundamentally important to health and moreover that: 'we need to be mindful of the potential health impact of the entire array of social, political and economic policy we humans develop, such as social security, child welfare, education, or the location of potentially polluting industries' (Link and Phelan, 2002, p. 732).

For example, in recent years the need to provide health and social care for an increasingly ageing population has worried many governments. The potential for individuals to outlive their financial resources, for intergenerational antagonism and for problems with quality of life in older age are also concerns. In the American Geriatrics Society conference on 'Creating Very Old People', Louria (2005) argued that improving the health of an ageing population will require a broad systems approach to health that includes the following features:

*   changes in retirement age

*   strengthening (and replacing) social security systems

*   mandating the requirement to save during working age.

Many commentators have also expressed concerns with increasing environmental degradation and the impact of this on both physical and mental health. For example, a study of depression and neighbourhood in New York City (Galea et al., 2005) found a strong association between depression and poor quality built environment; researchers concluded that more attention should be paid to physical environment and urban planning within public health promotion. Other psycho-social research has also identified a relationship between environment and mental health or wellbeing. For example, it is well documented that certain spaces and places can promote a fear of violence and crime. Frumkin (2001), however, suggests that the focus should be on the salutogenic effects of a closer relationship to nature, rather than on traditional public health concerns. Drawing on the biophilia thesis (the notion that human beings have an innate affinity with nature), Frumkin focuses on the four domains of nature and the way in which each of these can enhance health (see Box 3.8).

Box 3.8 The four domains of nature

Animals

Pet ownership may improve physical and mental health.

Plants

It is suggested that plants make places more pleasant and convivial, reduce stress and, possibly, promote healing. Horticultural therapy is widely practised in occupational therapy.

Landscapes

Natural landscapes are thought to reduce stress. Some research on this has been carried out in dental care and prisons.

Wilderness

This refers to being **in** the landscape, rather than just viewing it. Wilderness therapy has been used with people with mental health problems.

(Adapted from Frumkin, 2001)

Thinking point think of one example of where the domains of nature could be used to improve public health in a setting with which you are familiar.

If you think about some of the settings that are familiar to you, it is easy to see how some of these ideas are evident in everyday practice. For example, many schools have a class pet such as a hamster or goldfish.

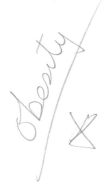

Some schools have 'wilderness areas', 'wildflower meadows' or a community allotment, and may organise trips to city farms, or similar locations. Many pay special attention to achieving a convivial environment both within school buildings and on school grounds. However, although some researchers have argued in favour of the biophilia thesis, the evidence is mixed, and others have argued that nature has no positive effect on health and wellbeing.

Environmental degradation, coupled with shifting balances between production and consumption, can also have a considerable impact on physical health. For example, in relation to obesity, it is easy to see how the placing of commerce and leisure in out-of-town locations and the need to commute to schools and workplaces places an over-reliance on the car for both children and adults alike (Gard and Wright, 2005). Lack of children's play facilities and open spaces, coupled with concerns with neighbourhood safety, also mean that children are less likely to engage in physical activity and more likely to participate in sedentary hobbies such as watching television or electronic gaming (see Chapter 12).

The issue of sustainability is also important here in that the unsustainable use of natural resources is a fundamental threat to human health. For example, for a healthy diet, most would agree that the local availability of affordable healthy foods must be improved. For sustainability, these foods should also be locally produced (so as to reduce food miles and energy consumption) and organic (so as to reduce the use of chemical pollutants). At the *Third International Conference on Health Promotion* the *Sundsvall Statement on Supportive Environments for Health* (WHO, 1991) acknowledged the fundamental link between environment and global health and called for the creation of supportive environments and for public health action at a local level. The United Nations' 1992 Earth Summit developed a programme of action on sustainable development: *Agenda 21* is a comprehensive plan of action to be taken globally, nationally and locally. It sets out twenty-seven principles to guide and underpin the action programme. These initiatives, and others, have had a significant influence on the UK-wide agenda on health and the environment, and in March 2005 all of the countries in the UK signed up to a shared framework for sustainable development (DEFRA, 2005). Box 3.9 considers actions at a number of different levels.

Box 3.9 The potential for environmental health action

Consumer action: fitting double glazing or loft insulation; purchasing 'fair trade' food and clothing

> **Citizen action:**   starting a local campaign; joining a community allotment
>
> **Household action:**   reducing energy and water consumption; recycling paper and glass
>
> **Community action:**   setting up a recycling project; establishing a skills-exchange scheme
>
> **Professional action:**   working in a sustainable way; supporting local sustainable projects
>
> **Local authority action:**   enabling public participation in environmental priority settings; setting and enforcing sustainability targets
>
> **Organisational action:**   assessing the potential for energy saving; purchasing from sustainable sources
>
> **National and international action:**   setting policy frameworks; encouraging change at lower levels.

Thinking point   consider your own environmental health actions.

A wide range of social, political and economic policies, at local, national and international levels, has a role to play in the social and environmental conditions that influence the health of individuals and communities.

3.5 Conclusion

As you have seen throughout this chapter there are considerable health inequalities in both morbidity and mortality. These inequalities have been largely persistent across time and have, in fact, widened. You have also seen how health chances differ according to age, gender, ethnicity and socio-economic status.

Psycho-social, lifecourse and neo-materialist explanations can be useful in analysing the relationships between inequalities and the factors that influence health. There is a clear relationship between concepts and definitions of health and the factors that are thought to influence health and disease. The Lalonde Report was influential because it recognised that health was more than healthcare and proposed that a multifactoral approach would be the best way to promote public health. Building on this, and drawing on the influential framework proposed by Dahlgren and Whitehead (1991), this chapter has considered how each of the five layers they identify can influence health. A multifactoral explanation would consider the role played by biology and genetics, lifestyle and behaviour, living and working conditions, social and community networks, and the wider social conditions in which individuals are located – not in isolation – but in relation to one another.

References

Acheson, D. *et al.* (1998) *Independent Inquiry into Inequalities in Health Report*, The Stationery Office, London.

Age Concern Scotland (2005) *Older People in Scotland*, Age Concern, Scotland.

Albert, B. (2007) 'Disability Rights, Genetics and Public Health', in J. Douglas, S. Earle, S. Handsley, C. E. Lloyd and S. Spurr (eds) *A Reader in Promoting Public Health: Challenge and Controversy*, Sage in association with the Open University, London.

Bagnall, G., Longhurst, B. and Savage, M. (2003) 'Children, Belonging and Social Capital: The PTA and the Middle Class Narratives of Social Involvement in the North West of England', *Sociological Research Online*, Vol. 8(4), http://www.socresonline.org.uk/8/4/bagnall.html [last accessed 4th April 2006].

Barker D.J.P. (1989) 'Growth in utero, blood pressure in childhood and adult life, and mortality from cardiovascular disease', *British Medical Journal*, Vol. 298, pp. 564–7.

Bartley, M. (2004) *Health Inequality – An Introduction to Theories, Concepts and Methods*, Polity, Cambridge.

Bello, N. and Mosca, L. (2004) 'Epidemiology of coronary heart disease in women', *Progress in Cardiovascular Diseases*, Vol. 46(4), pp. 287–95.

Bourdieu, P. (1986) 'The forms of capital', in J. Richardson (ed.), *Handbook of theory and research for the sociology of education*, Macmillan, New York.

Bourdieu, P. (1999) *The Weight of the Social World*, Polity, Cambridge.

Boyce, W. F. (2002) 'Influence of health promotion bureaucracy on community participation: a Canadian case study', *Health Promotion International*, Vol. 17, No. 1, pp. 61–68.

Chadwick, E. (1842) [1965] *Report on the Sanitary Condition of the Labouring Population of Great Britain*, edited and with an introduction by M.W. Flinn. Edinburgh University Press, Edinburgh.

Chartered Institute of Personnel and Development (2005) *Absence Management: A survey of policy and practice*, [http://www.cipd.co.uk/subjects/hrpract/absence/absmagmt.htm] [last accessed 4th April 2006].

Coleman, J. (1988) 'Social capital in the creation of human capital', *American Journal of Sociology*, Vol. 94(supplement), pp. S95–S120.

Dahlgren, G. and Whitehead, M. (1991) *Policies and strategies to promote social equity in health*, Institute of Futures Studies, Stockholm.

Davey-Smith, Chaturvedi, N., Harding, N., Nazroo, S. and Williams, R. (2000) 'Ethnic inequalities in health: a review of UK epidemiological evidence', *Critical Public Health*, Vol. 10(4), pp. 375–408.

Davison, C., Frankel, S. and Davey-Smith, G. (1992) 'The limits of lifestyle: re-assessing 'fatalism' in the popular culture of illness prevention', *Social Science and Medicine*, Vol. 34(6), pp. 675–85.

Department for Environment, Food and Rural Affairs (DEFRA) (2005) *One future - different paths: The UK's shared framework for sustainable development*, DEFRA, London.

Department for Work and Pensions (DfWP) (2005) Press Release: Government to appoint national director for occupational health, 26th September, http://www.dwp.gov.uk/mediacentre/pressreleases/2005/sep/cphs005b.asp [last accessed 4th April 2006].

Department of Health and Social Security (DHSS) (1976) *Prevention and Health: Everybody's Business*, HMSO, London.

Department of Health and Social Security (DHSS) (1980) *The Black Report on Inequalities in Health*, HMSO, London.

Department of Health and Social Security (DHSS) (1987) *Promoting Better Health*, HMSO, London.

Department of Health (DoH) (2004) *Choosing Health: Making Healthier Choices Easier*, TSO, London.

http://www.dh.gov.uk/PublicationsAndStatistics/Publications/PublicationsPolicyAndGuidance/PublicationsPolicyAndGuidanceArticle/fs/en?CONTENT_ID=4094550&chk=aN5Cor [last accessed 4th April 2006].

Department of Health (DoH) ((2000) *Health Survey for England 1999: The Health of Minority Ethnic Groups*, The Stationery Office, London.

Department of Health (DoH) (1999) *Saving Lives: Our Healthier Nation*, London: The Stationery Office. http://www.ohn.gov.uk/ohn/ohn.htm.

Department of Health (DoH) (1992) *The Health of the Nation: A Strategy for Health in England*, HMSO, London.

Department of Trade and Industry (DTI) (2005) *Managing Change: Practical ways to reduce long hours and reform working practices*, HMSO, London.

Dew, K., Keefe, V., Small, K. (2005) 'Choosing' to work when sick: workplace presenteeism, *Social Science and Medicine*, Vol. 60(10), pp. 2273–282.

Earle, S. and Sharp, K. 'In defence of a woman's right to choose: Disability, abortion and feminist politics', in J. Douglas, S. Earle, S. Handsley, C. E. Lloyd and S. Spurr (eds) *A Reader in Promoting Public Health: Challenge and Controversy*, Sage in association with the Open University, London.

Ettorre, E. (2002) *Reproductive genetics, gender and the body*, Routlege, London.

Engels, F. (1845) [1999] *The Condition of the Working Class in England*, Oxford University Press, Oxford.

Featherstone, M. and Hepworth, M. (1988) 'The Mask of Ageing and the Postmodern Life Course', in M. Featherstone, M. Hepworth and B. S. Turner (eds) *The Body: Social Process and Cultural Theory*, Sage, London.

Fodor, J.G. and Tzerovska, R. (2004) 'Coronary heart disease: is gender important?' *The Journal of Men's Health and Gender*, Vol.1(1), pp. 32–7.

Frumkin, P. (2001) 'Beyond toxicity – Human health and the natural environment', *American Journal of Preventive Medicine*, Vol. 20(3), pp. 234–40.

Galea, S., Ahern, J., Rudenstine, S., Wallace, Z. and Vlahov, D. (2005) 'Urban built environment and depression: a multilevel analysis', *Journal of Epidemiology and Community Health*, Vol. 59(10), pp. 822–27.

Gard, M. and Wright, J. (2005) *The Obesity Epidemic: Science and Ideology*, Routledge, London.

Gibson, A. (2007) 'Does social capital have a role to play in the health of communities?' in J. Douglas, S. Earle, S. Handsley, C. E. Lloyd and S. Spurr (eds) *A Reader in Promoting Public Health: Challenge and Controversy*, Sage in association with the Open University, London.

Graham, H. (1993) *When Life's A Drag: Women, Smoking and Disadvantage*, HMSO, London.

de Groot, L.C.P.G.M., Verheijden, M.W. and de Henauw, S. (2004) 'Lifestyle, nutritional status, health and mortality in elderly people across Europe', *Journals of Gerontology*, Vol. 59A(12), pp. 1277–284.

Hassall, R., Rose, J. and McDonald, J. (2005) 'Parenting stress in mothers of children with an intellectual disability: the effects of parental cognitions in relation to child characteristics and family support', *Journal of Intellectual Disability Research*, Vol. 49(6), pp. 405–18.

Hawe, P. and Shiell, A. (2000) 'Social capital and health promotion: a review', *Social Science and Medicine*, Vol. 51(6), pp. 871–85.

Hemström, Ö. (2005) 'Health inequalities by wage income in Sweden: The role of work environment', *Social Science and Medicine*, Vol. 61(3), pp. 637–47.

Kaplan, G.A., Pamuk, E.R., Lynch, J.W., Cohen, R.D. and Balfour, J.L. (1996) 'Inequality in income and mortality in the United States: analysis of mortality and potential pathways', *British Medical Journal*, Vol. 312, pp. 999–1003.

Kawachi, I., Kennedy, B.P. and Lochner, K. (1997) 'Long live community. Social capital as public health'. *The American Prospect*, Vol. 35, pp. 56–59.

Lader, D. and Goddard, E. (2004) *Smoking-related behaviour and attitudes*, ONS, London.

Lalonde, M. (1974) *A New Perspective on the Health of Canadians – A Working Document, Ministry of Supply and Services*, Ottawa, http://www.hc-sc.gc.ca/hcs-sss/alt_formats/ hpb-dgps/pdf/pubs/1974-lalonde/lalonde_e.pdf [last accessed 4th April 2006].

Link, B.G. and Phelan, J.C. (2002) 'McKeown and the idea that social conditions are fundamental causes of disease', *American Journal of Public Health*, Vol. 92(5), pp. 730–32.

Lippman, A. (1991) 'Prenatal Genetic Testing and Screening: Constructing Needs and Reinforcing Inequalities', *American Journal of Law and Medicine*, Vol. 17(1/2), pp. 15-50.

Louria, D.B. (2005) 'Extraordinary longevity: Individual and societal issues', *Journal of the American Geriatrics Society*, Vol. 53(7), Suppl, pp. S317–19.

Lynch, J.W., Smith, G.D., Kaplan, G.A. and House, J.S. (2000) 'Income inequality and mortality: importance to health of individual income, psychosocial environment, or material conditions', *British Medical Journal*, Vol. 320, pp. 1200–204.

Macintyre, S. (1995) 'The public understanding of science or the scientific understanding of the public? A review of the social context of the 'new genetics'', *Public Understanding of Science*, Vol. 4 pp. 223–32.

McKay (2000) *Making the Lalonde Report – Towards a New Perspective on Health Project*, Health Network, CPRN.

McKeown, T. (1976) *The Role of Medicine: Dream, Mirage or Nemesis?* Nuffield Provincial Hospitals Trust, England.

Mitteness, L. S. and Barker, J. C. (1995) 'Stigmatizing a 'normal' condition: Urinary Incontinence in Late Life', *Medical Anthropology Quarterly*, Vol. 9(2), pp. 188–210.

O'Donnell, T. (2005) 'Social Class and Health', in E. Denny and S. Earle (eds) *Sociology for Nurses*, Polity, Cambridge.

Office for National Statistics (ONS) (2004a) *Gaps in income and wealth remain large*, http:// www.statistics.gov.uk/CCI/nugget.asp?ID=1005&Pos=2&ColRank=2&Rank=640 [last accessed 4 April 2006]

Office for National Statistics (ONS) (2004b) *Drinking to excess rising among women*, http:// www.statistics.gov.uk/cci/nugget_print.asp?ID=922 [last accessed 4 April 2006]

Office for National Statistics (ONS) (2005a) *Social Trends 35*, HMSO, London.

Office for National Statistics (ONS) (2005b) 'Sickness Absence from Work in the UK', *Labour Market Trends*, Vol. 113(4), pp. 149–58.

Office for National Statistics (ONS) (2005c) *Women Outliving Men*, http://www.statistics. gov.uk/cci/nugget.asp?id=168 [last accessed 4 April 2006].

Office for National Statistics (ONS) (2005d) *Smoking-related Behaviour and Attitudes, 2000*, HMSO, London.

Petchesky, R. P. (1986) *Abortion and Woman's Choice: The State, Sexuality, and Reproductive Freedom*, Verso, London.

Petchesky, R. P. (1980) 'Reproductive Freedom: Beyond a Woman's Right to Choose', *Signs*, Vol. 5(4), pp. 661–85.

Portes, A. (1998) *Social Capital: Its origins and applications*, Russell Sage, New York.

Putnam, R. D. (1995) 'Bowling alone: America's declining social capital', *Journal of Democracy*, Vol. 6, pp. 65–78.

Raeburn, J. and Rootman, I. (1989) 'Towards an expanded health field concept: conceptual and research issues in a new era of health promotion', *Health Promotion*, Vol. 3, pp. 383–92.

Rotter, J. B. (1954) *Social Learning and Clinical Psychology.* Prentice-Hall, New York.

Rowe, J. L., Montgomery, G. H., Duberstein, P. R. and Bovbjerg, D. H.(2005) 'Health Locus of Control and Perceived Risk for Breast Cancer in Healthy Women', *Behavioral Medicine*, Vol. 31(1), pp. 33–40.

Siegrist J., Peter, R., Junge, A., Cremer, P. and Seidel, D. (1990) 'Low status control, high effort at work and ischemic heart disease: prospective evidence from blue-collar men', *Social Science and Medicine*, Vol. 31(10), pp. 1127–134.

Sidell, M. (2007) 'Older people's health: applying Antonovsky's salutogenic paradigm' in J. Douglas, S. Earle, S. Handsley, C. E. Lloyd and S. Spurr (eds) *A Reader in Promoting Public Health: Challenge and Controversy*, Sage in association with the Open University, London.

Social Exclusion Unit (2004) http://www.socialexclusion.gov.uk/page.asp?pf=1&id=213 [last accessed 4 April 2006]

Ståhl, T., Rütten, A., Nutbeam, D., Bauman, A., Kannas, L., Abel, T., Lüschen, G., Rodriguez, Diaz J. A., Vinck, J. and van der Zee, J. (2001) 'The importance of the social environment for physically active lifestyle – results from an international study', *Social Science and Medicine*, Vol. 52(1), pp. 1–10.

Sullivan, A. (2001) 'Cultural Capital and Educational Attainment', *Sociology*, Vol. 35(4), pp. 893–912.

Tudor Hart J. (1971) 'The inverse care law'. *Lancet*, pp. 405–12.

United Nations (1992) *Earth Summit. Agenda 21: The United Nations Programme of Action from Rio*, UN Department of Information, New York.

van de Mheen H., Stronks, K. and Mackenbach, J.P. (1998) 'A lifecourse perspective on socio-economic inequalities in health: the influence of childhood socio-economic conditions and selection processes', *Sociology of Health and Illness*, Vol. 20(5), pp. 754–77.

Wall, E., Ferrazi, G. and Schryer, F. (1998) 'Getting the goods on social capital', *Rural Sociology*, Vol. 63(2), pp. 300–322.

Wang, C., Bowen, D.J. and Kardia, S.L.R. (2005) 'Research and Practice Opportunities at the Intersection of Health Education, Health Behavior and Genomics', *Health Education and Behavior*, Vol. 32(5), pp. 686–701.

Webster, C. and French, J. (2002) 'The Cycle of Conflict: the history of the public health and health promotion movements', in L. Adams, M. Amos and J. Munro (eds) *Promoting Health: politics and practice*, Sage, London.

Weidner, G. and Cain (2003) 'The Gender Gap in Heart Disease: Lessons from Eastern Europe', *Men's Health Forum*, Vol. 93(5), pp. 768–70.

Wheeler, B., Shaw, M., Mitchell, R. and Dorling D. (2005) *Life in Britain: Using Millennial Census data to understand poverty, inequality and place*, The Policy Press, Bristol.

World Health Organisation (WHO) (1991) *Third International Conference on Health Promotion*, 9–15 June, Sundsvall, Sweden.

Yeung, A.B. (2004) 'An Intricate Triangle – Religiosity, Volunteering, and Social Capital: The European Perspective, the Case of Finland', *Nonprofit and Voluntary Sector Quarterly*, Vol. 33(3), pp. 401–422.

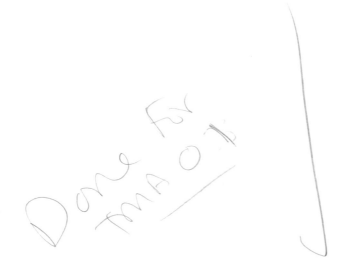

Chapter 4

Who promotes public health?

Jennie Naidoo and Sarah Earle

Introduction

Earlier chapters have focused on discussing the nature and scope of multidisciplinary public health, ways of understanding the concept of health, and the factors that influence health. However, promoting public health requires that actions are taken at local, regional, national and international levels by both individuals and agencies. This chapter considers some of the individuals, groups and agencies that promote public health at all of these levels, and begins with a discussion of whether health is everybody's business. Next, this chapter focuses on the range of agencies that either directly, or indirectly, promote public health at international, national, regional and local levels. The chapter then moves on to consider some of the individuals and groups who promote public health as part of their professional remit. Then, finally, the chapter considers the wider perspective, including the role of the media and those who promote public health in a voluntary, or a lay, capacity.

4.1 Promoting public health: everybody's business?

Identifying who promotes public health depends on how health is defined; the wider the definition of health, the broader the range of people and agencies who promote health. Adopting a construct of positive health and wellbeing that is socially and economically determined, rather than the narrow medical model of physical health, significantly increases the number of partners who, in different ways, promote public health. This is the guiding principle across the UK.

Thinking point adopting a broad definition of health, think about the people and agencies involved in promoting your health.

You may have included a wide range of people and agencies, from health staff such as health visitors and nurses, to lay people such as family members and friends. Perhaps, also, you may have thought about the role of the media, the government and the private sector. Although people with whom one has immediate face-to-face contact in the community probably spring to mind first as individuals who promote health, with reflection it is clear that unseen partners at regional, national or even international levels are also vital in terms of providing the policy and environmental context to support health. To a very large extent, policy frameworks and funding streams are responsible for the extent to which frontline staff are enabled to promote health and wellbeing. Most health promoters have other core functions that can easily take over all their work time and energy; without support and direction from employing organisations, the promotion of health and wellbeing can easily slip down the scale of priorities and even be lost altogether. Managers and financial directors can therefore be the most important health promoters in an organisation, even if they have no direct health function. However, they can also restrict the capacity of people who work to promote health.

The diversity of partners or stakeholders involved in promoting health is also related to the fact that multidisciplinary public health may be formal or informal, and direct or indirect. Formal methods of promoting health can be carried out in a planned manner by trained practitioners who may use theoretical frameworks to guide their input. Informal methods of promoting health can also be carried out spontaneously and reactively by lay people.

Thinking point — what are the implications of suggesting that promoting public health is everybody's business?

Identifying who promotes health depends on what aspects of public health promotion are being considered. Promoting public health includes the development and implementation of healthy policies, community development work, research and evaluation to develop an evidence base, initiatives in a range of settings, provision of information, and support for individuals. These diverse activities are undertaken by a range of agencies, practitioners and the general public, whose activities to promote health will now be considered.

4.2 Agencies promoting public health

There are many agencies at international, national, regional and local levels that promote health in diverse ways. Some of these agencies have a formal remit for promoting public health, but these are in a minority. More commonly, agencies have some other formal remit but, in practice, and if the wide range of factors that promote public health are considered (see Chapter 3), then their activities can often make a significant contribution to the promotion of good health in society. What follows is an account of some of the major agencies' roles in promoting health. Agencies are presented according to their level, starting with those at international level.

4.2.1 International policy-making organisations

These organisations make global policy in areas such as health and economics. Although far removed from the everyday experience of most people, such organisations do have an important impact on the social and physical environment. For example, it has been argued that free trade agreements that open up the privatisation of health services have the effect of widening health inequalities within developed nations such as the UK as well as between nations (Navarro, 1998). Such agreements therefore directly counteract public health policies and strategies that attempt to reduce health inequalities.

The World Health Organization (WHO) is committed to reducing inequalities both between and within countries and – as discussed in Chapter 1 – can be commended for championing health promotion, for example through its work on *The Ottawa Charter for Health Promotion* (WHO, 1986). It has also led the way with some innovative projects such as the first worldwide *Framework Convention on Tobacco Control* (WHO, 2003), which advocates measures to reduce the demand for tobacco through controls on advertising and promotion, pricing and taxation policies, and protection from exposure to environmental tobacco smoke. The WHO worldwide programme to eliminate polio has also been very successful in some countries, such as India, but has foundered in other countries, such as Angola, Afghanistan, the Democratic Republic of Congo, Sudan and Somalia, where continued conflict has meant mass immunisation programmes are impossible to implement. Despite its high profile and some impressive achievements, the WHO is usually viewed as a minor player compared to the global economic institutions discussed below. The WHO has also been criticised for failing to speak out on the issues that concern developing countries, and for lacking an independent voice (Smith, 2003).

Created in 1995 to facilitate free trade worldwide, the World Trade Organisation (WTO) has been criticised at many levels for seeking to privatise public services (including health services) and acting in the interests of major capitalist countries, most notably the USA. Some commentators argue that free trade benefits public health through economic growth and increased gross national product (GNP), though others would suggest that reliance on this trickle-down effect is ineffectual (McClean, 2003).

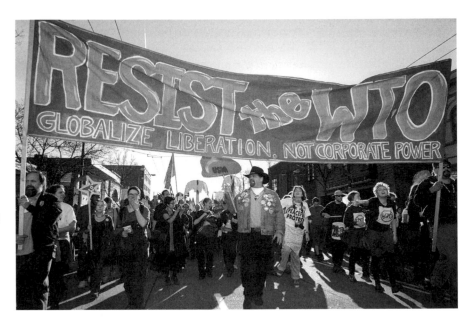

Figure 4.1   Protestors and rioters prevented the launch of a new trade round, demonstrating grassroots antagonism against the WTO, Seattle 1999 © Nick Cobbing / Rex Features

Created in 1944, the World Bank provides financial assistance for developing countries and is a major funder of health projects. The World Bank's key activities include investment in health and education, social development, environmental protection and the fostering of private business enterprise (for example, see Box 4.1). However, the effects of World Bank loans are mixed. Although loans enable health, education and development projects to take place, they have also resulted in countries being instructed to change food production methods, resulting in the increased use of pesticides and environmental degradation (Prowse, 2003). The long term impact may well be persistent major health and environmental problems (Prowse, 2003), as well as increased debt.

Box 4.1 Education Project in Turkey

Between 2002 and 2006, the World Bank loaned 300 million dollars to help fund an education project in Turkey. By 2015 the project aims to have:

- extended primary school education from five to eight years

- eliminated gender disparity in education

- halved the number of children living in extreme poverty.

(Adapted from: www.worldbank.org)

Also set up in 1944, the International Monetary Fund (IMF) now has 184 member nations. Voting rights of member countries depend on their economic performance and, hence, quota or subscription. This has led to the dominance of the IMF by the developed G7 countries, and especially the USA. This lack of democratic accountability has been criticised. For example, Woods (2001), in a critique of both the World Bank and the IMF suggests that the actions of both institutions need to become more transparent if they are to increase their accountability.

Key roles of the IMF are to promote economic stability and growth, to foster international trade, and to provide loans. Many loans to developing countries are dependant on the imposition of structural adjustment programmes (SAPs) designed to reduce government public expenditure and strengthen the economy. The combination of SAPs and debt repayment has forced many developing countries to reduce their spending on public services, including health and education services (McClean, 2003). There has been sustained criticism of the effects of IMF policy in terms of factors including public health from many commentators including non-government organisations (NGOs) (Prowse, 2003), for example, the campaign to end Third World debt.

NGOs such as Oxfam, Médecins Sans Frontières and Save the Children act as critics of international organisations' activities in developing countries, and are involved in innovative service delivery in partnership with local agencies. There are hundreds of thousands of NGOs across the world, large and small, involved in issues such as sustainable environmental development (for example, Greenpeace) and human rights (for example, Amnesty International), amongst others. Increasingly, NGOs are providing a resource for interventions and policies determined by the host countries (Prowse, 2003). Although many NGOs may lack the 'teeth' needed to bring about change, they are seen as increasingly influential in world affairs and are often consulted by governments and international agencies such as the UN.

4.2.2 National and regional organisations

Key agencies such as the Department of Health, the Department for Communities and Local Government (formerly Office of the Deputy Prime Minister (ODPM)) and the Department for Environment, Food and Rural Affairs (DEFRA), make and implement policies that determine the overall environment for health. These organisations, therefore, have a profound effect on the broad socio-economic and environmental factors that influence health. If adopting a social model of health, it is vital that such factors are considered. However, health is not always high up on some of these agencies' agendas and policies that impact on health may be adopted for other reasons (for example, economic ones). The Health Development

Agency (HDA) in England, established in 2000 to supersede the former Health Education Authority (HEA), focused on providing a resource for health professionals to promote health and an evidence base for public health; however, it had lost the former function of the HEA to promote health and health education directly to members of the public. The HDA has now been subsumed within the National Institute for Health and Clinical Excellence (NICE), which came into being on 1 April 2005, and has a much broader remit than its predecessor, the National Institute for Clinical Excellence. NICE's Centre for Public Health Excellence retains a focus on evaluating interventions and providing guidance for professionals. Health Scotland, created in 2003, provides a national focus for improving health and reducing health inequalities in Scotland. The Health Promotion Agency for Northern Ireland and the Welsh Assembly provide a similar function for Northern Ireland and Wales respectively.

The five agencies discussed below either have an explicit remit for health (the first three) or – if the broad range of factors that determine health are recognised – have a profound effect on health even if this is not their main purpose (the remaining two).

1   The role of the Food Standards Agency (FSA) is to protect public health and consumer interests in relation to food. It provides advice and information to the public and UK governments on food safety from 'farm to fork', as well as playing a role in monitoring and enforcing regulations and legislation in the food industry.

Thinking point   consider the ways in which the FSA can promote public health.

As part of their role, the FSA conducts food surveys (for example, on the level of nitrates in lettuce), they regulate food labelling and the use of GM and novel foods. For example, in 2004, the FSA authorised an application from Unilever for approval of phytosterol-esters to be included as a cholesterol-lowering ingredient in milk- and yogurt-type products.

2   The Health Protection Agency (HPA) is a UK-wide agency, established as a national expert co-ordinating body within the NHS in 2003. It has a remit for dealing with any health threat event, including disease epidemics, chemical fires, bombings and radiation exposures. The HPA operates at national, regional and local levels, integrating what were formerly a range of separate public health laboratories and health emergency planning services. The work of the HPA is organised within three centres:

The Centre for Infectious Diseases

The Centre for Emergency Preparedness and Response

The Centre for Radiation, Chemical and Environmental Hazards

3   The United Kingdom Public Health Association (UKPHA), formed in 1999 by the merging of three organisations, is an independent voluntary organisation that seeks to represent and support the public health movement in the UK. It works in partnership with a coalition of other national public health organisations: the Chartered Institute of Environmental Health, the Royal Institute of Public Health, the Royal Society for the Promotion of Health and the Faculty of Public Health. The UKPHA acts as an independent advocate of public health and has three priority areas: combating health inequalities, promoting sustainable development, and challenging anti-health forces. It has a multidisciplinary membership, bringing together individuals and organisations from all sectors. However, although the UKPHA represents a powerful lobbying force for multidisciplinary public health, it has not always had a focus on the professional skills required for public health and health promotion work (MacDonald, 2001).

You have now considered some of the main agencies with a specific remit for health. Next, you consider other agencies, beginning with the role of the Treasury.

4   The Treasury is the United Kingdom's economics and finance ministry. It has immense influence in directing the UK's economic and fiscal policy. Its aim is to raise the rate of sustainable growth, and thus achieve rising prosperity and a better quality of life with economic and employment opportunities for all. As such, it is a key player in promoting socio-economic growth and health. The Wanless Report (2002), commissioned by the Treasury to assess the resources required to provide high-quality health services in the future, was a key factor in securing investment in public health. The Wanless Report identified three possible models for investment in prevention and public health: 'slow uptake', 'solid progress' and 'fully engaged'. As discussed in Chapter 1, the Report advocated the adoption of the 'fully engaged' scenario, whereby people become more engaged in their own health, as the most cost-effective. The second Wanless Report on the progress of current policy (Wanless, 2004) found progress to be patchy and inconsistent. The NHS remains a sickness service rather than a health service. Other challenges for public health identified by the second Wanless Report include a public health workforce that is 'fit for purpose', an improved evidence base, and improved health literacy amongst the general population.

The Treasury is responsible for the investment in and reform of public services and for their delivery and performance. Accountability, transparency and performance in public services are monitored via Public Service Agreements (PSAs) and targets which are set for each government department. PSAs outline each department's aim, objectives and key outcome-based targets and form an essential part of the spending plans set out in Spending Reviews. For example, DEFRA's objectives and performance targets include the protection of rural, urban, marine and global environments (DEFRA, 2004).

5   The Department for Transport (DfT) aims to ensure that transport services are safe, secure and reliable and also that they safeguard the environment. Access to acceptable and affordable transport is an important factor in individual and communal wellbeing. The DfT is involved in many road safety campaigns targeting children, young people, and alcohol and drug users, amongst others. However, there is very little research on the effectiveness of such campaigns. For example, an international survey of twenty countries found that only two of these countries – Iceland and the UK – had commissioned research in the area of child road safety publicity (DfT, 2004). Furthermore, the evidence that does exist is mixed. For example, in a systematic review of randomised controlled trials of safety education for pedestrians, the authors conclude that although the Global Road Safety Partnership (and others) strongly recommend road safety education for all children worldwide, 'there is no reliable evidence supporting the effectiveness of pedestrian education for preventing injuries in children' (Duperrex et al., 2002, p. 1131).

Many government agencies, and responsibilities, have been devolved to Northern Ireland, Wales and Scotland. Devolution, or the delegation of power from a central government to local bodies, was granted to the Scottish Parliament in 1998 and to the National Assembly for Wales and the Northern Ireland Assembly in 1999. However, following crises in the peace process, the Northern Ireland Assembly was suspended in 2002. The Scottish Parliament and the Northern Ireland Assembly, the latter subject to its restoration, have primary legislative powers over many areas. This means they can pass their own laws on issues such as education, social care and environmental policies. The Welsh Assembly has secondary legislative powers only, meaning it is only able to vary some laws passed by the Houses of Parliament on issues which have been devolved to Wales. Health and education are examples of matters that are now the responsibility of devolved government. Issues that concern the UK or have an international focus, such as defence, foreign policy or economic policy, are reserved and dealt with at Westminster.

The Welsh Assembly is responsible for developing and implementing policies and programmes for all issues that have been devolved to Wales. The National Public Health Service for Wales brings together the former health authorities in Wales, the Public Health Laboratory Service in Wales including the Communicable Disease Surveillance Centre, and academic departments of public health. The aim is to bring together all available resources for public health and hence to work efficiently to promote public health.

In December 1999, the Department for Social Development was established as part of the Northern Ireland Assembly's Executive Committee. It has strategic responsibility for urban regeneration, community and voluntary sector development, social legislation, housing, social security benefits, pensions and child support. For example, the Northern Ireland Social Security Agency is responsible for assessing and paying social security benefits. Northern Ireland has primary and secondary legislative powers to run the NHS in Northern Ireland, although the Department of Health retains control over some areas, for example, abortion, genetics, medicine safety and oversight of medical professions.

The Scottish Parliament also has primary and secondary legislative powers to run the NHS in Scotland with the same exceptions outlined above, and has primary legislative powers over many areas that affect health such as environmental, housing and transport policies. In April 2003, the Public Health Institute in Scotland and the Health Education Board for Scotland were subsumed under Health Scotland, an NHS organisation that serves the whole of the public health community in Scotland. Its key responsibilities include leading the delivery of health improvement programmes, disseminating evidence, learning and good practice, and establishing the practical arrangements for working with key partners.

In England, eight Public Health Observatories (PHOs) were established in 2000, one for each NHS region. PHOs provide information and data about health at a local level and are linked together, with their equivalents in Ireland and Northern Ireland, Scotland and Wales, as the Association of Public Health Observatories (APHO), to form a network of knowledge, information and surveillance in public health. PHOs and the AHPO aim to strengthen public health input into a range of government initiatives. For example, the APHO has recently reported on the relationship between interpersonal violence and public health (McVeigh et al., 2005) and the impact of lifestyle on health (Crowther et al., 2005).

Since devolution, changes to the English regions have also taken place with increasing emphasis being placed on the role of the regions in promoting sustainability, improving services and meeting diverse regional needs. In 1999, the Regional Development Agencies (RDAs) were formally launched in eight English regions, and in 2000 the Greater London Authority was created as the ninth region. RDAs aim to co-ordinate regional economic development and regeneration under the scrutiny of the Regional Assemblies. These Assemblies, which operate within the same boundaries as the Government Offices in the Regions (GOs) and the RDAs, are co-ordinated by the English Regions Network.

Regional Assemblies are voluntary, multi-party agencies which comprise up to 70 per cent of local authority members and at least 30 per cent drawn from a range of regional stakeholders; these include higher and further education institutions, the Confederation of British Industry, the Trades Union Congress, the NHS, the small business sector, voluntary organisations and others.

Thinking point   how important is the role of regional agencies in promoting public health?

The English White Paper *Your Region, Your Choice* (Office of the Deputy Prime Minister, 2002) sets out plans to decentralise government and further strengthen the regions with the introduction of elected Regional Assemblies, notably in the North East, the North West, and Yorkshire and the Humber. These elected assemblies would have responsibility for many issues that impact directly on the public's health, including housing, transport, environmental protection, and fire and rescue. However, a referendum on a proposal to establish an elected Regional Assembly in the North East Region was turned down by the North East electorate in 2004.

National agencies play a vital role in public health by establishing policy, as well as setting and monitoring standards. Regional agencies are playing an increasingly important role in promoting public health in a way that takes into account regional diversity and inequality (ODPM, 2005). Each region has its own characteristics and priorities. For example, in the South West, priorities include rural affairs and the protection of World Heritage Sites such as the 'Jurassic Coastline' in Devon and Dorset. In contrast, in the East Midlands, priorities include reducing anti-social behaviour, reducing crime and the fear of crime. Since 2002, public health groups with a regional director of public health have been linked to each of the nine GOs. Local Strategic Partnerships (LSPs) are single non-statutory bodies that bring together local public, private, community and voluntary organisations, at a local level, working with communities to identify and tackle issues such as crime, unemployment, education, health and housing in a co-ordinated way. Local authorities are also duty-bound to prepare a Community Strategy to improve the wellbeing of an area and its people. LSPs play a significant role in developing the Community Strategy; they are key local processes which co-ordinate the public health work that occurs on the ground at a local level.

4.2.3 The role of local organisations

As the wide range of factors that influence health has been recognised, over many years, the role of local government in promoting public health has become increasingly visible (Allen, 2001). For example, *The Health of the Nation* (DoH, 1992) and *Saving Lives: Our Healthier Nation* (DoH, 1999) both recognised the involvement of local authorities in a wide range of services. More recently, *Choosing Health* (DoH, 2004), *Wellbeing in Wales* (Welsh Assembly Government, 2002) and *Partnership for Care*

(Scottish Executive, 2003) have all emphasised the role of local authorities in bringing about change to improve health, and reduce inequalities in health. Note that *Agenda 21* (UN, 1992), the comprehensive plan for sustainable development – which was mentioned in Chapter 3 – also singles out local government as having a special role to play.

In the UK, approximately 2 million people are employed by local authorities. The vast majority of these are teachers, but the rest include the police, firefighters, housing officers, social workers and environmental health officers, as well as other manual and non-manual employees. Uniquely, local authorities are directly accountable to their local area and they have both mandatory statutory duties (for example, drinking-water surveillance) and discretionary powers (for example, the provision of home improvement grants). However, it has been argued that over many years these discretionary powers have been eroded (Carter, 1996), and further changes have taken place post-devolution (Jeffery, 2002). The portfolio of services provided by local government has also changed over the years. For example, at one time councils were responsible for the provision of gas supplies, whereas this is no longer the case. Local authorities are responsible for the provision of services that include education, fire and rescue, housing, licensing, waste disposal and social services.

Locally, public health is not just promoted by local authorities but also by the Public Health Departments and Health Promotion Teams located within the NHS at a local level. Box 4.2 outlines some of the health promotion activities carried out by Health Promotion Teams. These teams can be organised as an integrated model whereby all staff are generalists, or can be based on a model incorporating people working within different specialisms.

Box 4.2 The work of Health Promotion Teams

- Involvement in public education campaigns
- Running a sex workers' forum
- Providing men's health information in barbers' shops
- Writing and distributing alcohol awareness packs
- Producing newsletters
- Providing sex education for schools
- Co-ordinating a virtual baby parenting scheme
- Offering CPD (Continuing Professional Development) with teachers/school nurses

- Promoting participation in sport and leisure for adults with learning difficulties

- Hosting a children's mental health conference

- Commissioning research on the social needs of people living with HIV/AIDS

As outlined in Chapter 1, Directors of Public Health no longer require medical training and some are now located within Primary Care Trusts (PCTs) or local Public Health Teams (in Wales), and others are appointed jointly between local authorities and the NHS. In England, *Choosing Health* (DoH, 2004) firmly endorses the idea of a health-promoting NHS with a strong emphasis on prevention and health – rather than treatment and disease – across all National Service Framework areas, and better partnerships between the NHS and local authorities and other agencies. Similar strategies are evident across the UK. It is interesting to note how the medical model of health is increasingly less influential than other models and approaches to health.

The next section continues to explore who promotes public health by focusing on some key professional groups.

4.3 Professional groups promoting public health

This section focuses on some of the groups who promote public health within the remit of their professional roles. The multidisciplinary public health workforce includes those who promote public health as the main part of their job – for example, public health practitioners such as health visitors and environmental health workers. It also includes people working within the wider public health workforce – for example, social workers, nurses and teachers. What follows is a brief outline of the responsibilities and duties of some of these professional groups.

4.3.1 Environmental health practitioners

Following on from the discussion of the role of local authorities in the previous section, the focus in this section is on the pivotal role of environmental health practitioners (EHPs). These practitioners work in both the private and public sectors, in generalist and specialist capacities; the majority work for local authorities. Environmental health specialisms include: housing, public health, food safety, occupational health and environmental protection. EHPs aim to protect people from current and future environmental hazards in their living and working surroundings. They have statutory health enforcement duties to ensure compliance with legislation in areas that include food safety, health and safety at work, and housing standards. There is some variation across the UK though; for example, in Scotland food hygiene premises must be inspected by Registered Food Safety Officers, whereas this is not the case in England, Wales and Northern Ireland.

EHPs also have an advisory role, working with households, business owners, managers and shopkeepers, amongst others. They work closely with other occupational groups such as Trading Standards Officers, Housing Officers and Planning Officers. Typical day-to-day tasks include:

- inspecting premises and advising on hygiene and safety issues
- following up complaints and investigating outbreaks of food poisoning or infectious diseases
- monitoring standards and taking enforcement action
- collecting samples for laboratory testing
- giving educational talks to groups of people in the community
- giving evidence in cases that come to court.

Many EHPs work reactively, often in difficult situations where they are trying to achieve a balanced outcome; in order to do so they must draw on a wide range of skills and knowledge. Lammin (2005) argues that it is time for an ethical debate to take place with respect to the work carried out by environmental health practitioners. She argues, for example, that it is sometimes difficult to apply the principles of beneficence, non-maleficence and justice to all people equally, and in all situations (for example, see Box 4.3).

Box 4.3 The dilemma of an environmental health practitioner

[A] couple with learning difficulties, who were living independently in the community, were the victims of a campaign of abuse from within their own family. As a result of this mistreatment, the couple feared the bully and others, and would not answer the door. Waste materials were thrown into the garden and subsequently built up and regular small arson attacks were carried out on piles of materials in the garden. Inevitably, the environmental health department received a complaint from a neighbour who was concerned about the rats being attracted to the gardens by the waste and the burnt remnants of belongings. The ethical dilemma is clear – does an EHP serve a notice on a victimised, stressed and confused couple when rats are

> discovered? The notice would resolve the rat problem but what of the harm to the individuals who are intellectually unable to cope with the situation they find themselves in and emotionally in a state of acute anxiety.
>
> (Lammin, 2005, p. 21)

4.3.2 Health professionals

Healthcare professionals, such as nurses, doctors and midwives, provide direct services to manage and treat health problems but they also provide preventive treatment to prevent illness from developing (for example, vaccination) and education and advice (for example, on how to wean infants or to ensure a safe home environment for frail older people). Healthcare staff have traditionally used a medical perspective dominated by biology and physiology; however this is changing and a more holistic view of health is now more commonly adopted by some individuals and groups (see box 4.4).

Box 4.4 Domestic violence in pregnancy

The Bristol Pregnancy and Domestic Violence Programme aims to equip midwives with the required knowledge and skills to ask women about domestic violence as a routine part of antenatal care. The programme provides in-service training and follow up support for midwives. Evaluation of the programme has shown increased confidence and willingness to enquire about domestic violence, although the presence of other family members and lack of time and resources meant midwives asked about domestic violence only 50 per cent of the time.

(Adapted from Salmon et al., 2004)

Generally healthcare staff enjoy a high degree of credibility and trust; that is, the lay public will believe their advice and will trust that it is given with no ulterior motive. However, this situation may be shifting due to the massive increase in the availability of information on the internet (though, given differential access and use, this is likely to impact differently across social groups). Studies also show that individuals often use information from the internet to supplement more traditional types of health information rather than as a replacement for it (Fox et al., 2005; Pandey et al., 2003). Scandals, for example, the Bristol baby hearts scandal, and the Shipman murders have also had an impact on public trust in health professionals and healthcare more generally. Writing in the *Guardian*, Robinson (2004), for example, argues: 'although doctors still command more trust than politicians, we are more mistrustful of health programmes than ever before. No wonder public confidence has hit rock bottom. Scarcely a day goes by without another health 'scandal' about babies' organs or misdiagnosis of abuse.'

Other healthcare workers, such as health visitors, public health doctors, public health specialists and health promotion practitioners also play a pivotal role in promoting public health. Public health specialists have undertaken further training to fulfil their expert role as leaders of public health. Although public health specialists are no longer required to have medical training, they must either pass the Faculty of Public Health examinations and training programme, or apply by portfolio to the UK Voluntary Register for Public Health Specialists (UKVRPS). Applicants to the register are assessed across the ten core standards for public health listed in Box 1.7 of Chapter 1. These skills may be acquired through a range of training and education programmes, including many that may not be designated as public health. It is their combined use and focus that marks them out as public health skills.

Health promotion specialists (HPSs) are a disparate and relatively small group of practitioners with diverse origins and roles. Although it is difficult to calculate their numbers, the Society of Health Education and Health Promotion Specialists (www.hj-web.co.uk/sheps/) suggest that there are approximately 2,000 health promotion specialists in the UK. There is no mandatory training or accreditation for HPSs, and many HPSs have qualified in health, education or social care before going on to become involved in public health promotion. However, many will have a specialist postgraduate qualification in health promotion or public health and some will have management qualifications.

HPSs may also be located in a variety of organisations and settings, including NHS authorities and trusts, local authorities and voluntary agencies. The role includes policy development, organisational change and development, community development work, development of health information materials, needs assessment, programme planning and evaluation of interventions, media advocacy, and health education with individuals and communities. Some HPSs focus on one project or topic while others cover a range of topics. The ten core standards for public health (see Box 1.7) are also relevant to the work of HPSs. The project report *Shaping the Future of Public Health* published by the Department of Health and Welsh Assembly Government (2005) makes recommendations for the future of health promotion and the role of HPSs, calling for:

- improved capacity for a sustainable workforce
- clear career pathways and recognition

- skills and competency development
- supervision, accreditation and regulation.

Allied health professionals (AHPs) form another very large group of professionals – including pharmacists, chiropodists and podiatrists, complementary and allied health practitioners, dieticians, psychologists, occupational therapists, orthoptists, physiotherapists, psychotherapists, radiographers and speech and language therapists – all of whom promote public health (Scriven, 2005). AHPs work with children and adults of all ages who are ill or have a disability or special needs, enabling people to manage and adapt to their condition, increase their mobility or communication skills, and gain or regain independent living skills. They work within a variety of settings including hospitals, clinics, schools, workplaces and people's homes.

Thinking point   how can allied health professionals become further involved in promoting public health?

Given the increasing number of people living with long-term conditions and the *Long-term (Neurological) Conditions National Service Framework* (NSF) (DoH, 2005a), the role of AHPs is likely to become more significant over time. For example, in Scotland, several AHPs have been appointed as Public Health Practitioners, and the Scottish Executive has committed itself to developing AHP consultant roles. Although AHPs fulfil distinct clinical roles, they play an important part in promoting public health. For example, physiotherapists can promote health through cardiac rehabilitation programmes (Jones and Hinton, 2005) and occupational therapists can promote the mental health of clients with rheumatoid arthritis (Adams and Pearce, 2005). The role of the community pharmacist has also become increasingly important in promoting public health through activities such as the provision of smoking cessation advice, free diabetes testing and use of the pharmacy as a credit union collection point (DoH, 2005b).

4.3.3 Social care workers

The boundary between health and social care is somewhat arbitrary, and many services provided by social and care workers promote health and wellbeing, for example, protecting children from abuse or supporting marginalised groups such as older people, disabled people and mental health survivors through services such as self-help activities, counselling and help with claiming benefits.

Social workers are located in Social Services departments within local authorities (although this is expected to be phased out as attempts are made to integrate health and social services), in Children's Trusts, intermediate care teams, community mental health teams and voluntary and charitable organisations.

There is considerable overlap between 'health' and 'social' care. This overlap is not surprising if a holistic view of health and wellbeing, which includes social contact, physical activity and good nutrition as well as mental, emotional and spiritual care, is used. This is particularly true of the care of older people with long-term conditions. However, for this group, the historic division between medical care provided free by the NHS, and social care provided on a means-tested basis by council social and care workers is complex and provides obstacles to the provision of seamless care designed to meet the needs of the person. This has been recognised, and the single assessment process, introduced in the National Service Framework for Older People (DoH, 2001), aims to ensure that a single assessment of older people's health and social care needs is undertaken. It is hoped that this will reduce duplication of assessment and lead to seamless care. But if budgets remain separate, it is difficult to see how seamless care will be achieved. However, in the English White Paper *Our Health, Our Care, Our Say* (DoH, 2006), plans have been announced for joint commissioning between PCTs and local authorities, with a streamlining of budgets and planning cycles, a wider role for Directors of Public Health and more joint health and social care appointments. The position in Northern Ireland is already different in that health and social care are provided together within the remit of its Department of Health, Social Services and Public Safety.

Thinking point consider which other occupational groups can promote public health.

Occupational groups whose primary concern is not health can also promote public health in a variety of ways. For example, education staff promote health through the provision of safe and enabling learning environments that encourage pupils and students to fulfil their potential. More directly, many education staff also provide information on health topics and enable students to discuss their attitudes towards health issues, thus supporting pupils' autonomy and empowerment. Leisure services staff are also responsible for promoting health. Such staff are responsible for promoting opportunities for physical exercise and providing a safe environment in which people can exercise. Targeted activities, such as women-only swimming sessions, encourage the participation of groups who might otherwise feel uneasy and excluded. Housing officers and police officers also promote public health as they have legal duties and responsibilities for ensuring public safety.

Regardless of who promotes health, working in collaboration is one of the most important aspects of promoting public health. It remains an important feature of success, both from the perspective of those working to promote public health as well as from those that benefit from it. Under LSPs, collaborative working takes place on all aspects of health, such as housing and environment, and with all client groups, for example, teenagers or people with mental health problems. Sure Start Children's Centres, which build on local Sure Start programmes, provide a good example of the way in which individuals and groups can work together to promote public health. Children's Centres are at the heart of the Government's collaborative strategy for children and families, with local authorities having strategic responsibility for the delivery of services that include: childcare, parental outreach and support for parents and carers who wish to retrain or take up employment.

4.4 The wider perspective

There can be many different partners within multidisciplinary public health. This section considers the wider perspective by focusing on the roles of the media and of voluntary workers and lay people.

4.4.1 Public health and the media

The influence of the media on people's knowledge, beliefs and attitudes is contested, but acknowledged by all to be significant (King, 2003). Public health has a long history of using the media to try to achieve behaviour change, with disappointing results (Gatherer et al., 1979; Sowden and Arblaster, 1998; Tones and Green, 2004). The simplistic model of information leading to attitude and behaviour change has been shown to be flawed (Wallack et al., 1993). However, the media can exert a powerful influence through disseminating simple information, raising awareness, and putting public health issues on the public agenda; some would argue that they can, if other enabling factors are present, change behaviour (Naidoo and Wills, 2000). Other research suggests that the shock tactics used in some health education messages result in unfavourable side effects (SIRC, 1999). For example, some people can experience 'warning fatigue' and become desensitised to health promotion messages. Others will develop what researchers call 'riskfactorphobia', where they will become increasingly anxious about the risks in their diet and lifestyle. Another possible side effect is the 'forbidden fruit effect', where individuals will seek to deliberately defy health warnings. One example of this was the UK's beef-on-the-bone scare in 1997 which prompted sales of rib-eye-beef to rocket.

The media can also serve to misinform the public through either intentional or unintentional coverage or sensationalist journalism. For example, there is considerable concern with the way in which the media represent mental health users as 'psychotic' and 'dangerous'. The media may also promote health scares, sometimes with disastrous consequences. For example, numerous contraceptive pill scares have led to considerable worry and anxiety and immediate rises in unwanted pregnancies and terminations (Furedi and Paintin, 1998; *The Lancet*, 2002). However, these are not the only biased sources of information. A former editor of the *British Medical Journal* has argued that medical journals are no more than 'an extension of the marketing arm of pharmaceutical companies', and that while medical trials are often seen as the most robust source of information, trials funded by drug companies rarely produce unfavourable results (Kmietowicz, 2005).

Although public health and advertising specialists are involved in planned campaigns, journalists and editors also have a role in promoting health in their coverage and appropriate presentation of health issues. 'Media advocacy' is the term used to describe the use of the media to generate public concern about the ways in which the legislative, economic or environmental context affects public health. Chapman and Lupton (1994) cite successful examples of the use of media advocacy in Australia to achieve tighter gun control and to prevent accidental drowning through the fencing in of garden pools.

4.4.2 Informal public health workers

Informal public health workers include lay people and voluntary workers who promote public health. The voluntary sector includes many charities and organisations that provide accessible services for vulnerable groups in society. For example, Care and Repair England is a charity that provides help and support with housing issues so that older and disabled people can live independently in their own homes for as long as possible. Research has shown that both older volunteers and the people they serve enjoy a better quality of life than those not involved in volunteering or voluntary groups (Wheeler et al., 1998), and that direct face-to-face contact appears to be most important in promoting health.

Lay networks of social support, such as neighbours and members of community or religious organisations, enhance social capital which, as already discussed in Chapter 3, is increasingly recognised as vital to good health and wellbeing (Bourdieu, 1986; Coleman, 1988; Putnam, 1995). Strengthening social capital is a key objective of a number of social interventions such as neighbourhood regeneration schemes and Health Action Zones (for example, see Box 4.5). Although many of these interventions are funded from public money, they depend on the participation of members of the public.

Box 4.5 Energy efficiency HAZ project, Armagh and Dungannon

The HAZ joined with key partners to improve energy efficiency in areas of rural isolation with higher than average concentrations of unfit dwellings. The project aimed to reduce domestic energy usage, lower the cost of fuel bills and contribute to a decrease in the levels of cold-related illness and early death. Energy efficiency zones were established with community workers as active promoters and facilitators of energy efficiency schemes and grants for homes.

(Adapted from http://www.adhaz.org.uk/)

Thinking point   how much of your daily routine is concerned with promoting health?

Lay people may promote health consciously or not be aware of their health promoting role. Consciously, lay people may seek to provide health knowledge and make healthy choices for themselves, their families and wider networks of relatives and friends. For example, parents may seek to provide healthy meals at home and encourage their children to take regular exercise as part of a conscious effort to promote the health of their family. The vast majority of the care provided for children, adults with disabilities, and older relatives is by family members. Providing such care in an informal family setting generally enables those who are cared for to maximise their potential for wellbeing and empowerment. Family members often act as mediators between sick individuals and primary healthcare providers, and between individuals in need of support and social care providers. As such, they are key players in determining when needs cannot be met informally but must be referred to professionals.

There is currently great emphasis within the NHS on working with families and lay people to identify and address needs. In 2003 the Commission for Patient and Public Involvement in Health (CPPIH) was established to promote greater lay involvement within health services. There are Patient and Public Involvement (PPI) forums in all NHS trusts and PCTs in England. However, in August 2006 the CPPIH will be abolished and replaced with a new body, and the PPI forums will be replaced by Local Involvement Networks (LINks). It is anticipated that these LINks will enable wider patient and public involvement in health. The NHS Plan (DoH, 2000) made a commitment to establish a Patient Advice and Liaison Service (PALS) in every Trust by 2002. PALS provide information, advice and support to patients, families and carers and are used, by Trusts, to monitor trends and identify gaps in service provision. Research suggests, however, that while PALS are making more than a tokenistic contribution to patient involvement in health, there is a limit to how far they can influence structural and cultural change within the NHS (Buchanan et al., 2005).

Not all health promotion by lay people is recognised as such. Family and friends provide an important social network that supports individuals and thereby indirectly promotes their health and wellbeing. Many women play a pivotal role in promoting family health, for example, through the purchase and preparation of meals, tending to the sick and through the surveillance of family members' health. It could even be argued that women's role in the family is one of the most important. However, some studies have identified the increasing role of fathers in day-to-day family practices (Gatrell, 2005).

Normal social interaction is health-promoting in effect, although few people would cite this as their explicit aim. Lay people also promote health by providing exemplars or role models, either consciously or not. For example, a neighbour may provide a good role model for healthy eating or regular exercise. Many theoretical frameworks of decision making on health stress the importance of significant others and role models (see Chapter 5). Generally, role models will be more effective the more similar they are in circumstances to the person. Although pop stars and sports heroes are important role models, especially for young people, in terms of aspirations, their circumstances are clearly removed from those of most people. Role models from within people's communities have added credibility because they can be seen to be 'just like me' in many respects. People might think 'If Fred down the road can quit smoking and get fit, so can I!'. *Choosing Health* (DoH, 2004) seeks to capitalise on this through the introduction of personal trainers. Personal trainers will be lay people who receive education and training for their role in persuading people, on a one-to-one basis, to adopt healthier lifestyles.

Political and policy processes may seem very remote to most people. However the general public can become involved in policy change in a variety of ways, from individual contact with their MPs or the media to organised lobbying on specific issues. Lobbying is the process of trying to influence policy makers in favour of a specific cause. Many organisations take on a lobbying role to try to promote public health policies and strategies. The widespread recognition that health is determined by a variety of socio-economic factors, many of which have a global dimension, means that lobbying for political, policy and economic outcomes is seen as legitimate public health promotion. For example, grassroots organisations such as the Pensioners' Forum play a part in campaigning on behalf of older people. Lobbying activities include the compilation of expert reports, mass action such as petitions or letter-writing campaigns, and using favourable public opinion polls and the mass media to publicise views.

A recent example of successful lobbying by a number of organisations (including Action on Smoking and Health (ASH), the British Medical Association, the Royal College of Physicians and the Faculty of Public Health) is the ban on smoking in public places in the Republic of Ireland, which has been widely hailed as a success. Introduced in 2004, the ban on smoking has attracted widespread support and not led to any major loss of business in the tourist and hospitality trades. England, Northern Ireland, Scotland and Wales have now followed suit.

Lipsky (1980), in his seminal work on street-level bureaucrats (or frontline workers), argues that many public service workers are in a position to exert a great deal of influence on how policy is implemented. This is due to several factors. First, such workers (including healthcare workers and social workers) typically work in environments where resources are scarce and where demand exceeds supply. Second, performance management in such areas is notoriously difficult as goals are general and difficult to measure. Third, clients or service users are typically non-voluntary, and do not have the means to take their service elsewhere if they do not like the service they receive. These elements conspire to give street-level bureaucrats a degree of power and autonomy in deciding how they will deliver services and to whom they will give priority. For example, writing specifically about disability, Hudson (1997) argues that street-level bureaucrats become authoritative figures who act to gate-keep services, thus rationing provision and being selective in the information they give to individual clients.

Street-level bureaucracy can also create a work environment that is stressful and in which difficult decisions must be made. As already outlined in Chapter 1, when resources are finite, the (re)distribution of resources is a moral, political and social issue.

Thinking point   can you think of other individuals or agencies who promote public health?

Employers can also promote public health. For example, as you have read in Chapter 3, work promotes health in many ways, providing an income, social networks, self-esteem and structure, and it is particularly important for maintaining good mental health. However, work can also contribute (both directly and indirectly) to illness and disease. Traditionally the focus has been on occupational illness rather than the opportunities offered by seeing workplaces as health-promoting. In a study of doctors working in stressful general practice environments, Stanley et al. (2005) draw on a salutogenic approach to explore how the workplace can prevent doctor 'burnout' (also see discussion on salutogenesis in Chapter 2). They argue that by providing in-service training, educational programmes, supervision and support, the workplace can promote health rather than cause stress.

So employers have an important role to play. Trade unions are also key partners in promoting occupational health by promoting health and safety and representing workers' interests.

Partnerships with the private sector are also necessary if promoting public health is to be everybody's business (for example, see DoH, 2004), for example, in relation to the nature and quality of customer information and advice on health. Retailers also have a role to play in the promotion and pricing of health products, and manufacturers can play a part in product development, labelling and customer information. Increased corporate social responsibility has also become increasingly important and, some would say, demanded by the public. Indeed, many believe that public demand will be a crucial factor in the role of the private sector within multidisciplinary public health (DoH, 2004; French, 2007). This is also underpinned by the *Bangkok Charter for Health Promotion in a Globalised World* (WHO, 2005), which not only highlights the direct impact of the corporate sector on health but calls for the promotion of health to be a requirement for good corporate practice.

The relative power of different individuals and groups must be considered with respect to how influential they can be in lobbying for change. Sheer critical mass is important, but social and economic differentials are also relevant. Adopting a wider perspective illustrates how public health action can involve an enormous range of individuals and organisations at different levels.

Conclusion

There is a delicate balance between a nation state that facilitates health and one that is open to accusations of being a 'nanny state' (too prescriptive) or socially irresponsible (negligent). Health needs to be on the state's agenda and positively facilitated in numerous ways which acknowledge the diversity of factors that influence health. Too much emphasis on individual responsibility for health is likely to be ineffective and may lead to 'victim blaming' when illness occurs. Such a focus leads to the loss of opportunities to promote public health through economic and social policy making. However, too prescriptive an approach to health will impinge negatively on individual liberty and free will. As you have seen in previous chapters, the issue of who is ultimately responsible for the promotion of health is contentious and relates to political, economic and ethical debates.

This chapter has considered the question: 'Who promotes public health?' by examining a number of agencies, organisations and individuals who promote health, in both a formal and informal, and direct and indirect, manner and in professional and lay capacities. This chapter has also discussed some key dilemmas associated with promoting health, such as what kind of skills are required for promoting public health, as well as considering the policy context in which individuals, organisations and agencies promote public health.

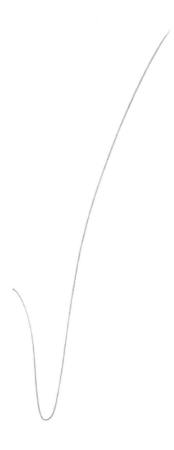

References

Adams, J. and Pearce, S. (2005) 'Occupational therapists and the promotion of psychological health in rheumatoid arthritis' in Scriven A., (ed.) *Health Promoting Practice: The Contribution of Nurses and Allied Health Professionals*, Basingstoke, Palgrave.

Allen, P. (2001) 'Health promotion, environmental health and local authorities', in Scriven A. and Orme J. (eds) *Health Promotion: Professional Perspectives* (2nd edn), Basingstoke/Milton Keynes, Palgrave/Open University Press.

Bourdieu, P. (1986) 'The forms of capital' in Richardson J., (ed.) *Handbook of Theory and Research for the Sociology of Education*, New York, Macmillan.

Buchanan, D., Abbott, S., Bentley, J., Lanceley, A. and Meyer, J. (2005) 'Let's be PALS: user-driven organizational change in healthcare', *British Journal of Management*, vol. 16, no. 4, pp. 315–28.

Carter, C. (1996) *Members One of Another: The Problems of Local Corporate Action*, York, Joseph Rowntree Foundation/York Publishing Services.

Chapman, S. and Lupton, D. (1994) *The Fight for Public Health: Principles and Practice of Media Advocacy*, London, BMJ Publishing.

Coleman, J. (1988) 'Social capital in the creation of human capital', *American Journal of Sociology*, vol. 94 (supplement), pp. S95–S120.

Crowther, R., Rolfe, L., Hill, A., Morgan, S., Rutter, H. and Watson, J. (2005) *Lifestyle and its Impact on Health*, Stockton on Tees, Association of Public Health Observatories.

Department for Environment, Food and Rural Affairs (DEFRA) (2004) *Public Service Agreement (PSA)* [online] http://www.hm-treasury.gov.uk/media//39947/sr04_psa_ch13.pdf (Accessed 8 September 2006).

Department of Health (DoH) (1992) *The Health of the Nation*, London, The Stationery Office.

Department of Health (DoH) (1999) *Saving Lives: Our Healthier Nation*, London, The Stationery Office.

Department of Health (DoH) (2000) *The NHS Plan*, London, The Stationery Office.

Department of Health (DoH) (2001) *The National Service Framework for Older People*, London, The Stationery Office.

Department of Health (DoH) (2004) *Choosing Health: Making Healthier Choices Easier – Public Health White Paper*, London, The Stationery Office.

Department of Health (DoH) (2005a) *The Long-Term Conditions (Neurological) National Service Framework*, London, The Stationery Office.

Department of Health (DoH) (2005b) *Choosing Health through Pharmacy: A Programme for Pharmaceutical Public Health 2005–2015*, London, The Stationery Office.

Department of Health (DoH)/Welsh Assembly Government (2005) *Shaping the Future of Public Health: Promoting Health in the NHS*, London/Cardiff, Department of Health/Welsh Assembly Government.

Department of Health (DoH) (2006) *Our Health, Our Care, Our Say: A New Direction for Community Services*, London, The Stationery Office.

Department for Transport (DfT) (2004) *Children's Road Traffic Safety: An International Survey of Policy and Practice, Road Safety Research Report No. 47*, London, Department for Transport.

Duperrex, O., Bunn, F. and Roberts, I. (2002) 'Safety education of pedestrians for injury prevention: a systematic review of randomised controlled trials', *British Medical Journal*, Vol. 324(1129) [doi:10.1136/bmj.324.7346.1129].

Fox, N.J., Ward, K.J. and O'Rourke, A.J. (2005) 'The "expert" patient: empowerment or medical dominance? The case of weight loss, pharmaceutical drugs and the internet', *Social Science and Medicine*, vol. 60, no. 6, pp. 1299–309.

French, J. (2007) 'The market-dominated future of public health' in Douglas, J., Earle, S., Handsley, S., Lloyd, C.E. and Spurr, S. (eds), *A Reader in Promoting Public Health: Challenge and Controversy*, London/Milton Keynes, Sage/The Open University.

Furedi, A. and Paintin, D. (1998) 'Conceptions and terminations after the 1995 warning about oral contraceptives', *The Lancet*, vol. 352 no. 9124, 25 July, pp. 323–4.

Gatherer, A., Parfit, J., Parker, E. and Vessey, M. (1979) *Is Health Education Effective?* London, Health Education Council.

Gatrell, C. (2005) *Hard Labour: The Sociology of Parenthood*, Buckingham, Open University Press.

Hudson, B. (1997) 'Michael Lipsky and street-level bureaucracy: a neglected perspective' in Hill M., (ed.) *The Policy Process: A Reader* (2nd edition), London, Harvester Wheatsheaf.

Jeffery, C. (2002) *Devolution: Challenging Local Government?* York, Joseph Rowntree Foundation.

Jones, J. and Hinton, S. (2005) 'Physiotherapists promoting health in cardiac rehabilitation' in Scriven A., (ed.) *Health Promoting Practice: The Contribution of Nurses and Allied Health Professionals*, Basingstoke, Palgrave.

King, M. (2003) 'Promoting public health: media constructions and social images of health in a post-modern society' in Costello J. and Haggart M., (eds), *Public Health and Society*, Basingstoke, Palgrave Macmillan.

Kmietowicz, Z. (2005) 'Medical journals are corrupted by dependence on drug companies', *British Medical Journal*, vol. 330:1169, doi:10.1136/bmj.330.7501.1169–b.

Lammin, S. (2005) 'Time for an ethical debate', *Environmental Health Journal,* January.

Lipsky, M. (1980) *Street-Level Bureaucracy: Dilemmas of the Individual in Public Services*, New York, Russell Sage Foundation.

McClean, S. (2003) 'Globalization and health' in Orme, J.et al. (eds) *Public Health for the 21st Century: New Perspectives on Policy, Participation and Practice*, Maidenhead, Open University Press.

MacDonald, G. (2001) *Making the Shift: A Report of Two Research Projects carried out for the Health Development Agency and the Society for Health Education and Promotion Specialists*, Birmingham/London SHEPS/HDA.

McVeigh, C., Hughes, K., Bellis, M.A., Ashton, J.R., Syed, Q. and Reed, E. (2005) *Violent Britain: People, Prevention and Public Health*, Liverpool, Centre for Public Health.

Naidoo, J. and Wills, J. (2000) *Health Promotion: Foundations for Practice* (2nd edn), Oxford, Elsevier.

Navarro, V. (1998) 'Neo-liberalism, 'globalization', unemployment, inequalities, and the welfare state', *International Journal of Health Services*, vol. 28, pp. 607–82.

Office of the Deputy Prime Minister(ODPM) (2002) *Your Region, Your Choice: Revitalising the English Regions*, London, ODPM.

Office of the Deputy Prime Minister (ODPM) (2005) *Realising the Potential of All Our Regions: The Story So Far*, London, ODPM.

Pandey, K.S., Hart, J.J. and Tiwary, S. (2003) 'Women's health and the internet: understanding emerging trends', *Social Science and Medicine*, vol. 56, no. 1, pp. 179–91.

Prowse, J. (2003) 'International influences on public health' in Watterson, A. (ed.) *Public Health in Practice*, Basingstoke, Palgrave.

Putnam, R.D. (1995) 'Bowling alone: America's declining social capital', *Journal of Democracy*, vol. 6, pp. 65–78.

Robinson, A. (2004) 'Cracks in public confidence', *Guardian*, 11 August 2004, [http://www.guardian.co.uk/g2/story/0,1280473,00.html] [Accessed 27 April 2006].

Salmon, D., Baird, K., Price, S. and Murphy, S. (2004) *An Evaluation of the Bristol Pregnancy and Domestic Violence Programme to promote the introduction of routine antenatal enquiry for domestic violence at North Bristol NHS Trust*, Bristol, Faculty of Health and Social Care, University of the West of England.

Scriven, A. (ed.) (2005) *Health Promoting Practice: The Contribution of Nurses and Allied Health Professionals*, Basingstoke, Palgrave.

Scottish Executive (2003) *Partnership for Care: Scotland's Health White Paper*, Edinburgh, Scottish Executive.

Social Issues in Research Centre (SIRC) (1999) 'The side effects of health warnings', *SIRC Bulletin*, 12 May, pp.1–3.

Smith, M.K. (2003) 'New WHO leader should keep health of the poor at the heart of the political agenda', *The Lancet*, vol. 361, no. 9351, p. 5.

Sowden, A.J. and Arblaster, L. (1998) 'Mass media interventions for preventing smoking in young people (review)', *The Cochrane Library*, Issue 1 2005, John Wiley.

Stanley, R., Matalon, A., Maoz, B. and Shiber, A. (2005) 'Keeping doctors healthy: a salutogenic perspective', *Families, Systems and Health*, vol. 23, no. 1, pp. 94–102.

The Lancet, (2002) 'A health scare in the mass media', *The Lancet*, Vol. 359 no. 9312, p. 1079.

Tones, K. and Green, J. (2004) *Health Promotion: Planning and Strategies*, London, Sage.

United Nations (1992) *Earth Summit. Agenda 21: The United Nations Programme of Action from Rio*, New York, UN Department of Information.

Wallack, L., Dorforman, L., Jennigan, D. and Themba, M. (1993) *Media Advocacy and Public Health: Power for Prevention*, Sage, London.

Wanless, D. (2002) *Securing Our Future Health: Taking A Long-Term View*, London, The Stationery Office.

Wanless, D. (2004) *Securing Good Health for the Whole Population: Final Report*. The Stationery Office, London.

Welsh Assembly Government (2002) *Wellbeing in Wales*, Cardiff, Office of the Chief Medical Officer.

Wheeler, J.A., Gorey, K.M. and Greenblatt, B. (1998) 'The beneficial effects of volunteering for older volunteers and the people they serve: a meta-analysis', *International Journal of Aging and Human Development*, vol. 47, pp. 69–79.

Woods, N. (2001) 'Making the IMF and the World Bank more accountable', *International Affairs*, vol. 77, no. 1, pp. 83–101.

World Health Organization (WHO) (1986) *Ottawa Charter for Health Promotion*, Geneva, WHO.

World Health Organization (WHO) (2003) *Framework Convention on Tobacco Control*, Geneva, WHO.

World Health Organization (WHO) (2005) *The Bangkok Charter for Health Promotion in a Globalised World*, Bangkok, WHO [online] http://www.who.int/healthpromotion/conferences/6gchp/bangkok_charter/en/ (Accessed 4 April 2006).

Chapter 5

Theoretical perspectives on promoting public health

Jane Wills and Sarah Earle

Introduction

Deciding how to promote the health of individuals, communities and populations is challenging, and different people will have different approaches. In part, this depends on how they define health itself, what they think are the factors contributing to a particular health problem, the extent to which they think individuals have responsibility for their own health, and how they perceive their role in all this. Theoretical perspectives on promoting public health also play a part. Theory can be used to analyse, predict or explain given phenomena and this chapter introduces you to some of the key theoretical perspectives on promoting public health. It begins by reconsidering, in Section 5.1, the eclectic nature of multidisciplinary public health and the subsequent range of explanations that can be applied to health problems and issues. Section 5.2 examines the theories that explain behaviour change in individuals and focuses on some of the barriers to, and facilitators of, change. Section 5.3 introduces theories of community change and, in Section 5.4, macro and micro theories of communication are discussed. Finally, the chapter considers alternative models of health promotion.

5.1 Understanding theory

Is it possible to promote public health without any knowledge, or understanding, of the theory that underpins practice? The answer to this question is probably 'yes'. However, to promote public health effectively, it is useful to develop your understanding of the different theories that underpin public health action and health behaviour. The first part of this section considers some of the approaches and perspectives on health – introduced in previous chapters – and shows how these different approaches influence the strategies adopted in promoting public health. The second part discusses the nature and role of theory in public health.

5.1.1 Promoting public health: an eclectic field

As discussed in earlier chapters, biomedicine defines health as the absence of disease. In modern western societies, a medical model of health predominates in which differences in health status are assumed to be biological or the result of individual lifestyles. However, this dominant approach is challenged by other approaches which suggest that lifestyle choices are socially shaped and that health and illness are also determined by structural variables: referred to as the behavioural and the socio-environmental approaches respectively. The dominant biomedical approach and the counter-approaches thus embrace divergent philosophical perspectives: the individualistic, which focuses on the person and assumes that people have 'agency' or the capacity for free will; and the collective or structural, which focuses on categories such as class and social and environmental factors.

Approaches to, or perspectives on, health influence not only the ways in which health issues are defined and prioritised, but also the choice of strategies and actions for addressing them. Figure 5.1 illustrates some of the priorities that might be targeted in the promotion of public health within each of the three main approaches introduced above.

Figure 5.1 Priorities for promoting public health		
Biomedical approach	**Behavioural approach**	**Socio-environmental approach**
Cardiovascular diseases	Smoking	Poverty
Cancers	Diet and nutrition	Unemployment
HIV/AIDS	Physical activity	Housing
Diabetes	Substance abuse	Social isolation
Obesity	Stress	Environmental pollution
		Hazardous living and working conditions

Thinking point   what strategies might you adopt to reduce heart disease if you took a behavioural approach?

Figure 5.2 illustrates some of the principal strategies that could be adopted by each of the three main approaches to health in order to reduce heart disease. Multidisciplinary public health embraces all these approaches, and the strategies are variously highlighted in policy and practice.

Figure 5.2   Three approaches to reducing heart disease

Health approach	Causes of problem	Principal strategies to address problem
Biomedical	Hypertension Family history Hypercholesterolemia	Treatment Drugs Low salt/low cholesterol dietary regimen
Behavioural	Smoking High fat diet Low level of physical activity High stress levels	Health education Health communication Self-help/mutual aid (e.g. smoking cessation) Policies to support lifestyle choices e.g. workplace catering, cycle routes
Socio-environmental	Living conditions Working conditions Social isolation	Policy change Advocacy Community mobilisation Self-help/mutual aid

5.1.2 What is theory?

Theories are organised sets of knowledge applicable in a variety of circumstances that may help us to analyse, predict or explain a particular phenomenon and the ways in which change takes place in individuals, communities, organisations and societies. In most disciplines the building of theory and progress towards an explanation for phenomena is an accepted part of study and research. Theory might thus help to answer different questions and may be:

- Descriptive: what is it ... ?

- Explanatory: why is it ... ?

- Predictive: what would happen if ... ?

- Prescriptive: what should be done ... ?

A developed theory of personal health behaviour may thus provide an explanatory framework accounting for the factors influencing a phenomenon, and the relationship between these factors.

The main elements of theories are known as concepts and the key concepts of a specific theory are known as constructs. Like theory, a model can also be descriptive, explanatory, predictive or prescriptive. Some scholars use the terms 'theory' and 'model' interchangeably.

Public health has been described as atheoretical (Smith, 1985; McKinlay, 1998). However, epidemiology, which seeks to understand the social distribution of disease (and has traditionally underpinned public health), incorporates many of the concepts and methods of disciplines such as sociology, psychology, economics, geography and biology, and so, arguably, cannot really be described as atheoretical. There have also been many attempts to formulate a theory of health promotion, but a large number of these (Tones, 1981; Ewles and Simnett, 1985; Tannahill, 1985) have been little more than models describing and categorising existing activity, even though some references to both theory and ethical principles can be found in them.

Broadly, the development of theory serves three purposes:

1   It bounds a discipline and contributes to processes such as professionalisation. For example, attempts have been made to systematise and organise knowledge as part of the development of the occupational standards for public health practice (Skills for Health, 2004).

2   It may help to separate one field from another: politically, philosophically and ethically. For example, it could be argued that the authority and legitimacy of health promotion might be strengthened through the development of a core theoretical framework to underpin practice.

3   At a more pragmatic level, theory may provide a guide to programme planning (National Cancer Institute, 2003; Nutbeam and Harris, 2004). For example, a theory can provide insight into how a practitioner is able to shape programme strategies to reach individuals, communities and organisations and have an impact on them.

This chapter will show how, in promoting public health, individuals may draw from many theories from different disciplines, depending on their focus. It can be argued that this diversity creates irresolvable tensions between conflicting ways of thinking about and measuring health, leading to different (and competing) kinds of public health action, and that it could therefore be a weakness because of the incompatibility of the theories that underpin public health work (Wills and Woodhead, 2004). However, this eclectic and inclusive nature of multidisciplinary public health can actually be a strength, because health and the factors that influence health are also diverse.

5.2 Theories explaining behaviour change in individuals

A number of theories help us to understand the determinants of health behaviour and how to identify the barriers to, and facilitators of, change. They focus on factors within individuals such as knowledge, attitudes, beliefs, motivation and self concept. In this way, they are both explanatory frameworks and also guides to programme design.

5.2.1 The Health Belief Model

The Health Belief Model (Becker, 1974) is one of the oldest theories designed to explain health behaviour. Developed to demonstrate why people would or would not participate in programmes to prevent or detect disease, the model is based on two constructs: threat appraisal and behavioural evaluation. There may be some variables (demographic, socio-psychological and structural) and specific cues to action, such as a doctor's advice that may cause a person to think about their health, but according to this model, individuals will act to protect or promote their health under the following circumstances:

- if they are susceptible to a condition or problem
- if the consequences of the condition are severe
- if the recommended actions to deal with the problem are beneficial
- if the benefits of taking action outweigh the costs or barriers.

For example, if the Health Belief Model were to be applied to prevent the spread of HIV/AIDS, individuals would be more likely to practise safer sex if they believed that:

- they were at risk of HIV infection by having unprotected sex
- the consequences of the infection were serious
- safer sex practices (e.g. condom use) were effective in reducing the risk of infection
- the benefits of safer sex practices in reducing the risk of infection outweighed the potential barriers to, and costs of, condom use, such as embarrassment, lessening of pleasure and potentially difficult communication with a partner.

The Health Belief Model suggests that behaviour change is a result of a process in which information is carefully scrutinised and weighed up before a decision is reached and that individual behaviour will be guided by the 'rationality' of protecting one's health.

Thinking point   can you think of any other factors that may motivate behaviour change?

Behaviour may be guided by other rationalities, such as coping or pleasure. The role of smoking in stress relief, for example, makes it appear sensible to many people to continue smoking even though it is known to be harmful. Perception of risk is an important concept in behaviour change theories. Application of the Health Belief Model could suggest that health risks should be personalised and heightened to encourage an awareness of a threat to health and thus beliefs of susceptibility. However, not only could this lead to the over-simplification of information, but it is not in itself a health-promoting action. Although the model offers no guide as to how to modify health beliefs, it can help practitioners to focus on possible facilitators of, and barriers to, individual behaviour change.

5.2.2 Theories of reasoned action and planned behaviour

The theories of reasoned action and planned behaviour (Ajzen and Fishbein, 1980) further developed understandings of behaviour change at the individual level by suggesting that people's *intention* to behave in a certain way is the key to whether they actually do so. Whether or not a person will change their behaviour is influenced by:

- **Attitudes towards that behaviour**, which are determined by the belief that a desired outcome will occur if a particular behaviour is followed and that the outcome will be beneficial to health. For example, people will be more likely to have a positive attitude towards exercise if they believe that it will make them feel and look better.

- **Subjective norms**, which relate to a person's beliefs about what others think they should do (normative beliefs) and to their motivation to comply with the wishes of others. For example, if a smoker feels that most people do not smoke and that most of those whom they value think it would be good for them to give up smoking, then they are more likely to develop subjective norms that favour giving up.

- **Perceived behavioural control**, which relates to a person's beliefs about their self-efficacy. For example, a young person living away from home for the first time may be more likely to eat vegetables if they have a higher degree of perceived behavioural control, or confidence, in their ability to purchase and cook fresh food.

These theories of reasoned action and planned behaviour can be useful in thinking about the information that might be needed from individuals in order to develop an intervention that meets their health needs. They highlight the importance of understanding a person's beliefs about an issue, whom that person sees as affecting these beliefs and, consequently, their behaviour, and what they see as the barriers to taking action that may promote their health. In particular, attention should be paid to what Tones (1997) describes as the 'pushes and pulls' of competing motivations on intentions to act. These theories are particularly concerned with the influence of 'significant others' – family, friends, peers and celebrities – on an individual's intention to act. They have underpinned campaigns that use celebrities to put forward certain health education messages. For example, the Department of Health's 2005 'flu jab campaign was supported by celebrities such as Joan Collins, Terry Wogan and Cliff Richard.

5.2.3 The Transtheoretical (Stages of Change) Model

The Transtheoretical (Stages of Change) Model was developed to explain how individuals move towards adopting behaviour that will maintain good health (Prochaska and DiClemente, 1984). It uses stages of change as its core construct and integrates processes and principles of change from different theories, hence the name 'Transtheoretical'. It is based on the assumption that behaviour change is an ongoing process, rather than a single event, and that people have varying levels of motivation or readiness to change. The model identifies five stages of change:

1 **Pre-contemplation**   At this stage individuals are not considering changing their behaviour, or are consciously intending not to change.

2 **Contemplation**   At this stage people consider making a change to a specific behaviour.

3 **Preparation**   At this stage people make a serious commitment to change, for instance over the forthcoming two months, and begin to make the necessary preparation to do so.

4 **Action**   At this stage individuals are explicitly making changes in their behaviour or environment.

5 **Maintenance**   This refers to sustaining the change over time.

The model is based on observations that people appear to move through these stages in a predictable way, although some move more quickly than others. People may also move backwards as well as forwards through the stages. In later versions of this model, Prochaska et al. (1994) described a final stage of 'termination' at which individuals who have changed experience no temptation to return to their old behaviour. This applies equally to those who 'self-initiate' a change and those responding to advice and encouragement to change. The Transtheoretical Model provides a useful way of tailoring interventions to the stage at which people are in the change process. As an example, Figure 5.3 links the stages of change to the related challenges and to the actions a public health practitioner would need to carry out in order to help an individual who wanted to lose weight.

Figure 5.3 Use of Stages of Change Model to promote weight reduction (Source: adapted from Nutbeam and Harris, 1998, p. 18, Table 2.1)

Stage of change	Challenge	Example of suggested action
Pre-contemplation	Awareness raising	Provide information on the health risks of being overweight
Contemplation	Recognition of the benefits of change	Encourage client to draw up a list of pros and cons of present behaviour
Preparation	Support to overcome barriers to weight loss	Give information on local support
Action	Programme of change	Work out a plan for weight loss and monitor progress
Maintenance	Follow-up and support	Organise routine follow-up

Thinking point do you consider that the Stages of Change Model explains behaviour in the real world?

Despite the lack of evidence supporting its practice or the validity of these stages of change (Brug et al., 2005), the Transtheoretical Model has been very popular. It has been applied in motivational interviewing and brief interventions, especially for smoking cessation and alcohol reduction. Bunton et al. (2000) claim that this reflects the neo-liberal ideologies of the 1980s and 1990s which emphasised individualised, risk-based approaches in low-cost settings. However, there are ethical concerns that application of the model leads to categorising people either as appropriate for interventions or 'not ready', thus exacerbating existing inequalities, as individuals in the latter category are likely to be those who are already least able to access the social, cultural or economic resources and support for making changes to their behaviour.

Behaviour change theories inevitably emphasise this role of the individual in making health choices. Therefore, when applied to programme planning, such theories tend to disregard the structural factors that shape and constrain individual choices. More generally, such theories illustrate the critique or stance of much multidisciplinary public health in that this problematises individuals rather than structures, and focuses on monitoring individual behaviours rather than on changing the society in which individuals live.

From this discussion it can be seen that theories explaining behaviour change in people are often unable to address the wider factors that influence health. However, Section 5.2.4 below will introduce you to the Health Action Model, which does attempt to take into account some of these other factors.

5.2.4 The Health Action Model

The theories of reasoned action and planned behaviour and the Stages of Change Model, like the Health Belief Model, are concerned with how people decide to behave in a certain way. The Health Belief Model fails to take into account the influence of family, friends or other role models, whereas the theories of reasoned action and planned behaviour put a great deal of emphasis on this. However, whatever it is that truly motivates people, both these approaches to understanding behaviour change in people assume that individuals make rational decisions. Certain behaviours, of course, cannot be described as rational; in particular, addictive behaviours, or engaging in unsafe sexual practices. The pursuit of pleasure and short-term gratification can seem much more attractive than rather vague and longer-term benefits such as 'good health'. The Health Action Model (Tones, 1988) (see Figure 5.4) tries to take account of strong motivating forces – such as hunger, pain, pleasure and sex – in order to understand why people act in seemingly irrational ways.

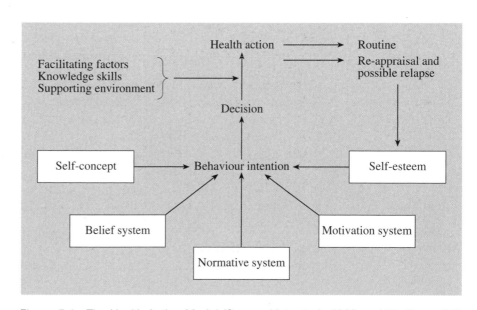

Figure 5.4 The Health Action Model (Source: Katz et al., 2000, p. 159, Figure 9.2)

Figure 5.4 shows that the Health Action Model identifies three general systems that influence behaviour: the motivation system, the belief system (as in the Health Belief Model) and the normative system (which represents the influence of social pressures on behaviour, such as conforming to peer-group norms). This model emphasises self-concept (identity) and self-esteem as important factors in the motivation for health behaviours, and points to the complexity of people's health behaviour generally. The model also illustrates how people's health behaviour is dependent, to a large extent, on the conditions of their lives, which, for many, are beyond their control. For example, Chapter 3 discussed research carried out by Graham (1993) on women and smoking, which showed that low-income lone mothers constituted the group most likely to smoke cigarettes. However, Graham also showed how this could be explained by understanding the context of these women's lives, which were lived in poverty and social exclusion.

5.3 Community change theories

As discussed in previous chapters, it is widely recognised that health is influenced by many factors and, subsequently, that to bring about change, a multifactoral approach is required. This understanding has shifted the focus of public health to broader 'system-level' interventions that focus on communities.

Thinking point spend a few minutes thinking about the different communities in which you are involved.

Most people are part of, or involved in, communities. Some people may be involved in professional communities, or workplace communities. It is also important to think about neighbourhoods as communities, as well as the idea of a 'global community'. Communities are seen as a central resource for change, as reflected in many community-based initiatives such as Sure Start and Health Action Zones. Community-level models are frameworks for understanding how social systems function and change, and how communities and organisations can be engaged. Understanding change in communities and organisations draws heavily on socio-ecological models of health which describe people as existing in complex social, cultural, economic and political environments, aspects of which (individually or through interaction) can enhance or damage health.

Bronfenbrenner (1979) describes human development as part of an ecological environment consisting of a set of 'nested structures' or systems which impact on each other: the micro system, focusing on the individual; the meso system, involving linkage with other settings in which the individual participates (e.g. school, workplace, or neighbourhood); the exo system, concerned with the impact of policies on the individual; and the macro system of public policy making.

The settings approach to promoting health, which links to Bronfenbrenner's meso system mentioned above, has been widely adopted by the World Health Organization (WHO) which suggests that health is created and lived by people within the settings of their everyday lives (WHO, 1986). Settings can normally be identified as having physical boundaries, a range of people with defined roles, and an organisational structure with its own culture and processes. The settings approach is rooted in this socio-ecological understanding of health and uses 'whole system' thinking and working (whole system thinking considers interconnections between systems and seeks to address simultaneously a range of problems).

In multidisciplinary public health there is an important conceptual difference between those generally small-scale activities which are provided in the community for individuals in a specific locality or a population sub-group, such as a breastfeeding support group, and those activities which involve people from the community in defining problems, targets and actions which are usually referred to as 'community development'. Community-based public health tends to work around local health issues and to a professionally determined agenda (a 'top-down' approach), while community development programmes may be large-scale and complex, incorporating many different activities underpinned by explicit values and principles of participation, equity, sustainability and partnership (a 'bottom-up' approach). Indeed, many recent UK-based heart health projects have adopted a community development approach.

Rothman (1987) developed a widely used typology that distinguishes between community-level initiatives, drawing attention to how these differ according to levels of community involvement and participation, the extent to which the agenda relates directly or indirectly to health, and whether they focus on addressing problems (and are therefore deficit based) or on building strengths (asset based). Rothman's typology consists of social planning, locality development and social action.

- **Social planning**   A community identifies local problems and uses a variety of resources and skills (budgeting, networking) to address those problems. Box 5.1 outlines a community-based initiative to tackle smoking in a low-income area in Scotland, which draws on the local identification of health problems.

Box 5.1 Breathing Space, Edinburgh, Scotland

Breathing Space is a community development initiative designed to tackle high levels of smoking in a low-income area of Edinburgh in Scotland. Local community groups had identified smoking as a priority health concern, which they had already begun to address through the implementation of no-smoking policies and smoking cessation support. The initiative aims to capitalise on local knowledge and encourage local involvement in the development of activities that would create a supportive environment in which to tackle smoking.

(Adapted from Ritchie et al., 2004, p. 53)

- **Locality development**   This is based on principles of mutual aid which stresses building capacity in the community and emphasises the community's own resources and assets (which, as mentioned above, may also be called community development). Figure 5.5 outlines the inputs, activities and structure of a capacity-building project in China funded by the World Bank. This project focuses specifically on enhancing knowledge and skills in order to increase staff and organisational capacity among front-line workers, managers and academics. In this case, the focus was on development among professionals, but much community development work involves lay people.

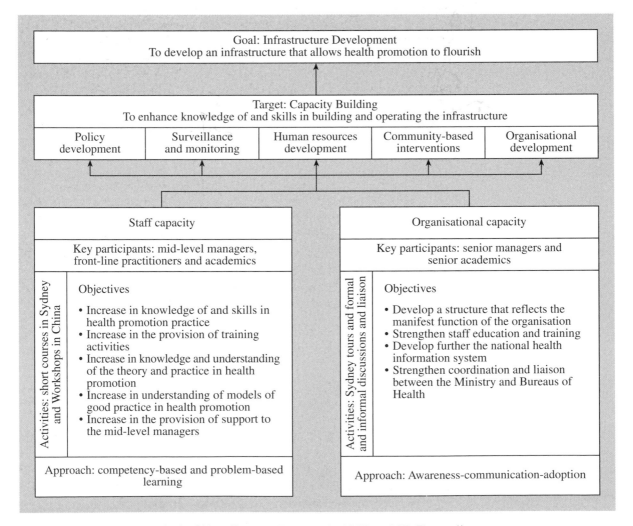

Figure 5.5   Building capacity in China (Source: Tang et al., 2005, p. 287, Figure 1)

- **Social action**   This aims to increase the problem-solving abilities of the community to achieve changes, and seeks to address the disadvantage experienced by oppressed groups. Box 5.2 provides an example of such an approach.

Box 5.2 Chicago Southeast Diabetes Community Action Coalition

A group of local residents and health and social care providers, together with a local university, founded the Southeast Diabetes Community Action Coalition in an area with very high rates of diabetes and associated levels of morbidity and mortality. The coalition used a participatory action research model to guide their capacity-building activities, which included training in diabetes, coalition building, research methods and action planning. These activities encouraged coalition members to reflect on the social causes of, and solutions to, high levels of diabetes in their community.

(Adapted from Giachello et al., 2003, p. 309)

Although working with communities is a central feature of promoting public health, there is no one theory of community change. Rather, theories derive from the broad ideological perspectives of the liberal/individualist versus the collectivist/socialist. These reflect different philosophical assumptions about the nature of societal change and the principal sources of health problems. The distinction between these perspectives informs many of the attempts to define and describe practice (see Beattie's 1991 model of health promotion; also, Caplan and Holland, 1990).

Popple (1995) describes pluralist, radical and socialist approaches to community work. Pluralist theories suggest that change in communities takes place as a result of the constant bargaining of competing interests. Thus, practice is about helping groups to overcome the problems in their neighbourhood by mutual support, developing skills and sharing activities, and creating communal coherence. In many cases, however, community work is something done to rather than with the community, and its intention is more to placate by using community energy and resources to supplement public services, rather than to empower. Radical and socialist theories have focused on understanding inequality within society. An understanding of power and control in relation to, for example, the use and ownership of information, the role and agenda of professionals, or the active discrimination against certain groups, informs this theoretical basis of community development work. This has long been associated with the work of Paulo Freire, who worked on literacy programmes with poor peasants in

Peru and Brazil and saw informal education as the political and social means of changing power relationships (Freire, 1970) (see also Chapter 1).

From this discussion it can be seen that, although community practice does not use a single model of community organisation, several concepts are central to the various approaches, as illustrated in Figure 5.6.

Figure 5.6   Community organisation

Concept	Definition	Example of application
Empowerment	Process of gaining mastery and power over oneself/one's community, to produce change	Give individuals and communities confidence, tools and responsibility for making decisions that affect them
Community competence	A community's ability to engage in effective problem solving	Work with community to identify problems; create consensus, and reach goals
Participation and relevance	Learners should be active participants, and work should 'start where the people are'	Help community set targets within the context of pre-existing goals, and encourage active participation
Issue selection	Identifying winnable, simple, specific concerns as focus of action	Assist community in examining how community members can communicate their concerns, and whether success is likely
Critical consciousness	Developing understanding of root causes of problems	Guide consideration of health concerns within broad perspective of social problems

(Sources: based on National Cancer Institute, 2003; Nutbeam and Harris, 2004)

Complex community interventions or social programmes, such as Sure Start or Health Action Zones, consist of these multiple activities with several layers of organisation. The theory underpinning such interventions can be hard to discern and is, in any case, often ignored in evaluations because the focus is on the inputs and the results, not on why change may have taken place. Health Action Zones and Healthy Living Centres, however, have been evaluated by evaluation strategies known as 'theory of change' and realistic evaluation (Pawson and Tilley, 1997). These strategies focus on the mechanisms of change in the belief that social programmes are based on implicit or explicit assumptions about how and why such programmes work. The task of the evaluation is to help practitioners understand and work with these theories and their assumptions, with the aim of examining the extent to which theories about social programmes hold (Hills, 2004). However, in a recent report based on six international case studies, Coote et al. (2004) found that large community-based initiatives, far from being theory driven, are often designed on the basis of informed guesswork and expert hunches and are driven by political imperatives.

5.4 Communication theories

Communication is at the heart of public health action. For example, governments and their agencies may need to communicate health information messages to the public, communities may need to communicate their requirements to a variety of agencies, and individuals may need to communicate health messages both in professional capacities and as lay people. Communication is an everyday activity and the skills involved may seem to be deceptively simple. However, communicating in a way that is health enhancing is not simply a matter of getting the message across; even in the briefest of encounters, it involves building relationships and recognising the power relations that exist between people and groups.

Thinking point   consider the different health messages that are communicated to you.

Levy (1997) has identified ten 'top' suggestions for good communication in public health:

1   Listen: this is an essential part of communication.
2   Capture attention by taking advantage of, and creating, opportunities to communicate.
3   Prepare well: being expert in your communication takes careful preparation.
4   Communicate with passion and if you care deeply about an issue, let others know about it.
5   Give communication a human face: relate stories about real people and real situations.
6   Think globally, communicate locally: communicate in such a way that global – or national – issues are related to local issues, situations and benefits.
7   Communicate in multiple ways: to get a message across, use a variety of media.
8   Communicate with all groups in society.
9   Empower individuals and communities to become engaged in public health issues.
10   Evaluate the impact of your communication. What could you do to improve future communication?

There are many types, forms and levels of communication, and different ways of theorising about them. This section explores both macro and micro levels of communication.

5.4.1 Mass media communication

Mass media campaigns and media resources, such as leaflets and posters, form a central part of much public health action and are described later in this chapter with reference to Beattie (1991) as 'health persuasion'. Communication theories help us to understand the ways in which such information is processed, from the time it is received to its impact on behaviour. Traditional models have focused on conceptualising and analysing mass communication as:

- Who?
- Says what?
- To whom?
- In what way?
- With what effect?

Research from the 1950s and the advent of television has shown that the characteristics (attractiveness, credibility, similarity) of those providing information impact on its effectiveness.

Thinking point   consider whether a celebrity role model, an 'expert' or a lay person would be most persuasive in influencing health behaviour.

Sources of information that are liked and are deemed to have specific expertise are more likely to improve recall and initiate attitude change (for a useful summary of attitude and communication theories see Bennett and Murphy, 1997). On the one hand, therefore, people are influenced by the person associated with an image or a source they admire, hence the widespread use of celebrity role models to promote health messages. On the other hand, however, when recommendations are made for a change, expert knowledge is seen as the most credible.

Models designed to explain health behaviour, such as the Health Belief Model, suggest that perception of threat is a factor prompting attitudinal or behavioural change. Indeed, many people believe that health communications about issues such as smoking, drink-driving or drug use should include frightening images that make people sit up and take notice. Yet studies of communication suggest that fear-arousing messages may actually encourage resistance among audiences and denial that the message applies to them, and may even contribute to positive attitudes to the very behaviour they are trying to counter (Montazeri, 1998), as in the case of the

1987 drug education campaign 'Heroin Screws You Up' (see Figure 5.7). On the other hand, people with little involvement in the issue –those who are not drug users, for instance – may respond to such emotional appeals. Similar questions were raised in Chapter 4 in the discussion of public health and the media.

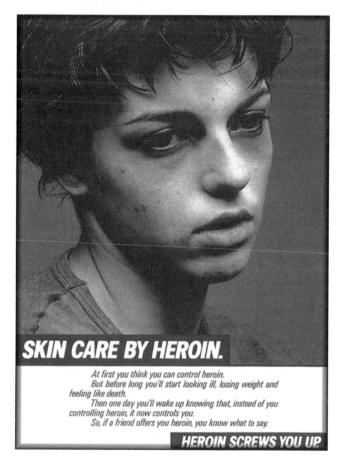

Figure 5.7 'Heroin Screws You Up': images such as these, which were intended to instil fear, were used as pin-ups by teenage girls who found the images 'sexy' and 'cool'

You now examine two of the theories that help to explain communication within social systems: diffusion of innovations and social marketing.

5.4.2 Diffusion of innovations

The diffusion of innovations theory (Rogers, 1995) helps to explain the spread, and adoption, of new ideas within a community and, like other ways of understanding behaviour change (such as the Transtheoretical Model), it suggests that people go through a series of stages before they adopt a new idea: initial awareness and increased knowledge; persuasion and interest in trying out the innovation; a decision to test out the innovation; and, finally, adoption.

The theory is based on observations that the legitimisation of an innovation within a community typically follows an S-shaped trajectory, with a small, initial uptake by 'innovators', normally from higher socio-economic groups, followed by 'early adopters' and then the 'early majority' for whom the utility of the innovation must be clear. These are eventually followed by the 'late majority', who tend to gain information from those around them, and finally the 'laggards', who tend to be more isolated and thus traditional in behaviour (see Figure 5.8). Change thus occurs in these groups more as a result of conformity to social norms and compliance with the majority, rather than as a result of an assessment of the costs and benefits of the innovation itself, its ease of adoption or perceptions about its immediate effects.

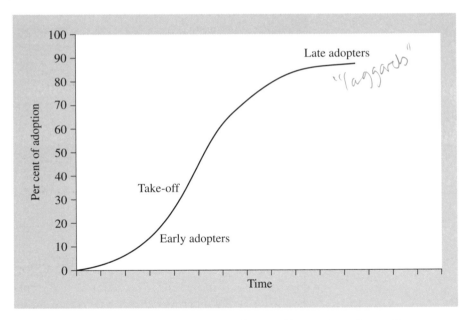

Figure 5.8   The S-shaped curve of the diffusion of innovations theory (Source: Adapted from Rogers and Scott, 1997, Figure 2)

According to Bennett and Murphy (1997), although diffusion of innovations theory seems to help explain the spread and adoption of new ideas, it is not fully understood. Application of the model would suggest that, although the mass media may be influential in raising awareness and in the early diffusion of ideas, an opinion leader or a 'change agent' plays an essential role in the communications process in spreading information and in stimulating and facilitating change, especially to late adopters. Peers, rather than experts, are more likely to be appropriate change agents. What also becomes clear from the model is that different social systems will adopt ideas at different rates, and that isolated 'traditional' communities are the least likely to adopt any innovation.

5.4.3 Social marketing

Social marketing is the process by which behaviour is influenced by the promotion of the acceptability of a social idea (see French, 2007). Kotler and Zaltman (1971) defined it as the adaptation of commercial marketing techniques to the analysis, planning and execution of programmes. Social marketing has a consumer orientation in emphasising the need to understand the interests and requirements of the target audience and ensuring through market research that any service or message is acceptable to that group. Part of the marketing strategy is market segmentation – a principle that people are not simply part of a population sub-group with an identity associated with socio-economic or demographic variables (age, class, location, and so on), but may also be divided according to readiness for change (as mentioned in relation to the Transtheoretical, or Stages of Change Model discussed in Section 5.2.3 above), or psychological variables such as personality type.

Social marketing, like generic marketing, works on the principle of mutual exchange – that is, that the 'seller' (e.g. a health practitioner) has something to offer the 'buyer' (the target audience) that is of benefit to them. Like any exchange there are costs, although these are not necessarily financial (for instance, they may include time, effort, embarrassment or discomfort), and perceived benefits associated with the idea, service or product. The benefits, however, are not material (examples might include better body image, being socially accepted and feeling fitter). The Health Belief Model also includes this element of a cost–benefit equation as part of theorising behaviour change.

However, social marketing is more difficult than the marketing of a commercial product. Marketing is based on a strategy of 'the marketing mix' which refers to four 'Ps': product, price, place and promotion. Yet the health 'product' itself, be it a behaviour or an idea, is intangible. It can involve changing intractable behaviours where the benefits may seem distant or unobtainable; and the 'price' to pay to obtain health, in terms of inconvenience, embarrassment or discomfort, can seem very high. The challenge for social marketing is to reach people in the places where they might be receptive to a 'health product', using channels and means that are acceptable. This is far more complex than simply placing an advertisement or a poster.

In summary, social marketing and the theories of individual behaviour change discussed earlier in this chapter also inform understandings of mass communication in the following ways:

- The beliefs and attitudes of the receiver will affect the impact of any communication.

- Individuals are part of social systems, and social norms can influence the adoption of ideas and new behaviours.

- For a person to be favourably disposed to a message and consequent behaviour change will depend on how they perceive the source of the message.
- A health message needs to acknowledge the costs and benefits of making a change in behaviour.

5.4.4 Interpersonal communication

Communication theories exploring interpersonal interactions tend to fall into several categories. Social psychological approaches address the clarity, openness and effectiveness of the messages. They look at the quality of the interpersonal relationship and whether mutual understanding is achieved, particularly with regard to both parties understanding one another's agendas, attitudes, expectations and goals. In addition, they take into account awareness of external social factors; for example, the setting in which the interaction takes places and the socio-economic status of both parties. Psychological theories relate to cognition, information processing and interpersonal interactions (and conflict between communicating parties).

Thinking point   what are some of the purposes of communication?

Communication takes place in many forms; it can be verbal and non-verbal and can serve a variety of purposes, for example:

- to control, influence or direct others
- to express either positive or negative emotions
- to reflect, share or ask for feedback
- to provide information.

Although there is considerable overlap between the four areas listed above, they illustrate the form, content and function of interpersonal communication.

Traditionally, interpersonal health communication was thought of as a one-way process, but it is now more commonly seen to be a two-way exchange between individuals, and to recognise shared power relations and collaborative approaches to public health (Duggan, 2006). The context in which health communication takes place can affect the style of exchange, however. For example, writing about communication between midwives and women, McCourt (2006) shows that, in clinical settings, more hierarchical forms of interaction are typical, whereas in community settings, more conversational approaches are used.

Research on interpersonal communication tends to focus on the *process* of communication and has shown that such communication can affect health outcomes (Duggan, 2006). The skills required to communicate effectively are often assumed and taken for granted, yet listening and questioning are probably two of the most important skills in public health work with individuals. Good listening – which refers to actively listening and comprehending what is being said – is a skill that can be learned and improved. Buckman and Kason (1992) suggest that the golden rule is to allow the other person to speak without interruption. Attentive listening includes:

- observing the speaker (if this is possible)

- ensuring eye contact is appropriate and acceptable

- concentrating on both words and non-verbal behaviour

- thinking about what is being said and how it is being stated

- being, looking and sounding interested

- indicating one's attention with body language (e.g. nodding)

- vocalising occasionally (e.g. 'hmm' or 'tell me more')

- being open-minded

- tolerating short silences.

The ability to use questions to promote communication is linked closely to listening and is equally important for developing a rapport with another person. To indicate careful listening, you might request clarification or amplification of the other person's views. Attentive listening to answers to questions will foster appropriate and sensitive responses. Questions can be framed in particular ways in order to open channels of communication or reduce interactions. A frequently used strategy is to employ questions to reflect back what the other person has said as confirmation of listening to, understanding and valuing the communication. This technique is widely used in counselling and coaching. Different types of questions are also used in research and you can read about these in later chapters.

Thinking point   can you identify any of the barriers to good listening?

Being aware of how well you listen can enable you to reflect on your own performance. It is always possible to improve listening and other communication skills by removing the barriers to good listening and communication. Figure 5.9 lists some of the potential barriers to effective listening.

Figure 5.9	Potential barriers to effective listening
Location of cause	Reasons
The listener	Negative attitude to the speaker or subject Impatient to speak oneself Fixed ideas on the subject being discussed Stress or anxiety about the subject or one's understanding Blocking an unpleasant message, or selective attention Not hearing due to physical difficulties Limited knowledge of language being spoken
The speaker	Poor oral presentation Insensitivity to feedback Appearance Preconceived ideas and stereotypes
The environment	Noise Discomfort Lack of privacy

Differences in gender, age, ethnicity, cultural and religious background, class and sexuality could also influence interpersonal communications. However, other barriers also exist. Semantics – or the meaning of words – can also lead to misinterpretations and misunderstandings. For example, in her work on diabetes in British South Asian communities, Lloyd (2007) argues that, although Asian support workers can positively improve health outcomes, there are conceptual, cultural and linguistic challenges to communication. In most health situations, the use of 'specialist' language (medical or technical terms) can also lead to ineffective communication.

The most effective health communication makes appropriate and timely use of specialist and everyday language, depending on the context of the communication. For example, when communicating with colleagues or like-minded individuals, specialist language is often appropriate. Research suggests that interprofessional education can be an important part of improving communication between groups of practitioners by establishing common values, changing attitudes and developing mutual understanding and respect (Priest et al., 2005). However, when practitioners communicate with lay people, or when lay people communicate with one another, specialist language may not always be appropriate, and everyday language may be more effective. Of course, just as it is important not to use language that may be too technical, it is also important not to patronise by using language that is too simplistic. When communicating with older people, for example, it is important not to use patronising 'elderspeak' (Bethea and Balazs, 1997). Increasing levels of health literacy among some groups also has implications for interpersonal communication in health.

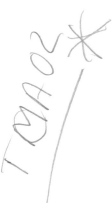

5.5 Models of health promotion

So far in this chapter you have explored theories that provide explanations for change and how such theories are located within particular disciplines and, thus, within particular ways of seeing the world. As outlined in this and previous chapters, multidisciplinary public health encompasses numerous approaches, all of which are informed by different disciplines. One response to this diversity is to identify and map discrete 'approaches' to practice in models which would represent the field. In this section the focus is on models of health promotion.

5.5.1 Normative models

Normative models of health promotion seek either to map or to represent reality, or to provide a blueprint from which to copy. An influential example of the mapping of health education practice was developed by Ewles and Simnett in 1985 and then further refined (1992, 1999, 2003) to create five approaches (see Figure 5.10). Different types of health-promoting activity were seen as important in each approach. In developing this framework, Ewles and Simnett (2003) argue that there is no 'right' approach to promoting health and that individuals need to work out for themselves how best to go about promoting health by drawing on their own values and (if one exists) their own professional code of conduct. Although the different approaches are seen as having distinctive priorities and objectives, and as reflecting very different views of patients/clients, there is an underlying assumption that, if practitioners are acting in good faith, then any of these approaches is valid.

The framework offers a clear and useful account of different ways of thinking about promoting public health. It also draws on practice experience as the basis from which to distil the five approaches and in doing so attempts to illuminate the dilemmas of health promotion. It does not tell us much, though, about what might motivate practitioners to select one approach rather than another. The 'medical' approach is seen as involving clinical intervention, but the other approaches are described in terms of particular activities and values which are not occupationally specific. However, the professional training of particular groups in the health and social care sectors are likely to predispose them to work within one approach rather than another. A 'societal change' approach might be seen as appropriate by an environmental health worker, for example, but rejected as irrelevant by an occupational therapist working on a hospital ward. It could also be argued that the approaches are not discrete. For example, a community health project might include aspects of the educational approach (providing health information) and societal change (lobbying for a local baby clinic or safe play areas), as well as being client-centred. More importantly, it does not tell us much about how practice

	Aim	Health promotion activity	Important values	Example: smoking
Medical	Freedom from medically defined disease and disability	Promotion of medical intervention to prevent or ameliorate illhealth	Patient compliance with preventive medical procedures	*Aim:* freedom from lung disease, heart disease and other smoking-related disorders. *Activity:* encourage people to seek early detection and treatment of smoking-related disorders.
Behaviour change	Individual behaviour conducive to freedom from disease	Attitude and behaviour change to encourage adoption of 'healthier' lifestyle	Healthy lifestyle as defined by health promoter	*Aim:* behaviour changes from smoking to not smoking. *Activity:* persuasive education to prevent non-smokers from starting and persuade smokers to stop.
Educational	Individuals with knowledge and understanding enabling well-informed decisions to be made and acted upon	Information about cause and effects of health-demoting factors. Exploration of values and attitudes. Development of skills required for healthy living	Individual right of free choice. Health promoter's responsibility to identify educational content	*Aim:* clients will have understanding of the effects of smoking on health. They will make a decision whether or not to smoke and act on that decision. *Activity:* giving information to clients about the effects of smoking. Helping them to explore their own values and attitudes and come to a decision. Helping them to learn how to stop smoking if they want to.
Client-centred	Working with clients on the clients' own terms	Working with health issues, choices and actions with which clients identify. Empowering the client	Clients as equals. Clients' right to set agenda. Self-empowerment of client	Anti-smoking issues are only considered if clients identify them as a concern. Clients identify what, if anything, they want to know and do about it.
Societal change	Physical and social environment which enables choice of healthier lifestyle	Political/social action to change physical/social environment	Right and need to make environment health enhancing	*Aim:* to make smoking socially unacceptable, so that it is easier not to smoke. *Activity:* no-smoking policy in all public places. Cigarette sales less accessible, especially to children, promotion of non-smoking as social norm. Limiting and challenging tobacco advertising and sports sponsorship.

Figure 5.10   Five approaches to health promotion (Source: Katz et al., 2000, pp. 82–3, Table 5.1)

changes or how people might modify or transform practice. It simply describes existing practice that can be observed and reported, not 'what might be'.

Tones and Tilford (2001) identified 'educational', 'preventive', 'empowerment' and 'radical' approaches to promoting health and acknowledged that each has its merits, before concluding that they viewed empowerment as the central focus of health education and health promotion. Health education is seen as a driving force empowering lay and professional people by raising their consciousness of health issues, policies and choices. Through health education, communities and health professional bodies can prepare themselves for change and begin to effect the transformation in public policy that will address social and environmental inequalities and improve health (see Figure 5.11). However, this also works in reverse: environmental and social circumstances exert their own influence on individuals and communities. They may also, by these means, influence health education messages.

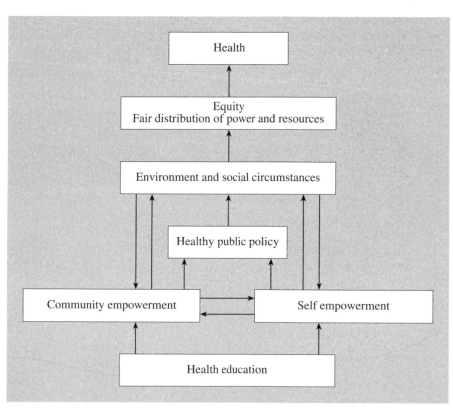

Figure 5.11   Tones's model of health education, empowerment and health promotion (Source: Katz et al., 2000, p. 85, Figure 5.1)

Thinking point   how else might health education be viewed as empowering?

A different model was proposed by Tannahill (1985), which demonstrates the wide range of possibilities for health promotion by incorporating prevention, health education and health protection in overlapping spheres (see Figure 5.12). Prevention (1) focuses on services such as immunisations, cervical screenings, hypertension case-finding and the use of nicotine chewing gum to aid smoking cessation. Health education (5) is aimed at influencing behaviour on positive health grounds and seeks to help individuals, groups or whole communities to develop positive health attitudes and skills. Health protection (6) deals with regulations and policies such as the implementation of a workplace smoking policy in the interests of providing clean air or the commitment of public funds to the provision of accessible leisure facilities. Health promotion not only incorporates all the domains described above, but also the overlapping areas. Preventive health education (2) includes educational efforts to influence lifestyle in the interests of preventing illhealth, as well as efforts to encourage the uptake of preventive services. Preventive health protection (3) addresses policies and regulations of a preventive nature, such as fluoridation of water supplies to prevent dental caries. Health education aimed at health protection (7) involves raising awareness of, and securing support for, positive health protection measures, among both the public and policy makers. All three dimensions come together as health education, prevention and health protection overlap (4) in efforts to stimulate a social environment conducive to the success of preventive health protection measures; for example, intensive lobbying for seat-belt legislation. The categories are not rigidly separate compartments, but in reality are often combined. For example, most public health measures are of a preventive nature and are aimed at empowering individuals to adopt healthy lifestyles.

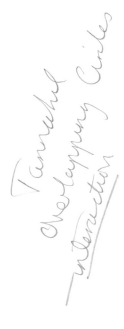

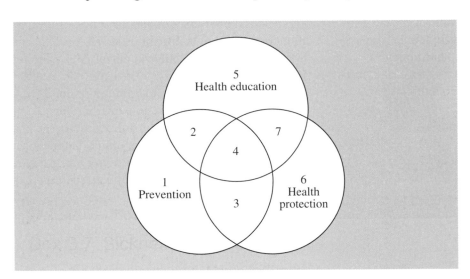

Figure 5.12   A model of health promotion (Source: Katz et al., 2000, p. 86, Figure 5.2)

Tannahill's model highlights the potential overlap between prevention and positive action, viewing effective health education as an essential building block for securing change. Contemporary health promotion work, it suggests, does not focus exclusively either on prevention and disease reduction or on structural and social change. A progressive primary healthcare team, for example, might offer a combination of health education (such as a well woman clinic), preventive services (such as immunisation) and disease management (such as asthma or diabetes education). It might also be involved in outreach work in schools and play a small part in publicising and supporting specialist health promotion campaigns.

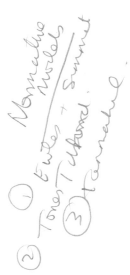

The model offers many combinations of approach, but it does not make explicit the political or social values underlying each approach, or reveal any preferences as to methods.

5.5.2 Analytical models

Explicit in all the models outlined above is an acknowledgement of how securing better health is bound up with addressing fundamental questions about social inequality. Yet they are still essentially describing how health promotion happens rather than commenting on the values and conflicts that underpin it. A consensus, that all approaches are valid depending on the context and that they are interrelated and work most effectively in combination with each other, is implied. No one approach is seen to take or should take priority. Although this inclusive strategy is reassuring, it may be that recycling descriptions of current practice is ultimately unproductive and does not stimulate anyone to go much beyond the status quo. Analytical models, on the other hand, go beyond the present boundaries of health promotion practice and provide a commentary on practice. By making explicit the links between core values and principles and different kinds of practice, a greater understanding of the philosophy and priorities of promoting public health may be derived (Naidoo and Wills, 2000).

A structural and conceptual map of health promotion can be developed to highlight the assumptions and frameworks underpinning different ways of engaging in practice (Beattie, 1984). It has been adapted (Beattie, 1991) to inspect the theoretical underpinnings of health promotion (see Figure 5.13). Its most important feature is the positioning of various accounts of health promotion within a broader socio-cultural framework. This model is explicitly saying that health promotion is embedded in wider social and cultural practices, in ideologies and political struggles. It is not something apart from the rest of society; indeed, it reflects in its territory struggles over power, control, autonomy and authority. The strength of this model lies in acknowledging that tensions exist between those who claim to provide objective definitions of health and those who would want to provide more subjective, relativist accounts, as well as tensions between those who feel that health can be promoted from within the existing social order, and those who feel that many problems with health occur only as a result of the existing social order which therefore needs to be challenged and replaced.

The typology is generated by means of two axes: mode of intervention (whether authoritative or negotiated) and focus of intervention in a society (whether individual or collective) (see again Figure 5.13). In this model social values are seen as driving practice, so that a 'health persuasion' approach to health promotion reflects a paternalist and individual-oriented philosophy. Individualism may not necessarily imply paternalism, however,

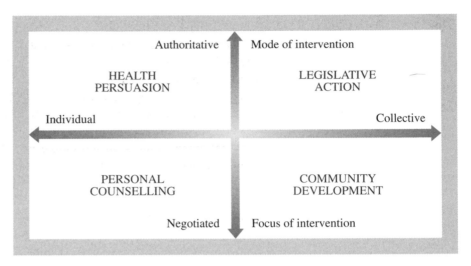

Figure 5.13   Beattie's model of health promotion (Source: Katz et al., 2000, p. 91, Figure 5.3)

and the model highlights a 'personal counselling' approach based on negotiation. The 'social change' approach of Ewles and Simnett (2003) assumes a concomitant philosophy of collective action, but Beattie's model demonstrates that collective action can be participative, non-participative, community-based or paternalist. Such an analysis helps to tease out some of the complexities underlying health action.

Beattie's model is not bounded by current practice and can be used to generate new approaches. Figure 5.14 gives an example of Beattie's model applied to promoting older people's health, where health is widely defined.

Figure 5.14 Beattie's model and promoting the health of older people	
Health persuasion Education about medication Falls advice 'Sloppy slipper' campaign	**Legislative action** Nutrition policies for nursing homes Winter heating allowance Transport services Flexible employment policies Housing hazard assessments
Personal counselling Pre-retirement courses Visiting services	**Community development** Lobby groups on pensions

Beattie's model enables reflection on the social and political perspectives underlying health promotion approaches. Beattie (1991) suggests that underpinning the 'conservative' model of health persuasion is a biopathological model of health which sees health promotion as attempting to repair deficits. Underlying a radical, community development approach to health promotion are assumptions about empowerment and equity and the mobilisation of communities to effect change. Underlying Beattie's model, personal counselling is an individual non-directive approach in which people are assumed to be free to determine their own lives, and underlying what Beattie terms the reformism of legislative action are assumptions about the role of the state in protecting public health. It was noted earlier, and elsewhere, that prevention and health protection are part of a more traditional, medical approach which focuses on the individual and on the treatment of disease, whereas more radical approaches are linked to healthy public policy strategies.

Other models have also attempted to link public health action to social and political structures, and to frameworks of social knowledge; note how they draw on some of the distinct models of health outlined in Chapter 2, Section 2.3. For example, Caplan and Holland's model of health promotion (Caplan and Holland, 1990; Caplan, 1993) plots theories of society (conflict or consensual) against ways of knowing about the social world (subjective or objective) (see Figure 5.15). The resulting quadrants represent different forms of health promotion which are not dissimilar from those set out in the five approaches offered by Ewles and Simnett (1999) (see again Figure 5.10).

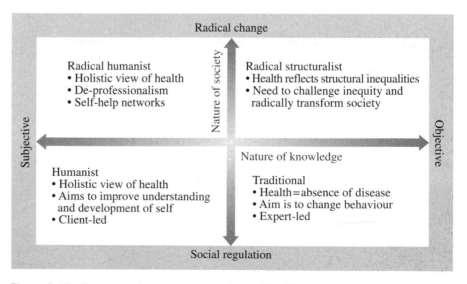

Figure 5.15   Four paradigms or perspectives of health promotion (Source: Katz et al., 2000, p. 93, Figure 5.4)

Conclusion

This chapter has explored some of the theories that inform health promotion and public health. Some of these, such as those concerning cognition and behaviour are fairly well-established, while others concerning community organisation and development are less well-formed or tested. As Nutbeam and Harris (2004, p. 75) suggest, they represent the art of health promotion as much as they represent the science, but given the need to increase the evidence base for multidisciplinary public health, it is important to draw out and discuss the theories that underpin public health action.

Models are different ways of conceptualising an emerging field. Although they clearly show links between different disciplinary frameworks – social theory, political theory, social psychology, and so on – they are often not explanatory or predictive. Although there are similarities in the mapping of different approaches to promoting health, there are significant differences in their philosophical and epistemological bases.

Given the many different factors that influence health, there is no single theory that can be applied to practice and there is no 'right' approach to promoting public health. An individual's view of the causes of health and illhealth will be influenced both by their personal values and by wider socio-cultural values, and this will lead to different approaches to promoting health being privileged or discounted. This chapter has shown how some of the frameworks that influence public health action may be built from evidence, whereas others are normative and represent different ideological or ethical positions, such as individual responsibility or the pursuit of social justice. The next chapter draws on the material contained in this, and previous, chapters to focus on the health of children and young people.

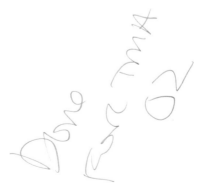

References

Ajzen, I. and Fishbein, M. (1980) *Understanding Attitudes and Predicting Social Behaviour*, Englewood Cliffs, NJ, Prentice Hall.

Beattie, A. (1984) 'Health education and the science teacher', *Education and Health*, January, pp. 9–15.

Beattie, A. (1991) 'Knowledge and control in health promotion: a test case for social theory' in Gabe, J., Calnan, M. and Bury, M. (eds) *The Sociology of the Health Service*, London, Routledge.

Becker, M. (1974) 'The Health Belief Model and personal health behaviour', *Health Education Monographs*, vol. 2, no. 4, pp. 324–473.

Bennett, P. and Murphy, S. (1997) *Psychology and Health Promotion*, Buckingham, Open University Press.

Bethea, L.S. and Balazs, A.L. (1997) 'Improving intergenerational health care communication', *Journal of Health Communication*, vol. 2, no. 1, pp. 129–37.

Bronfenbrenner, U. (1979) *The Ecology of Human Development: Experiments by Nature and Design*, Cambridge, MA, Harvard University Press.

Brug, J., Conner, M., Harre, N., Kremer, S., McKellar, S. and Whitelaw, S. (2005) 'The transtheoretical model and stages of change: a critique', *Health Education Research*, vol. 20, no. 2, pp. 244–58.

Buckman, R. and Kason, Y. (1992) *How to Break Bad News: A Guide for Health Care Professionals*, Basingstoke, Macmillan.

Bunton, R., Baldwin, S., Flynn, D. and Whitelaw, S. (2000) 'The stages of change model in health promotion: science and ideology', *Critical Public Health*, vol. 10, no. 1, pp. 55–70.

Caplan, R. (1993) 'The importance of social theory for health promotion: from description to reflexivity', *Health Promotion International*, vol. 8, no. 2, pp. 147–57.

Caplan, R. and Holland, R. (1990) 'Rethinking health education theory', *Health Education Journal*, vol. 49, no. 1, pp. 10–12.

Coote, A., Allen, J. and Woodhead, D. (2004) *Finding out What Works: Building Knowledge about Complex Community-Based Initiatives*, London, Kings Fund.

Downie, R.S., Fyfe, C. and Tannahill, A. (1990) *Health Promotion: Models and Values*, Oxford, Oxford University Press.

Duggan, A. (2006) 'Understanding interpersonal communication processes across health contexts: advances in the last decade and challenges for the next decade', *Journal of Health Communication*, vol. 11, no. 2, pp. 93–108.

Ewles, L. and Simnett, I. (1985) *Promoting Health*, Wiley, Chichester.

Ewles, L. and Simnett, I. (1992) *Promoting Health* (2nd edn), London, Scutari.

Ewles, L. and Simnett, I. (1999) *Promoting Health* (4th edn), Edinburgh, Baillière Tindall.

Ewles, L. and Simnett, I. (2003) *Promoting Health* (5th edn), Edinburgh, Baillière Tindall.

Freire, P. (1970) *Pedagogy of the Oppressed*, New York, Seabury Press.

French, J. (2007) 'The market-dominated future of public health?' in Douglas, J., Earle, S., Handsley, S., Lloyd, C.E. and Spurr, S. (eds) *A Reader in Promoting Public Health: Challenge and Controversy* , Sage in association with The Open University, London.

Giachello, A.L., Arrom, J.O., Davis, M., Sayad, J.V., Ramirez, D., Nandi, C. and Ramos, S. (2003) 'Reducing diabetes health disparities through community-based participatory action research: the Chicago Southeast Diabetes Community Action', *Public Health Reports*, vol. 188, no. 4, pp. 309–23.

Graham, H. (1993) *When Life's a Drag: Women, Smoking and Disadvantage*, London, HMSO.

Hills, D. (2004) *Evaluation of Community-Level Interventions for Health Improvement: A Review of Experience in the UK*, London, Health Development Agency.

Katz, J., Peberdy, A. and Douglas, J. (2000) *Promoting Health: Knowledge and Practice* (2nd edn), Basingstoke, Palgrave Macmillan/Milton Keynes, The Open University.

Kotler, P. and Zaltman, G. (1971) 'An approach to planned social change', *Journal of Marketing*, vol. 35, pp. 3–12.

Levy, B.S. (1997) 'Communicating public health: a "top 10" list', *Nation's Health*, vol. 27, no. 1, p. 2.

Lloyd, C.E. (2007) 'Researching the views of diabetes service users from South Asian backgrounds: a reflection on some of the issues' in Lloyd et al. (eds) (2007).

Lloyd, C.E., Handsley, S., Douglas, J., Earle, S. and Spurr, S. (eds) (2007) *Policy and Practice in Promoting Public Health*, London, Sage/Milton Keynes, The Open University.

McCourt, C. (2006) 'Supporting choice and control? Communication and interaction between midwives and women at the antenatal booking visit', *Social Science and Medicine*, vol. 62, no. 6, pp. 1307–318.

McKinlay, J.B. (1998) 'Paradigmatic obstacles to improving the health of populations–implications for health policy', *Salud Publica Mex*, vol. 40, no. 4, pp.369–79.

Montazeri, A. (1998) 'Fear-inducing and positive image strategies in health education campaigns', *International Journal of Health Promotion and Education*, vol. 36, no. 3, pp. 68–75.

Naidoo, J. and Wills, J. (2000) *Health Promotion: Foundations for Practice* (2nd edn), Edinburgh, Baillière Tindall.

National Cancer Institute (2003) *Theory at a Glance: A Guide For Health Promotion Practice*, US Department of Health & Human Services [online], http://www.nci.nih.gov/PDF/481f5d53-63df-41bc-bfaf-5aa48ee1da4d/TAAG3.pdf (Accessed 24 July 2006).

Nutbeam, D. and Harris, E. (1998) *Theory in a Nutshell: A Practitioner's Guide to Commonly Used Theories and Models in Health Promotion*, Sydney, National Centre for Health Promotion.

Nutbeam, D. and Harris, E. (2004) *Theory in a Nutshell: A Practical Guide to Health Promotion Theories* (2nd edn), Sydney, McGraw Hill.

Pawson, R. and Tilley, N. (1997) *Realistic Evaluation*, London, Sage.

Popple, K. (1995) *Analysing Community Work: Its Theory and Practice*, Buckingham, Open University Press.

Priest, H., Sawyer, A., Roberts, P. and Rhodes, S. (2005) 'A survey of interprofessional education in communication skills in health care programmes in the UK', *Journal of Interprofessional Care*, vol. 19, no. 3, pp. 236–50.

Prochaska, J.O. and DiClemente, C.C. (1984) *The Transtheoretical Approach: Crossing Traditional Boundaries of Therapy*, Homewood, IL, Dow Jones Irwin.

Prochaska, J.O., Norcross, J.C. and DiClemente, C.C. (1994) *Changing for Good*, New York, William Morrow and Company.

Ritchie, D., Parry, O., Gnich, W. and Platt, S. (2004) 'Issues of participation, ownership and empowerment in a community development programme: tackling smoking in a low-income area in Scotland', *Health Promotion International*, vol. 19, no. 1, pp. 51–9.

Rogers, E.M. (1995) *The Diffusion of Innovation* (4th edn), New York, Free Press.

Rogers, E.M. and Scott, K.L. (1997) *The Diffusion of Innovations Model and Outreach from the National Network of Libraries of Medicine to Native American Communities* [online], http://nnlm.gov/archive/pnr/eval/rogers.html (Accessed 9 November 2006).

Rothman, J. (1987) 'Three models of community organisation practice' in Cox, F., Erlich, J., Rothman, J. and Tropman, J. (eds) *Strategies of Community Organisation*, Itaska, IL, Peacock Publishing.

Scriven, A. and Orme, J. (eds) (1996) *Health Promotion: Professional Perspectives*, Basingstoke, Macmillan.

Skills for Health (2004) *National Occupational Standards for the Practice of Public Health Guide*, Bristol, Skills for Health.

Smith, A. (1985) 'The epidemiological basis of community medicine' in Smith, A. (ed.) *Recent Advances in Community Medicine*, Edinburgh, Churchill Livingstone.

Tang, K.C., Nutbeam, D., Kong, L.W. and Ruotao, Y.J. (2005) 'Building capacity for health promotion – a case study from China', *Health Promotion International*, vol. 20, no. 3, pp. 285–95.

Tannahill, A. (1985) 'What is health promotion?', *Health Education Journal*, vol. 44, no. 4, pp. 167–8.

Tones, B.K. (1981) 'Health education: prevention or subversion', *Royal Society of Health Journal*, vol. 101, no. 3, pp. 114–17.

Tones, B.K. (1988) 'Devising strategies for preventing drug misuse: the role of the health action model', *Health Education Research*, vol. 2, no. 4, pp. 305–17.

Tones, B.K. (1995) 'Health education as empowerment' in Health Education Authority, *Health Promotion Today*, London, Health Education Authority.

Tones, B.K. (1997) 'Health education: evidence of effectiveness', *Archives of Disease in Childhood*, vol. 77, no. 3, pp. 189–91.

Tones, B.K. and Tilford, S. (2001) *Health Promotion: Effectiveness, Efficiency and Equity* (3rd edn), London, Stanley Thornes.

Wills, J. and Woodhead, D. (2004) 'The glue that binds – articulating values in multidisciplinary public health', *Critical Public Health*, vol. 14, no. 1, pp. 7–15.

World Health Organization (WHO) (1986) *Ottawa Charter for Health Promotion*, Ottawa, World Health Organization.

Chapter 6

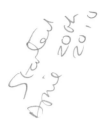

Focusing on the health of children and young people

Sarah Earle

Introduction

Childhood is a key stage in promoting public health since childhood disadvantage is thought to impact significantly on adult health (Graham and Power, 2004). The behaviours and habits formed early on in life are also thought to continue into adult life. Policy and practice reflect both these concerns and seek to challenge disadvantage and social inequality, tackle health-damaging behaviours, and empower children, young people and families, in order to promote public health. Before exploring these issues, this chapter begins by considering the social context of children's and young people's lives. Next, Section 6.2 explores the politics of children's health by thinking about how a healthy child or childhood comes to be defined, and examines the rationale for promoting the health of children and young people. It also develops some of the issues addressed in Chapter 3 by focusing on diversity and inequality in the health of children and young people. Then, drawing on some of the ideas developed in Chapter 2, Section 6.3 examines concepts of health and ways of ensuring that the voices of children and young people can be heard. Finally, the chapter examines the scope of multidisciplinary public health action by exploring the areas of childhood injury prevention, mental health in schools and sexual health promotion.

6.1 Children and young people in a social context

The classic work of Ariès (1962) is probably the most commonly cited in the area of childhood studies. While not without critics, Ariès argued that the concepts of 'child' and 'childhood' did not truly exist before the late seventeenth century when new ideas about 'children' and 'childhood' began to emerge. This era has been described as a 'new world' for children (Plumb, 1975). Ariès argued that, before the mid-eighteenth century, children were treated very much as adults and were expected to dress, behave and act in the way of adults. However, it is the twentieth century that has been described as the century of the child, in which ideologies of a child-centred society took centre stage in policy and practice (James and Prout, 1997). Mason (2005) suggests that the construction of childhood is closely related to the development of policies and practices. He argues that, in western societies, childhood has historically been sharply contrasted with adulthood; children are seen to be in a time of 'becoming', dependence and incompetence.

Although notions of childhood as a time of becoming are still prevalent, in more recent times an alternative approach has been put forward. This approach challenges the concept of children 'becoming' adults and sees children very much as 'beings' with experiences and views of their own. James and James argue that:

> the idea of childhood must be seen as a particular cultural phrasing of the early part of the life course, historically and politically contingent and subject to change ... how we see children and the ways in which we behave towards them necessarily shape children's experiences of being a child and also, therefore, their own responses to and engagement with the adult world.
>
> (James and James, 2004, p. 13)

In the literature, much has been made of the differences between children in the west and those in developing countries. For example, in parts of Northern Tanzania, changes in subsistence and labour have led to a reduction in fertility, with subsequent consequences for children's lives and the way in which childhood is understood (Hollos, 2002). It is important to recognise that 'children' and 'childhood' are not homogeneous terms and that they can be understood only in relation to diversity and difference. Distinctions must, therefore, be made between 'modern' and 'traditional' childhoods. It is also important to recognise multiple 'childhoods' and to be mindful of the way in which western concepts can assume a privileged status.

Thinking point   how would you define the terms 'child' and 'young person'?

Understandings of children and childhood change over time and space and cannot be regarded as objectively real. Of course, although it is important to consider the social context of children's lives, childhood is more than a social phenomenon, and the biological, physical and psychological dimensions should not be denied. Whereas childhood and adulthood are defined in relation to each other, it is much harder to define young adulthood. At what age does a child become a young person? When does a young person become an adult? In many ways, the answers to these questions are irrelevant as there cannot really be a fixed age at which these transitions take place. In practice, children and young people develop according to a range of factors, including chronological age, cognitive skills, gender, their position in the family and a wide range of other biopsychosocial concerns. However, the transition from child (and young person) to adult is relevant in relation to the provision of services, age of consent, and rights and responsibilities, although even these are not static. For example, across the UK, the age for transition from child to adult care varies. As a result, regardless of individual need, access to particular services is organised according to chronological age.

Children's cognitive development, and subsequent capacity to make autonomous decisions, is highly relevant to how services are delivered and the extent to which the views of children and young people are taken into account. For instance, there is considerable debate in the literature, and on the ground, about the age at which a child should be permitted to refuse medical treatment. Currently (in 2007), young people aged sixteen and seventeen can legally consent to medical treatment but cannot legally refuse treatment. Under the age of sixteen, they can give consent only if they are judged to be competent to do so. Children and young people are afforded the rights of adults at different ages and according to different criteria. For example, the current age at which one can vote in the UK is eighteen, but many people believe that this should be lowered to sixteen. One is allowed to drive a car at the age of seventeen and to buy cigarettes at sixteen, but again, many people would like to see these ages extended to eighteen.

The terms 'child' and 'young person' are not unproblematic descriptors; they raise questions about definition and the validity of the competencies, rights and responsibilities ascribed to them. Thus, promoting the health of children and young people must take into account the social context of their lives. The next section examines this debate further by exploring the politics of children's and young people's health.

6.2 The politics of children's and young people's health

The concept of health is changing and contested. This section examines the politics of children's and young people's health by exploring their concepts of health. The section also considers issues of diversity and health inequalities.

6.2.1 A healthy child?

Although the idea of a 'healthy child' is often presented as factual and uncontested, the characteristics of child health are not neutral but constructed through social and political considerations. Sometimes these considerations are driven by powerful interests. For example, Mayall suggests that:

> What the medical profession, the nursing profession and other allied professions choose to study, highlight, test for, survey for, define as worthy of their attention, will be determined by a range of social and economic factors, including their own interests. These will include issues of public health, understandings of the appropriate respective inputs of doctors, nurses and other professionals as against mothers, fathers and other 'lay' people, models of what childhood is and how it should be lived ...
>
> (Mayall, 1996, p. 23)

This is, of course, not limited to the construction of health knowledge, but can be applied to other forms of knowledge too.

The politics of infant feeding provides a good example of how children's health is structured by social and economic factors. Current World Health Organization (WHO) guidelines recommend exclusive breastfeeding for the first six months of life, and conclude that breastfeeding is advantageous for women and children as well as for society as a whole (WHO, 2001). Although rates of breastfeeding are variable, and especially low in the UK, breastfeeding is fervently promoted by midwives, health visitors and others as both natural and desirable (Earle, 2003). This contemporary emphasis on breastfeeding is in sharp contrast to the practices in infant feeding in the 1950s and 1960s when women were encouraged by health professionals to bottle feed using infant formula milk. At this time, formula milk was seen as health-enhancing, producing stronger, healthier and happier babies and mothers. However, in the late 1970s universal concern was expressed about the use of formula milk. Particular concern arose from the unethical marketing of formula milk in developing countries for which the physical, practical and social costs of infant formula were untenable. Since then, organisations such as Babymilk Action (see, for example, http://www.babymilkaction.org) have campaigned against the irresponsible sale and marketing of infant formula, most notably in the boycott against Nestlé, which now has the support of twenty countries.

Thinking point   can you think of any other ways in which definitions of child health have varied over time?

At one time a fat child was seen as a healthy child. Indeed, in some countries and cultures this idea persists. However, many would now argue that the reverse is true and that a fat child is generally regarded as an unhealthy child (see also Chapter 12). Ideas about what is 'healthy' or 'unhealthy' have changed over time, and what is known to be 'true' about child health is subject to shifting and competing interpretations.

6.2.2 Diversity, inequalities and child health

Children and young people are often expected to be healthy, and deviation from this is seen as unusual. However, there are striking differences in the health chances of different groups of children and young people. Low birth weight is an important indicator of birth outcomes. It is also strongly associated with both immediate and long-term illhealth in infancy, childhood and later life. Figure 6.1 shows the infant mortality rate by registration and father's socio-economic status. From this you can see that mortality is highest for babies who are sole registered and that there is a considerable difference between socio-economic groups.

[handwritten margin notes: "In the UK, in this day and age" and "where from"]

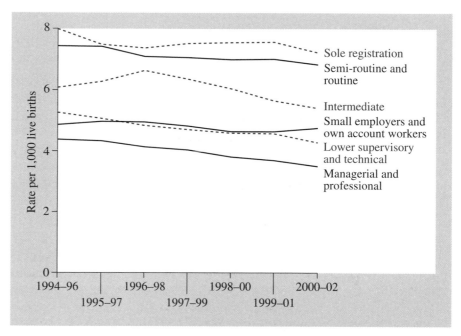

Figure 6.1 Infant mortality rate by sole registration and father's socio-economic status, England and Wales, 2002 (Source: ONS, 2004a, p. 72, Figure 6.4)

Birth weight distributions also differ between ethnic groups. Babies whose mothers were born in the 'New Commonwealth' (an association of independent states) have higher rates of low birth weight than others. Those whose mothers were born in East Africa or the Caribbean are more likely than others to be of very low birth weight (see Figure 6.2). Arguably, although there are objectively real differences in mortality and morbidity between different groups, it must be recognised that western norms, regardless of their suitability, have become the yardstick for measuring birth weight, and 'normal' growth and development, in all ethnic groups. A comparative study of ethnicity and birth weight in over 800,000 babies born in Norway, Pakistan, Vietnam and North Africa between 1980 and 1995 (Vangen et al., 2002) concluded that differences in perinatal mortality between ethnic groups could not be explained by differences in mean birth weight. (Anthropometry, or the study of the measurement of the human body, is discussed further in Chapter 12.)

Figure 6.2 Low birth weight live births by mother's country of birth and birth weight of babies, 2000 (Source: Macfarlane et al., 2004, p. 33, Table 8.8)

England — Numbers and percentages

	All	Not stated	Under 1,500	1,500-2,499	Under 2,500	Under 1,500	1,500-2499	Under 2,500
	Numbers					Percentages of stated birth weights		
All	604,441	1,020	7,536	38,191	45,727	1.2	6.3	7.6
United Kingdom	510,835	766	6,206	31,475	37,681	1.2	6.2	7.4
Outside the United Kingdom	93,606	254	1,330	6,716	8,046	1.4	7.2	8.6
Irish Republic	4,050	14	41	222	263	1.0	5.5	6.5
Other European Union	11,105	24	107	631	738	1.0	5.7	6.7
Rest of Europe	7,362	33	76	315	391	1.0	4.3	5.3
Australia, Canada and New Zealand	3,635	3	34	174	208	0.9	4.8	5.7
New Commonwealth	47,249	118	822	4,262	5,084	1.7	9.0	10.8
Bangladesh	7,482	13	79	702	781	1.1	9.4	10.5
India	6,650	9	112	767	879	1.7	11.5	13.2
Pakistan	13,561	18	220	1,295	1,515	1.6	9.6	11.2
East Africa	3,959	13	75	386	461	1.9	9.8	11.7
Southern Africa	1,907	10	23	103	126	1.2	5.4	6.6
Rest of Africa	6,537	38	207	482	689	3.2	7.4	10.6
Far East	1,538	0	16	86	102	1.0	5.6	6.6
Mediterranean	1,148	3	16	78	94	1.4	6.8	8.2
Caribbean	2,681	9	55	210	265	2.1	7.9	9.9
Rest of the New Commonwealth	1,786	5	19	153	172	1.1	8.6	9.7
Rest of the World and not stated	20,205	62	250	1,112	1,362	1.2	5.5	6.8

Birth weight (grams)

The impact of environment on children's health provides another example of the relationship between health, diversity and difference. The environmental factors that influence children's health can be defined as those aspects of a child's life determined by interactions with physical, chemical, biological and social factors. Particular environmental threats may include passive smoking, lead poisoning, indoor and outdoor air pollution, and pesticide exposure. Not all children are equally affected by poor environmental health: Figure 6.3 shows some of the inequalities between the richest and poorest countries of the world. Inequalities also exist more locally within a country, in that the poorest children are more likely to be exposed to environmental threats caused by inadequate housing, poor nutrition and limited access to healthcare.

Thinking point   how might these environmental threats be reduced or eradicated?

Many individuals, organisations and agencies are involved in reducing or eradicating the threat of environmental degradation. Chapter 3 outlined the potential for environmental health action, including the potential for change at individual or local levels, as well as that which can be achieved nationally or internationally through policy and legislation.

6.2.3 Why focus on the health of children and young people?

As noted at the beginning of this chapter, childhood is an important target for public health action since health behaviours and disadvantage in childhood are thought to continue into adult life. Drawing on the lifecourse perspective outlined in Chapter 3, Graham and Power (2004) show how childhood disadvantage can compromise adult health, by providing a framework for thinking about policies to improve the health of children from poorer backgrounds. Figure 6.4 suggests ways in which parental background can influence the health of children from birth through to leaving school. It also shows how the developmental health of children (physical, emotional, cognitive), their educational and social trajectories and their health behaviours can lead to poor adult health. The concept of foetal programming (Barker, 1989) is also part of a lifecourse approach, and suggests that maternal poverty can affect foetal development (see Chapter 3).

Much public health promotion targeted at children thus aims to prevent poor health developing in adulthood. Some aspects of promoting health, however, also aim to improve the health of children and young people, or prevent injury and illness. This distinction does, to some extent, reflect the distinction between children as 'becomings' in contrast to 'beings'

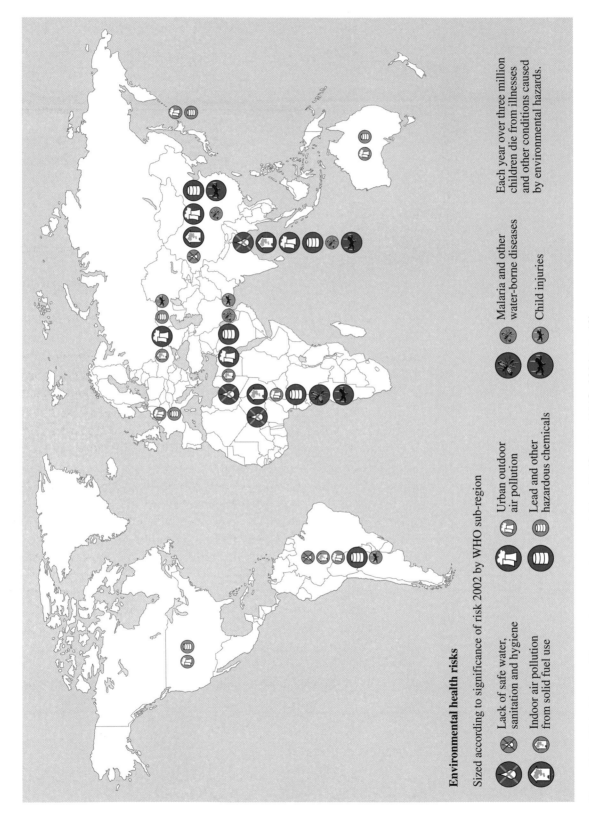

Environmental health risks

Sized according to significance of risk 2002 by WHO sub-region

Lack of safe water, sanitation and hygiene

Indoor air pollution from solid fuel use

Urban outdoor air pollution

Lead and other hazardous chemicals

Malaria and other water-borne diseases

Child injuries

Each year over three million children die from illnesses and other conditions caused by environmental hazards.

Figure 6.3   Global inequalities and poor environmental health (Source: WHO, 2004a, p. 13)

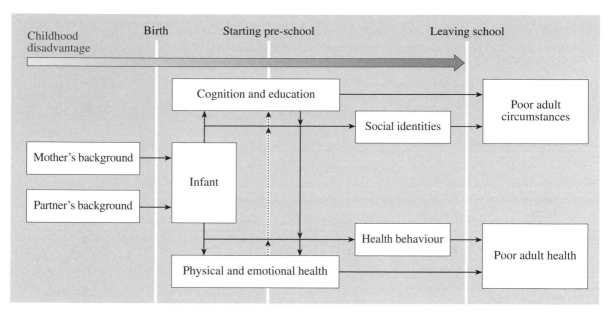

Figure 6.4   Lifecourse framework linking childhood disadvantage to poor adult health (Source: Graham and Power, 2004, p. 676, Figure 7)

 (Mason, 2005). Viner and Macfarlane (2005) suggest that there are five main reasons for focusing on the health of children and young people.

1   **Health behaviours continue into adult life**   It is thought that health behaviours are laid down during childhood and young adulthood and that they often continue into adulthood. This is a compelling reason for developing targeted and specific interventions for children and young people (e.g. smoking prevention).

2   **Immediate effects of health behaviours**   Whereas some health behaviours may have potential long-term effects, others may have more immediate effects and, thus, may need to be addressed regularly and in a timely way (e.g. road traffic safety awareness).

3   **Worrying trends in morbidity and mortality**   Statistics show worrying trends for both physical and mental illness among children and young people. Such trends indicate that urgent attention is required with regard to issues such as suicide, sexual health and obesity.

4   **Developmental issues**   With dynamic and continued development of every kind, children's health needs change continuously and so, too, does their need for the suitable delivery of public health promotion.

5   **Clustering of health risk**   There is evidence to suggest that health risk behaviours tend to cluster, especially in young adulthood. For example, those who smoke are also more likely to drink alcohol or use drugs. Public health promotion would be wise to focus on the cluster of health-risk behaviours.

Thinking point   can you think of other reasons for promoting the health of children and young people?

Although Viner and Macfarlane (2005) offer a useful rationale for promoting children's health, they adopt a restricted view of child health which focuses on individuals and their risk-taking behaviour. Others would suggest that a more comprehensive approach is needed, which acknowledges cultural and structural factors as well as individual behaviours. For example, a study of smoking among ten- and eleven-year-olds in Northern Ireland (Rugkåsa et al., 2001) highlights the significance of culture, revealing that smoking is a negotiation of status within children's culture. Drawing on the work of the social theorist Bourdieu (1989), the authors argue that children may smoke cigarettes in order to communicate certain images about themselves, thus setting themselves apart from other children (see Box 6.1). While both approaches are valid, the latter draws on a rationale focusing more on the notion of children as social beings, within the context of both their own normative cultures and wider structural factors. However, both approaches may inform multidisciplinary public health action with children and young people.

Box 6.1 Children's views on smoking in Northern Ireland

- Smoking as a form of communication:

  'I thought that if I started to smoke I'd be all big and that. I could make myself look older if I smoked.'
  [Female; smoker]

- Smoking as the basis of identity and solidarity:

  'I think they smoke because they don't want to be left out. They want to act cool.'
  [Female; non-smoker]

- Smoking as an adult activity:

  'Young people are destroying their health straight away ...'
  [Female; non-smoker]

  (Adapted from Rugkåsa et al., 2001, pp. 137, 135)

6.3 Making sense of health and illness

Chapter 2 explored the ways in which adults define health and considered some of the similarities and differences between these definitions. In this section we explore how children and young people define health, and consider how and why these definitions may vary from those of adults.

However, before focusing on this, it is useful to think about some of the ways in which children's voices can be heard.

Children's knowledge has often been unrecognised, trivialised or ignored. If children are seen as passive, dependent and incompetent, then they cannot know, understand or contribute to knowledge about their own health needs. However, children and young people acquire health knowledge from a variety of sources: in informal settings at home and in the playground, as well as from television programmes and advertisements. They also acquire it formally though health promotion and education and through prevention strategies within the school setting and at breakfast clubs, for example. In early childhood, the role of the family as the primary means of socialisation is particularly important. As a child grows older, other individuals, such as peers, become significant.

Children also learn about health and illness through their own experiences of these. Many children and young people are involved in caring for others. The role of children as carers for siblings or parents with long-term conditions, who are disabled or dependent on drugs or alcohol, has increasingly come to be recognised. For example, the Young Carers' Initiative (2006), a Children's Society project, urges health and social care workers to give choice, trust and respect to young carers with such responsibilities.

Until recently, researchers had not always valued children's own views of their health and had relied on the views of parents; this was especially true in the case of younger children. However, it is now recognised that even children as young as five years old can describe both physical and mental states, and that children from the age of eight can report on all aspects of their health experiences (Rebok et al., 2001). Many different methods are used in research with children; for example, pictorial scales, draw and write/tell techniques, sensory walks, interviews and focus groups. Choice of method will depend on the aims of the research as well as on the age group of the children involved.

The Children's Research Centre, based at The Open University in the UK, has developed an innovative method of researching children whereby children themselves are trained as social researchers and are then able to carry out their own research. The children participate in a ten-week interactive programme focusing on four aspects of the research process: research design, data collection, data analysis and dissemination. They learn to draw on other people's research findings and are guided on research ethics. The children are then able to carry out research in subjects of their own choosing. Two examples of these include the development of an exercise questionnaire by James Wright (2006), aged ten, and a study on the effect of death on children by Paul O'Brien (2006), aged twelve. In support of this type of research, Grover (2004) urges researchers and policy makers to ensure that children are active collaborators in telling their own stories, rather than just the passive objects of research.

Thinking point   in comparison with adults, how might children and young people make sense of health?

There is increasing interest in lay concepts of health and illness and, although little research in this field has been carried out on children and young people, some studies do exist. In general, these have shown that young children often associate health with eating good food, exercising, feeling good, and being fit, full of energy and able to do the things they want to do. In short, evidence suggests that children in the UK share with health educators a view that health is primarily about certain kinds of behaviour. According to Hill and Tisdall (1997), primary school-aged children tend to focus on three main issues:

1   food and nutrition
2   exercise
3   dental hygiene.

Like those of adults, children's concepts of health and illness show patterns, as well as discrepancies, in understanding. Research also shows that, as with adults, children and young people can show a marked difference between their knowledge of health and their actions. For example, although a child may understand that foods such as carrots and broccoli are 'healthy', they may not be willing to eat them. In some households, of course, some of these foods will not be available. In a study of Scottish schoolchildren (Inchley et al., 2001), which formed part of the WHO 'Cross-national health behaviour of school-aged children' (HBSC) study, data showed that nutritional messages have improved awareness of diet. (Another, well-known example of such a message might be the Department of Health's '5 A DAY' campaign: DoH, 2003.) However, in spite of this, the figures indicate that one-third of Scottish schoolchildren do not eat fruit on a daily basis and approximately half do not eat vegetables every day.

Thinking point   how might you account for the discrepancy between what children know about health and their health behaviours?

The discrepancy between what children know about health and their health behaviours raises questions about the efficacy of the campaign messages that target children and young people through health education and by using social marketing techniques. Theories explaining behaviour change in individuals are also relevant here. For example, the Health Belief Model could be used to explore individual barriers to behaviour change, and theories of reasoned action and planned behaviour could be used to examine the intention to change. The Health Action Model and theories of community change could be used to explore the wider context and the external barriers that influence the relationship between knowledge about health and health behaviours (see Chapter 5).

Many studies have shown that children's concepts of health become more concrete with age. For example, a study of children and young people in Germany, aged between five and sixteen years (Schmidt and Fröhling, 2000), showed that, when interviewed, younger children were less able to describe the characteristics of specific diseases. When asked to describe a person with AIDS, young children between the ages of five and eight years often gave irrelevant answers such as: 'Like someone who is drunk', and slightly older children gave descriptions of an unspecific patient role: for example, 'Laying in bed'. However, children aged between twelve and sixteen years were able to give more concrete answers such as: 'Someone who gets one illness after the other', and more abstract responses such as: 'AIDS is an illness which comes from the HIV virus' (Schmidt and Fröhling, 2000, p. 232), from which we can note how, as children reach young adulthood, they are more likely to draw on a biomedical model of health.

Concepts of risk – defined as the probability of something happening – are also important to children and young people's understanding of health, once again echoing the perceptions of health educators. Although young people, in particular, are perceived as enormous risk-takers, research shows that most are in fact often anxious and cautious about risk-taking (Hill and Tisdall, 1997), although this differs according to gender and age. Beck (1992) argues that risk is an increasing feature of contemporary societies in which decision-making becomes individualised, and risk and danger are created and recreated as socially constructed realities. Drawing on Beck's work on the 'risk society', many commentators have argued that issues concerning children's personal safety and risk have become a key concern for the new millennium (Backett-Milburn and Harden, 2004).

The importance of good mental health is also recognised by children. For example, when asked about health, young children will mention the importance of relaxing and maintaining good relationships with others (Rebok et al., 2001). In a study of Pakistani Muslims in Bradford (Bashford et al., 2002), fifty children and young people were asked to comment specifically on how they viewed mental health. Using a focus group method, the children and young people were asked to identify things they saw as being 'mentally healthy'. The answers were grouped across seven domains: views of others, ability, identity, physical health and attributes, feelings, mental ability and behaviour (see Box 6.2).

Box 6.2 Mental health: views of Pakistani Muslim children and young people

Views of others
'No one ever saying you are mental'

Ability
'Able to do anything'

Identity
'Knowing who you are'

Physical health and attributes
'Being normal, eating well, being active'

Feelings
'Feeling good about yourself, calm and relaxed'

Mental ability
'Being brainy at school'

Behaviour
'Being offered drugs and saying no'

(Adapted from Bashford et al., 2002)

The Green Paper, *Every Child Matters* (DfES, 2003), set out a commitment to improve the wellbeing of children and identified broad agreement on five key outcomes:

1   **being healthy**: enjoying good physical and mental health and living a healthy lifestyle
2   **staying safe**: being protected from harm and neglect and growing up able to look after themselves
3   **enjoying and achieving**: getting the most out of life and developing broad skills for adulthood
4   **making a positive contribution**: to the community and to society and not engaging in antisocial or offending behaviour
5   **economic wellbeing**: overcoming socio-economic disadvantages to achieve their full potential in life.

In England, this was followed by *Every Child Matters: Next Steps* (DfES, 2004a) and then by *Every Child Matters: Change for Children* (DfES, 2004b). In 2004 the Children Act also established the role of the Children's Commissioner, whose role is to promote an awareness of the views and interests of children in relation to the five outcomes listed above. The *Change for Children* programme is underpinned by a commitment to better service integration and partnership. The vehicle taking this forward has been identified as the Children's Trust, which aims to bring together all services for children and young people with a focus on improving outcomes. Children's participation is integral to the model of Children's Trusts. The National Service Framework (NSF) for Children, Young People and Maternity Services is a major part of the *Change for Children* programme. The participation of children is also important within the children's NSF as it aims to give children, young people and their parents increased information, power and choice, and seeks to involve them in service planning. Of course, although participation in research, planning or service evaluation is a laudable aim, in practice it can be hard to get children and young people to participate, and the youngest, most vulnerable and most socially excluded groups are the least likely to do so.

6.4 Promoting the health of children and young people

Promoting the health of children and young people covers many dimensions concerning both their physical and mental health. These activities range from the provision of pre-conceptual care and the promotion of healthy lifestyles, to the prevention of crime and antisocial behaviours, among others. The remaining sections of this chapter focus on three specific issues which will enable you to consider a range of contemporary concerns: childhood injury prevention, promoting positive mental health in schools and promoting the sexual health of children and young people.

6.4.1 Childhood injury prevention

Unintentional injury poses one of the biggest threats to life for children and young people in the UK. It is the leading cause of death and a major source of illness and disability. In 2003, injury accounted for 369 deaths among those aged under sixteen years in England and Wales (ONS, 2004b). In Scotland, thirty-one children died from unintentional injuries in 2003 (ISD Scotland, 2004a), and in Northern Ireland, eight children died from unintentional injuries in the same year (NISRA, 2003).

The term 'unintentional injury' is now more commonly used than the term 'accident' because accidents are seen to be somewhat unpredictable and unavoidable, whereas injury is seen as predictable and preventable. However, injury is not equally distributed: the poorest children are more likely to be injured, more likely to be seriously injured and more likely to be taken to hospital for treatment. For example, in Scotland, the rate of emergency admission following injury in a road traffic crash is almost double for children living in the most deprived areas (ISD Scotland, 2004b). There are also gender differences, with boys being almost twice as likely to be injured than girls, in all four countries of the UK.

Injury prevention has been recognised as a key target area within Sure Start, with a target of reducing by 10 per cent the number of children, aged 0–4 living in Sure Start local programme areas and Children's Centre areas, who are admitted to hospital as an emergency (Sure Start, 2006) (see Chapter 4 for a discussion of Sure Start Children's Centres). In recent years, fatal deaths from childhood injuries have begun to decrease and many initiatives are now underway with the aim of reducing further the number of unintended injuries. A Sure Start initiative in Berwick, a rural borough in England, focusing on injury prevention in the home is summarised in Box 6.3. This is an interesting initiative which places parents at the centre of its provision for very young children.

> ## Box 6.3 Sure Start in Berwick borough: safe steps in the home
>
> Summary of provision:
>
> - low-cost safety equipment available to all carers of children, managed by a parent worker
> - a six-week home safety course developed by a local parent
> - first aid and resuscitation sessions offered with certificate
> - car seat checks
> - interactive safety sessions running at local baby groups across the borough.
>
> (Adapted from Berwick Borough, 2006)

Thinking point what practical or ethical dilemmas do such initiatives raise?

Sure Start and other similar initiatives are valuable, but they raise practical and ethical dilemmas for practice. Although resources are made available to the most socially deprived areas, children and families living outside these areas – who might also benefit from these resources – do not have access to them. Arguably, this is unfair and can also raise dilemmas for practitioners who are mindful of promoting social justice.

In general, health protection and injury prevention in childhood takes one of two forms. The first type *prevents hazardous events from occurring*; for example, child-resistant packaging can prevent a child from accidentally ingesting medication or a toxic household substance. The second type *prevents injury once a hazardous event has taken place*; for example, the use of a bicycle helmet can prevent head injury when a crash occurs. Sleet et al. (2003) suggest that legislation and regulation play an important role in preventing childhood injuries and that they have been extremely successful. However, Licence (2004) argues that a broader approach is needed which requires intervention across the five areas set out in the Ottawa Charter for Health Promotion (WHO, 1986). These five areas were set out in Box 1.5 in Chapter 1. To remind you about them, they are listed again briefly in Box 6.4 below.

Box 6.4 Injury prevention and the Ottawa Charter

- **Healthy child public health policy**

  For example, through controls on the advertising and availability of health-damaging products.

- **A healthy environment**

  For example, ensuring that the environment encourages and facilitates a physically active lifestyle.

- **Strong community action**

  For example, to harness the resources of lay people to provide support for parents and to lobby for change.

- **Development of personal skills**

  For example, to develop positive parenting skills.

- **Reorientation of health services**

  For example, by addressing health promotion needs in collaboration with other agencies, or within other settings.

  (Adapted from WHO, 1986)

Thinking point can you think of other examples of interventions to prevent childhood injuries under each of the areas set out by the Ottawa Charter?

Other examples might include road traffic awareness interventions, or the building of safe play areas. It is often difficult to assess whether intervention strategies to prevent childhood injury actually work. Public health promotion in childhood focuses on both short- and long-term impact, although few studies report anything other than short-term outcomes (Licence, 2004). A review of injury intervention initiatives funded by the Health Development Agency (Towner et al., 2005) highlighted the complexity of evaluation in this field, but suggested that interventions should focus on universal as well as targeted approaches. The same review also recommended further qualitative research, arguing that parents and children often had specialised local knowledge of issues relating to risk, safety and danger.

6.4.2 Promoting positive mental health in schools

The mental health of children and young people has come under increasing scrutiny in the last few years. Bullying has received particular attention and is now recognised to cause both short- and long-term damage to physical and mental health (Hill and Tisdall, 1997). Those who are bullied are more likely to suffer from a poor self-image and are more likely to have, or develop, a mental health problem. In some instances, bullying has also been identified as a contributory factor in cases of suicide, more common in males than females. Victims of bullying are also more likely to find it difficult to concentrate in school or may absent themselves. It is worth noting that, although bullying is most certainly detrimental to health, not all bullying behaviours are equally damaging (Hoel et al., 2004).

Promoting health within a school context has become an important focus for promoting positive mental health among children and young people. Although, as Simpson and Freeman (2004, p. 341) have argued, health promotion in schools often adopts 'a naïve and narrow approach that fails to negotiate the gap between policy and practice, and the chasm between normative claims to knowledge and genuine understanding'. Drawing on the work of the European Network of Health Promoting Schools, in 1995 the WHO's Global School Health Initiative was launched to promote health through schools. Health promoting schools aim to promote health by focusing on three domains of activity:

1   the formal health curriculum

2   the school environment

3   school/community interactions.

As discussed in Chapters 3 and 4, multidisciplinary public health occurs in a range of settings, and a settings approach seeks to enable different social environments to maximise their health promoting potential. This whole-school approach requires traditional health education to be set within a wider framework which supports attitudes and practices that are conducive to good health, thus promoting positive health through change. The National Healthy Schools Programme in England, the Health Promoting Schools Initiative in Northern Ireland, the Welsh Network of Healthy School Schemes, and the Scottish Health Promoting Schools Unit, all work within the three domains outlined above.

Since 1999, schools have been required to operate an anti-bullying policy and many have adopted a whole-school approach. One such initiative is Schoolwatch, a pupil-organised initiative developed by South Wales Police, now operating in over 100 primary schools in South Wales. The initiative allows pupils to improve their environment by taking responsibility for their behaviour and their actions through the implementation of activities such as a 'bully box' in which to report incidents, playground patrols, a friendship garden, conservation areas and community projects. Compared with non-participants, Schoolwatch schools have reported declining incidents of bullying and that pupils are feeling happier and more valued (Warton and Barry, 1999). There are many other methods of managing bullying in schools; for example, assertiveness training, mediation and befriending.

Research suggests that homophobia can form an important part of bullying behaviour, although it often goes unrecognised. In an English study, Adams et al. (2004) noted that, whereas equal opportunities policies mentioned sexual orientation, anti-bullying policies rarely specified homophobic behaviour as a cause for concern. Another British study highlighted that teachers were aware of homophobic bullying but were confused, unable or unwilling to address the needs of lesbian and gay pupils (Warwick et al., 2001).

More recently, concerns have been expressed about the bullying of refugee children. In Scotland, the Anti Bullying Network asked teachers about bullying incidents involving refugee children, and they found that some problems occurred repeatedly (see Box 6.5).

Box 6.5 Bullying and refugee children in Scotland

- Refugee children may be mistrustful of authority and reluctant to report bullying.

- Some children are traumatised when they arrive.

- Children whose countries of origin have been at war sometimes display enmity towards each other.

- Learning, emotional, social or other problems may go unrecognised for some time because children arrive without records.

- Many refugee children have been used to a rigid, traditional system of discipline and may find it difficult to adapt to a more relaxed school ethos.

- Some cultural practices are different. One teacher said that he had to reprimand some older refugee boys (and some Scottish boys) because of their attitudes towards their female peers.

- Refugee parents need to be helped to understand that they have a role in working with teachers and pupils to tackle racism and bullying.

(Adapted from Anti-Bullying Network, undated)

Aside from initiatives that deal with bullying, many schools have introduced initiatives focusing on other aspects of mental health. The concept of 'emotional literacy', although controversial, also has some contemporary currency. It refers to the understanding and management of both 'caught' and 'taught' emotional skills. One school in Edinburgh has implemented an emotional literacy programme which encourages children to recognise their feelings and seeks to develop their emotional vocabulary (see Box 6.6).

Box 6.6 Wellbeing and emotion at Forthview Primary School, Scotland

- A 'feeling book' is available for children to write about how they feel. It is read out at a candlelit, quiet assembly.

- The Quiet Room, a snug, sensory space, is available to staff, parents and pupils to engage in personal and group reflection.

- Partnership with parents is encouraged in a range of ways; for example, by encouraging parents into school to play with children at the start of the day.

(Adapted from Scottish Parent Teacher Council, 2004)

Many theories have been put forward to explain children's emotional health, including those focusing on the role of schooling, the role of the home and the role of social groups. Most recently, some of these theories have been challenged by an interest in behavioural genetics as well as by theories of resilience which draw on a salutogenic approach. Buchanan (2000) suggests that the emotional health of children and young people is influenced by four intersecting domains which form an interacting ecological framework: the 'person', the 'family', 'the school/community' and the 'wider environment'.

6.4.3 Promoting the sexual health of children and young people

Good sexual health is widely acknowledged to be an important aspect of overall health (DoH, 2001). Although sexual rights are not stated in law, as a result of the United Nations Convention on the Rights of the Child (UNCRC) (UN, 1989) the human rights agenda has had a significant impact on access to information, education and sexual health services. The World Health Organization also states that all persons should have the right to the highest attainable standard of health in relation to sexuality, including access to sexual and reproductive healthcare services, information and education (WHO, 2004b).

The consequences of poor sexual health are various. They can be dangerous and irreversible and young people are thought to be at particular risk, especially those who are already experiencing social exclusion. Some of these consequences include chlamydia, HIV and unintended pregnancy, as well as the psychological consequences of sexual coercion and abuse (DoH, 2001).

Until relatively recently, sexual health was defined in relation to reproductive health. However, attention is now given to the overall promotion of sexual wellbeing as an area in its own right (WHO, 2004b). In the UK, sexual health is of increasing concern and this has been reflected through policy development across all four countries. Although the focus is now moving from a narrowly defined preventative approach to a social model of health which recognises the role of poverty and social exclusion, considerably more attention has been paid to disease prevention (of chlamydia, for example) and to the prevention of teenage pregnancy. The Social Exclusion Unit's Teenage Pregnancy Report (Social Exclusion Unit, 1999) showed that the UK has one of the highest rates of teenage pregnancy in western Europe: three times as high as France, and six times as high as the Netherlands. A recent update has shown that rates are still high, but are now in decline (Teenage Pregnancy Unit, 2005). The National Teenage Pregnancy Strategy sets out to halve the teenage pregnancy rate in England by 2010, and to increase the participation of teenage mothers in education, training or work by 60 per cent by the same date. Although it has been widely criticised, it has been commended for adopting an inclusive approach; for example, considerable work has been carried out on the needs of looked after children (children in care) and care leavers. Research suggests that young people who are looked after often have greater need for sexual health promotion than their peers, but often receive less attention (Corlyon, 2004). Box 6.7 outlines one initiative focusing on the sexual health needs of young people in residential and foster care.

Box 6.7 'X-perience' Surrey County Council

The first 'X-perience' Project accessed young people in residential care, while 'X-perience 2 and 3' contacted those in foster care. In all three programmes, young people between the ages of 14 and 16 were sent a letter inviting them to a residential course and asked to return an application form. Their carers/Residential Social Workers were informed about the programme, although it was preferred if young people referred themselves and attended because they wanted to. Two weeks prior to the residential course, the young people were invited to a planning evening where they were asked which health topics they would like to work on during the course – enabling young people to participate in their own health education. Sexual health was requested as a topic.

The residential course ran over 2 nights with almost two full days of workshops. The workshops were run by health promotion specialists, although other professionals were invited to contribute if the young people requested a topic in which they did not specialise. The workshops involved the young people as much as possible through mediums such as drama and art.

Training, focusing on the health of young people, was also offered to Residential Social Workers and foster carers – to complement the work of the residential programme and enable carers to offer young people advice and support after the course ...

The service was developed in response to a 'gap' in the provision of health advice and support for looked after children. The young people who attended the courses suggested that they had never been offered this type of service before, especially those in foster care. The programme received positive feedback from all involved. It gave young people the chance not only to learn about their health, but also to network with other young people in similar situations.

The success of the course is attributed to the fact that it allowed the young people to define what should be involved; meeting their actual needs rather than their perceived needs. Enabling them to choose the content also ensured that they were interested in the material delivered.

(Teenage Pregnancy Unit, 2003, pp. 5–6)

Culture and the regulation of sexuality

Traditionally, children's sexual identities have either been denied or subject to considerable regulation and surveillance. It is an area of identity surrounded by cultural taboos in which children are 'innocent' beings who must be protected from dangerous others. Discourses of childhood and sexuality have silenced children's voices and assumed a heterosexual homogeneity which does not exist in practice. For lesbian and gay young people these cultural taboos can be particularly problematic. Organisations and campaigns, such as Education for All (Stonewall, 2006), work to challenge homophobia in schools.

The regulation of sexuality also poses particular difficulties for disabled children and young people who are already both infantilised and asexualised (Douglas-Scott, 2004). As Shakespeare et al. (1996) have argued, disabled people are expected neither to reproduce nor be reproduced. Disabled sexual identity is often framed within discourses of risk and the need for protection from abuse. Although disabled children, especially those who have learning disabilities, are at a higher risk of physical and sexual abuse (Cambridge, 1999), such discourses do little to empower disabled children and young people to explore and express their sexual identities.

Sex and sexual health are also gendered experiences. For example, girls and young women are thought to learn about sex primarily in terms of risk and danger, to learn that people will make judgements about their sexual behaviour, and often to learn to absorb and act out the images and behaviours that boys and young men expect of them. On the other hand, boys and young men generally learn that 'being a man' means taking risks, and that masculinity can mean creating the impression that they are always ready for sex; they may also learn to think about sex and relationships only in terms of their own needs (HEA, 1998).

Thinking point   to what extent do you believe that these gendered stereotypes still exist?

According to Wilton (1994), these gendered stereotypes are not simply of academic interest but, within the context of sexual health and HIV/AIDS in particular, are literally issues of life and death. Studies carried out in Manchester and London (Holland et al., 1998), with young people aged between sixteen and twenty-one, highlighted that young women and young men experience sex and relationships very differently. For example, young women can find negotiating safe sex within the confines of a 'steady' heterosexual relationship difficult. One young woman said:

> Tony doesn't really like using them [condoms]. That used to annoy me, the fact that he knew we were going out and that we would probably end up [having sex without a condom].
>
> (Holland et al., 1998, p. 137)

Young men, on the other hand, feel that they have more freedom and that the double standards of sex and morality do not apply to them. For example, one young man said:

> If blokes do it they're studs; if women do it they're slags.
>
> (Holland et al., 1998, p. 179)

In what they term 'the male in the head', Holland et al. (1998) suggest that, although young people are able to subvert, resist and ignore gendered sexual stereotypes, masculine meanings and male sexual 'desires' are still privileged over those of girls and young women.

Sex education at school and in the home

Traditionally, the provision of information about sex and relationships was regarded as the domain of the home (and, to a lesser extent, the Church). However, by the 1940s, schools began to take increasing responsibility for sex education, partly in acknowledgement of the fact that parents were not properly equipped to provide children with the necessary information about sexual health (Simpson and Freeman, 2004). By the 1980s, school-based sex education was well established within the curriculum, though not without professional, parental and political concerns.

In spite of these concerns, schools are thought to be well placed to provide sex and relationships education (SRE). This is because, first, teachers are already well trained to facilitate learning, and the majority of teachers, parents, children and young people support the role of schools in delivering sex education; second, SRE enables students to develop a range of transferable skills that can be used in other areas of life and which, within a school setting, can be taught in such a manner as is appropriate to the age and stage of pupil development; and, last, because most children and young people attend school, schools are well placed to provide SRE (Young, 2004).

Of course, some children and young people will find the school setting an inappropriate place for SRE and may find teachers too authoritarian. For example, a national survey of sexual behaviour and lifestyles in Northern Ireland revealed that young people found sex education moralistic and value driven, with little room for mature, constructive or respectful debate (Rolston et al., 2005). Teachers may also lack the skills or knowledge needed to promote positive sexual health effectively. In some schools SRE is delivered by children themselves or, more commonly, by outside agencies. In the randomised intervention study on peer-led SRE – known as the RIPPLE study – thirteen- and fourteen-year-olds were given lessons by sixteen- and seventeen-year-old school students. These lessons took place in twenty-nine schools in central and southern England. There appear to have been some positive results, in that students reported that they liked the peer-led classes more and that they thought the peer educators had more relevant experience and respect, had similar values to themselves, used familiar language, were less moralistic about the subject than the teachers, and made their sessions more fun. However, there were mixed results and some schools refused to participate at all (Stephenson et al., 2004).

Thinking point think back to your own experiences of sex education. What could your school have done better?

Within the context of the National Healthy Schools Standard (DfES, 1999) (in England), and now in relation to the five outcomes of *Every Child Matters* (DfES, 2004b), schools provide SRE within the broader remit of personal, social and health education (PSHE). However – over and above what is provided within the national curriculum – this provision is non-statutory in primary schools and, given other curricular pressures, SRE continues to be a low priority. Even in secondary schools, where the provision of SRE is a statutory requirement, an OFSTED (2005) report found that some schools do not offer PSHE in any form. The politics of sexual health also influences the way in which SRE is delivered and can confuse teachers about how best to promote good sexual health in schools.

Box 6.8 gives an extract from an article published in the *Guardian* newspaper, in which Kate Hilpern summarises some of the challenges faced by parents today.

Box 6.8 Let's talk about sex, baby

Three sad facts about sex education in Britain: one, too many of our young people are told too little, too late and what they are told is too biological; two, young people don't want to hear about sex from peers or teachers – they want their parents to tell them; and three, parents are the last people to talk to them about it, particularly sons. Why is it that otherwise conscientious parents are failing their children in this way?

'I didn't want to acknowledge that Greg, who's 15, wasn't a child any more,' says Mandy Ashton, 39. 'And anyway, I don't know anything about boys and puberty. I'm a single mother with no brothers. When Greg asked me about changes to his genitalia, I didn't know how to answer him. I was so mortified that I asked him not to mention it again.'

According to Simon Blake, director of the Sex Education Forum, more than 50% of British parents would like guidance on how to talk to their kids about sex but don't know where to get it. As a result, 10% of girls start menstruating before being told anything about it, young homosexuals rarely get any support, and boys often feel they get the wink, wink, nudge, nudge approach and learn nothing. So what help is out there for parents such as Mandy Ashton, who simply don't know where to start?

The short answer is, not much ...

[...]

Dr Miriam Stoppard, author of several books on sex education, believes the biggest mistake 'suddenly clued-up parents' make is going too abruptly into discussions of sex. 'The only way sex education within the family really works is to talk about it from the moment the child is born,' she says. 'Equally important is picking the right time – meaning their "ready time" not yours.'

> Kerry McCall, a 40-year-old mother of five, knows exactly what she means. Unlike Mandy Ashton, McCall does talk to her kids about sex but they don't always listen. 'I was telling the 11-year-old some stuff the other day that I'd prepared carefully, and he suddenly asked if I'd got a "wiggly tuft". I was horrified, but then I realised he wasn't listening and was talking about Pokémon.'
>
> (Hilpern, 2000)

An increasing number of sexual health initiatives are being developed, aimed at supporting parents. For example, in Scotland, Healthy Respect (Scottish Executive, 2005) is a government-funded long-term initiative to improve the sexual health of young people; part of this initiative includes working with parents to develop age-specific materials. Speakeasy, a community development project first developed in Northern Ireland by the Family Planning Association, is another initiative involving parents (see Box 6.9). It is based on the rights of children and young people to have information and support regarding their sexuality, and on an acceptance that learning about sexuality, like learning in general, is a lifelong process. Speakeasy is now running in Northern Ireland and England.

Box 6.9 Speakeasy project

Parents are encouraged to provide positive sex education in the home and take on the role of sex educator by taking six to eight weekly workshops focusing on:

- skills relating to talking to children about sex

- knowledge of sexual health

- personal attitudes and values towards sex education.

A very positive external evaluation of the project highlighted:

- improved relationships between parent and child

- improved relationships with partner

- enhanced individual confidence around parenting

- increased level of personal knowledge

- community capacity building.

(Adapted from Family Planning Association, 2006)

Public health has adopted a predominantly preventative approach to sexual health, but empowering children and young people to expect and develop positive sexual relationships should also be a fundamental part of multidisciplinary public health. The provision of improved sex education is an important aim and requires collaboration between different agencies, organisations and individuals. However, sex education can only go so far in promoting positive sexual health unless children and young people have appropriate life skills. Avert, an international HIV- and AIDS-based non-governmental organisation (NGO), argues that sex education should work to develop the general life skills that enable children and young people to enjoy positive sexual health (Avert, 2006).

Conclusion

Promoting the health of children and young people is a complex task involving a wide range of settings and individuals. Although the views of children and young people have sometimes been marginalised, or ignored, there is an increasing impetus at all levels to ensure that children's voices are heard. Research suggests that the majority of children are able to express their views on matters relating to health and illness, and that different research methods may be appropriate for children and young people of diverse ages.

This chapter has focused on just three specific public health issues, but there are many others. Although the young are always perceived to be the healthiest people in society, there are considerable differences in their health, according to gender, age, ethnicity and sexuality. Good health is not equally distributed among children and young people, but tackling inequality requires a multidisciplinary approach, including health protection, prevention, education and promotion, as well as the development of capacity and skills in individuals and communities. There are many initiatives that seek to promote the health of children and young people. By involving them and seeking to understand issues of diversity and the politics of children's health – and by drawing on theoretical models and approaches to practice – these initiatives are more likely to achieve their aims.

References

Adams, N., Cox, T. and Dunstan, L. (2004) '"I am the hate that dare not speak its name": dealing with homophobia in secondary schools', *Educational Psychology in Practice*, vol. 20, no. 3, pp. 259–69.

Anti-Bullying Network (undated) *Welcoming Newcomers! Newsletter*, Edinburgh, Anti-Bullying Network [online], http://www.antibullying.net/newcomers1.htm (Accessed 28 April 2006).

Ariès, P. (1962) *Centuries of Childhood*, London, Jonathan Cape.

Avert (2006) http://www.avert.org/ (Accessed 21 August 2006).

Backett-Milburn, K. and Harden, J. (2004) 'How children and their families construct and negotiate risk, safety and danger', *Childhood*, vol. 11, no. 4, pp. 429–7.

Barker, D.J.P. (1989) 'Growth in utero, blood pressure in childhood and adult life, and mortality from cardiovascular disease', *British Medical Journal*, vol. 298, pp. 564–67.

Bashford, J., Kaur, J., Winters, M., Williams, R. and Patel, K. (2002) 'What are the mental health needs of Bradford's Pakistani Muslim children and young people and how can they be addressed?', *Healthy Minds: A Child & Adolescent Mental Health Research Project*, Lancaster, Centre for Ethnicity and Health, University of Lancaster; also available online at: http://www.uclan.ac.uk/facs/health/ethnicity/reports/healthyminds.htm (Accessed 27 October 2006).

Beck, U. (1992) *Risk Society: Towards a New Modernity*, London, Sage.

Berwick Borough (2006) *Safe Steps* [online], http://www.safesteps.co.uk/home/index.htm (Accessed 21 August 2006).

Bourdieu, P. (1989) *Distinction*, London, Routledge.

Buchanan, A. (2000) 'Present issues and concerns' in Buchanan, A. and Hudson, B. (eds) *Promoting Children's Emotional Well-Being*, Oxford, Oxford University Press.

Burtney, E. and Duffy, M. (eds) (2004) *Young People and Sexual Health: Individual, Social and Policy Contexts*, Basingstoke, Palgrave Macmillan.

Cambridge, P. (1999) 'The first hit: a case study of the physical abuse of people with learning disabilities and challenging behaviours in a residential service', *Disability and Society*, vol. 14, no. 3, pp. 285–308.

Corlyon, J. (2004) 'Sex, pregnancy and parenthood for young people who are looked after by local authorities' in Burtney and Duffy (eds) (2004).

Department for Education and Skills (DfES) (1999) *National Healthy Schools Standard* [online], http://www.standards.dfes.gov.uk/sie/si/SfCC/goodpractice/nhss/ (Accessed 21 August 2006).

Department for Education and Skills (DfES) (2003) *Every Child Matters*, Cm 5860, Norwich, The Stationery Office.

Department for Education and Skills (DfES) (2004a) *Every Child Matters: Next Steps*, Norwich, The Stationery Office.

Department for Education and Skills (DfES) (2004b) *Every Child Matters: Change for Children*, Norwich, The Stationery Office.

Department of Health (DoH) (2001) *The National Strategy for Sexual Health and HIV*, London, Department of Health.

Department of Health (DoH) (2003) *5 A DAY: Just Eat More (fruit & veg)*, London, Department of Health.

Douglas-Scott, S. (2004) 'Sexuality and learning disability' in Burtney and Duffy (eds) (2004).

Earle, S. (2003) 'Is breast best? Breastfeeding, motherhood and identity' in Earle, S. and Letherby, G. (eds) *Gender, Identity and Reproduction: Social Perspectives*, London, Palgrave Macmillan.

Family Planning Association (2006) http://www.fpa.org.uk/about/projects/index.htm (Accessed 21 August 2006).

Graham, H. and Power, C. (2004) 'Childhood disadvantage and health inequalities: a framework for policy based on lifecourse research', *Child: Care, Health and Development*, vol. 30, no. 6, pp. 671–8.

Grover, S. (2004) 'Why won't they listen to us? On giving power and voice to children participating in social research', *Childhood*, vol. 1, no. 1, pp. 81–93.

Health Education Authority (HEA) (1998) *The Implications of Research into Young People, Sex, Sexuality and Relationships*, London, Health Education Authority.

Hill, M. and Tisdall, K. (1997) *Children and Society*, London, Longman.

Hilpern, K. (2000) 'Let's talk about sex, baby', *Guardian*, 28 June [online], http://education.guardian.co.uk/parents/story/0,,337476,00.html (Accessed 28 April 2006).

Hoel, H., Faragher, B. and Cooper, C.L. (2004) 'Bullying is detrimental to health, but all bullying behaviours are not necessarily equally damaging', *British Journal of Guidance and Counselling*, vol. 32, no. 3, pp. 367–87.

Holland, J., Ramazanoglu, C., Sharpe, S. and Thomson, R. (1998) *The Male in the Head: Young People, Heterosexuality and Power*, London, The Tufnell Press.

Hollos, M. (2002) 'The cultural construction of childhood: changing concepts among the Pare of northern Tanzania', *Childhood*, vol. 9, no. 2, pp. 167–89.

Inchley, J., Todd, J., Bryce, C. and Currie, C. (2001) 'Dietary trends among Scottish schoolchildren in the 1990s', *Journal of Human Nutrition and Dietetics*, vol. 14, no. 3, pp. 207–16.

ISD Scotland (2004a) *Unintentional Injuries: Injuries by Age Group and Sex* [online], http://www.isdscotland.org/isd/info3.jsp?pContentID=3066&p_applic=CCC&p_service=Content.show& (Accessed 28 April 2006).

ISD Scotland (2004b) *Unintentional Injuries: Injuries in Children – Road Traffic Accidents (RTAs) by Deprivation* [online], http://www.isdscotland.org/isd/info3.jsp?pContentID=3068&p_applic=CCC&p_service=Content.show& (Accessed 28 April 2006).

James, A. and James, A.L. (2004) *Constructing Childhood: Theory, Policy and Social Practice*, London, Palgrave Macmillan.

James, A. and Prout, A. (eds) (1997) *Constructing and Reconstructing Childhood: Contemporary Issues in the Sociological Study of Childhood* (2nd edn), London, Falmer.

Licence, K. (2004) 'Promoting and protecting the health of children and young people', *Child: Care, Health and Development*, vol. 30, no. 6, pp. 623–35.

Macfarlane, A., Stafford, M. and Moser, K. (2004) 'Social inequalities', Chapter 8 in Office for National Statistics, *The Health of Children and Young People*, London, Office for National Statistics [online], http://www.statistics.gov.uk/children/downloads/inequalities.pdf (Accessed 28April 2006).

Mason, J. (2005) 'Child protection policy and the construction of childhood' in Mason, J. and Fattore, T. (eds) *Children Taken Seriously in Theory, Policy and Practice*, London, Jessica Kingsley.

Mayall, B. (1996) *Children, Health and the Social Order*, Buckingham, Open University Press.

Northern Ireland Statistics and Research Agency (NISRA) (2003) *The Registrar General's Annual Report for Northern Ireland 2003*, Belfast, Northern Ireland Statistics and Research Agency.

O'Brien, P. (2006) *How Does Death Affect Children?* [online], http://childrens-research-centre.open.ac.uk/research-doc/ How_does_death_affect_children.doc (Accessed 20 August 2006).

Office for National Statistics (ONS) (2004a) *Focus on Social Inequalities* (ed. P. Babb, J. Martin and P. Haezewindt), London, The Stationery Office [online], [http://www.statistics.gov.uk/downloads/theme_compendia/fosi2004/ SocialInequalities_full.pdf (Accessed 28 April 2006).

Office for National Statistics (ONS) (2004b) *DH3 – Mortality Statistics – Childhood, Infant and Perinatal Deaths 2003*, London, The Stationery Office.

OFSTED (2005) *Personal, Social and Health Education in Secondary Schools*, London, Department for Education and Skills [online], http://www.statistics.gov.uk/downloads/theme_health/Dh3_2003/DH3no36.pdf (Accessed 28 April 2006).

Plumb, J.H. (1975) 'The new world of children in eighteenth-century England', *Past and Present*, vol. 67, no. 1, pp. 64–95.

Rebok, G., Riley, A., Forrest, C., Starfield, B., Green, B., Robertson, J. and Tambor, E. (2001) 'Elementary school-aged children's reports of their health: a cognitive interviewing study', *Quality of Life Research*, vol. 10, no. 1, pp. 59–70.

Rolston, B., Schubotz, D. and Simpson, A. (2005) 'Sex education in Northern Ireland schools: a critical evaluation', *Journal of Sex Education*, vol. 5, no. 2, pp. 217–34.

Rugkåsa, J., Kennedy, O., Barton, M., Abaunza, P.S., Treacy, M.P. and Knox, B. (2001) 'Smoking and symbolism: children, communication and cigarettes', *Health Education Research*, vol. 16, no. 2, pp. 131–42.

Schmidt, L.R. and Fröhling, H. (2000) 'Lay concepts of health and illness from a developmental perspective', *Psychology and Health*, vol. 15, pp. 229–38.

Scottish Executive (2005) *External Evaluation of Healthy Respect, A National Health Demonstration Project: Final Summary Report* [online], http://www.scotland.gov.uk/Publications/2005/03/20909/55354/ (Accessed 21 August 2006).

Scottish Parent Teacher Council (2004) *Success Stories III: An Illustration of the Rich Diversity of Classroom and School Practice in Scotland*, Edinburgh, Scottish Parent Teacher Council.

Shakespeare, T., Gillespie-Sells, K. and Davies, D. (1996) *The Sexual Politics of Disability: Untold Desires*, London, Cassell.

Simpson, K. and Freeman, R. (2004) 'Critical health promotion and education – a new research challenge', *Health Education Research: Theory and Practice*, vol. 19, no. 3, pp. 340–8.

Sleet, D.A., Schieber, R.A. and Gilchrist, J. (2003) 'Health promotion policy and politics: lessons for childhood injury prevention', *Health Promotion Practice,* vol. 4, no 2, pp. 103–8.

Social Exclusion Unit (1999) *Teenage Pregnancy*, London, The Stationery Office.

Stephenson, J., Strange, V., Forrest, S., Oakley, A., Copas, A., Allen, E., Babiker, A., Black, S., Ali, M., Monteiro, H. and Johnson, A. (2004) 'Pupil-led sex education in England (RIPPLE study): cluster-randomised intervention trial', *The Lancet*, vol. 364, no. 9431, pp. 338–46.

Stonewall (2006) http://www.stonewall.org.uk/eduation_for_all/ (Accessed 21 August 2006).

Sure Start (2006) *Accidents and Injuries: Target* [online], http://www.surestart.gov.uk/surestartservices/healthrelated/healthandfamilysupport/accidentsandinjuries/target/ (Accessed 21 August 2006).

Teenage Pregnancy Unit (2003) *Teenage Pregnancy and Looked After Children/Care Leavers: Examples of Innovative Practice*, London, Department for Education and Skills.

Teenage Pregnancy Unit (2005) *Teenage Pregnancy Strategy Evaluation*, London, Department for Education and Skills.

Towner, E., Dowswell, T., Errington, G., Burkes, M. and Towner, J. (2005) *Injuries in Children Aged 0–15 years and Inequalities*, London, Health Development Agency.

United Nations (UN) (1989) *Convention on the Rights of the Child*, UN General Assembly Document A/RES/44/25, United Nations.

Vangen, S., Stoltenberg, C., Skjaerven, R., Magnus, P., Harris, J.R. and Stray-Pedersen, B. (2002) 'The heavier the better? Birthweight and perinatal mortality in different ethnic groups', *International Journal of Epidemiology*, vol. 31, no. 3, pp. 654–60.

Viner, R. and Macfarlane, A. (2005) 'ABC of adolescence: health promotion', *British Medical Journal*, vol. 330, pp. 527–9.

Warton, K. and Barry, S. (1999) *Schoolwatch: An Evaluation*, London, Home Office, Research, Development and Statistics Directorate.

Warwick, I., Aggleton, P. and Douglas, N. (2001) 'Playing it safe: addressing the emotional and physical health of lesbian and gay pupils in the UK', *Journal of Adolescence*, vol. 24, no. 1, pp. 129–40.

Wilton, T. (1994) 'Silences, absences and fragmentation' in Doyal, L., Naidoo, J. and Wilton, T. (eds) *AIDS: Setting a Feminist Agenda*, London, Taylor & Francis.

World Health Organization (WHO) (1986) *Ottawa Charter for Health Promotion*, Geneva, World Health Organization.

World Health Organization (WHO) (2001) *The Optimal Duration of Exclusive Breastfeeding: Results of a WHO Systematic Review*, Geneva, World Health Organization.

World Health Organization (WHO) (2004a) *Inheriting the World: The Atlas of Children's Health and the Environment*, Geneva, World Health Organization.

World Health Organization (WHO) (2004b) *Progress in Reproductive Health Research*, No. 67, Geneva, World Health Organization.

Wright, J. (2006) *The Exercise Questionnaire* [online], http://childrens-research-centre.open.ac.uk/research-doc/The_Exercise_q_ames_Wright.doc (Accessed 20 August 2006).

Young Carers' Initiative (2006) *Professionals: Social Services* [online], http://www.youngcarer.com/showPage.php?file=1111442025.htm (Accessed 20 August 2006).

Young, I. (2004) 'Exploring the role of schools in sexual health promotion' in Burtney and Duffy (eds) (2004).

Part II
Researching multidisciplinary public health

Modern multidisciplinary public health is influenced, both implicitly and explicitly, by personal and social values. Public health practice is also underpinned by ethical principles which inform both action and inaction. Moreover, contemporary practice is increasingly influenced, and underpinned, by research in health and public health promotion. Part II of this book provides a systematic analysis of the methodology and some of the methods used in researching health, as well as an analysis of the planning, evaluation and dissemination of public health promotion initiatives.

Drawing on some of the arguments discussed in Part I, Chapter 7, 'Researching health', explores how the research process is understood within lay, biomedical and social scientific discourses. In doing so, this chapter considers how research can be evaluated and how it might inform public health promotion. Chapter 8, 'Studying the population's health', focuses on key quantitative methods of inquiry as ways of investigating the health of groups within the population. The use of demography and epidemiology in promoting public health are explored, including survey research, questionnaire design and use, and the preparation and use of quantitative data. This is followed by a critical analysis of quantitative methods as applied to health issues and public health promotion.

Chapter 9, 'Qualitative research towards public health', explores the potential for qualitative methods in researching health, and their impact on public health promotion. Methods discussed include semi-structured interviewing, focus groups and participant and non-participant observation. Research also underpins the planning of public health promotion, which is the focus of the following chapter. Chapter 10, 'Using research to plan multidisciplinary public health interventions', examines how research evidence is used in planning interventions and critically analyses the use of planning models. In Chapter 11, 'Evaluating public health interventions', the focus is on the evaluation of public health initiatives. Here, the chapter provides a discussion of the politics of evidence-based public health promotion, critically discussing the role of both qualitative and quantitative methods. Chapter 11 also discusses the reporting and dissemination of evaluation findings.

The final chapter in Part II and in the book – Chapter 12, 'Understanding obesity' – draws together the material presented in Part II, using the example of obesity. The chapter examines definitions of obesity and critically reflects on the construction of obesity as a global public health problem. It also explores how research on obesity is gathered and interpreted and how interventions to prevent obesity and promote public health can be planned and evaluated.

Chapter 7

Researching health

Clive Pearson, Judy Thomas and Cathy Lloyd

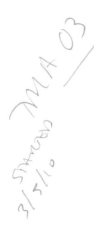

Introduction

Health research takes place in many different settings and is carried out by a wide range of people. Some have professional expertise in research, others have varying degrees of research experience, and some have none. Research does not occur in a vacuum, but is influenced by the political agenda of the time and by personal and professional preferences and perspectives, and is informed by different bodies of knowledge. How these bodies of knowledge inform the research process is one of the considerations of this chapter. There are countless sources of information about health available to us – books, magazines, television, radio, the internet and also each other. They all contain vast amounts of information on many different health-related topics, but not all knowledge is considered equally valid, and not all could be said to be health promoting. So, what counts as knowledge about health and how does this translate into public health research?

This chapter considers the following questions. What is the status of different kinds of knowledge about how to promote public health? How is knowledge gathered? And how are the methods used to do so justified? These questions are important because the answers provided inform public health practice in profound ways. What is known about promoting public health and how it is researched should be at the very heart of effective practice, no matter the level or setting in which practice takes place.

The chapter is in two parts. The first is concerned with the knowledge base of research. Section 7.1 considers different bodies of knowledge and leads into Section 7.2 which considers the relationship of these to researching health. Three different types of knowledge are considered: lay, biomedical and, finally, social science knowledge. Section 7.3 considers the role of research in promoting public health and looks specifically at the role of both lay people and professionals in this process. The second part of this chapter takes a more practical approach and considers how to search for (Section 7.4) and critically evaluate (Section 7.5) different types of knowledge and information relevant to promoting public health. The final section (Section 7.6) moves on to consider the design of research, and helps you to think about the different methods available for use in doing research.

7.1 Bodies of knowledge

What people know about health – what is held to be the 'truth' about health – is known because there are bodies of knowledge about health in a society or culture, into which people tap, either consciously or unconsciously. The term 'culture' is used here to indicate the beliefs and practices of a group of people or of a society as a whole. Clearly, *some* elements of knowledge about health do not come from any organised body of knowledge, but result from, for example, the subjective experience of pain and physical distress, and the personal knowledge people have about themselves (see Chapter 2). But even these experiences are mediated by other forms of knowledge drawn from and organised within a culture. It is not possible to talk about personal experiences of health or interpret those experiences without using the language and forms of debate current in existing bodies of knowledge within that culture.

Those bodies of knowledge are often in conflict about ways of doing research, as well as about issues around practice. It is the struggle between these bodies of knowledge, and the people and organisations who support and benefit from them, that creates alternative 'truths' about promoting public health. For example, there are significantly different explanations from within different bodies of knowledge as to who should intervene to encourage people to stop smoking. Smoking can be seen as a moral flaw, a psychological craving, a physical addiction, or a result of social pressure from peers or advertising, and any interventions that might be planned will reflect these understandings. Smoking can be discouraged by education, medical intervention, hypnotism or banning advertising. The explanation and intervention that is dominant in a culture depends on which is the most convincing body of knowledge, which has the most compelling and well-funded research, which has the most powerful professional groups allied to it, and which has the support of the bulk of government funding.

Thinking point   given recent changes in government policy with regard to smoking, what explanation for smoking has become the most dominant?

Although for many years cigarette manufacturers have been active with regard to the knowledge disseminated about the effects of smoking and individual responsibility for health actions, there has been a shift in the

balance of the relative importance of different explanations for smoking and if, how and when to intervene to discourage it. The resultant changes in law are coming into effect in the four nations of the UK at the time of writing (in 2006). What is being suggested here is that knowledge of health is not just about the accumulation of facts, but is influenced by power: the power of agencies and groups to define what that knowledge consists of, and the power to have those definitions acted upon.

One of the most influential understandings of how knowledge and power are linked is the French philosopher Michel Foucault's notion of discourse. Discourse is a set of ideas, statements and practices which provide a way of representing a particular kind of knowledge. For example, the ways in which people experience their own bodies can be classed as healthy or unhealthy according to how medical knowledge is produced – or constructed – and applied, often through official agencies. Foucault offers a fundamental challenge to the idea that knowledge is discovered. For him, 'truth is not a collection of insights or information floating about, parts of which are sooner or later revealed or discovered, nor does it lie deep within us waiting to be freed. Truth is produced through discourse ... and its production is imbued with relations of power' (Bleier, 1984, p. 195).

Foucault cites the example of the creation of 'hysteria' as a medical condition in nineteenth-century medical discourse, and the ways in which 'hysterical women' were 'treated' by doctors and, later, psychologists (Bleier, 1984). Other bodily experiences have, in turn, been medicalised, in that they have been explained and represented through medical discourse. Masturbation, for instance, for much of the twentieth century was seen as a medical problem requiring medical treatment. Another example of medicalisation has been the changing discourse around pregnancy and childbirth in western societies, and the dominance of the medical model with regard to the care and 'treatment' of women in labour.

7.2 The knowledge base of research

Just as the word 'health' is subject to varying definitions from within different models, 'research' too does not have a single meaning, nor does it consist of a simple set of practices which, if used properly, will reveal the truth. Existing bodies of knowledge or discourses understand and define research in different and often contradictory ways. Three key bodies of knowledge, from the point of view of researching public health, are lay knowledge, biomedical knowledge and social science knowledge. These are summarised in Figure 7.1 and considered in greater detail below.

Figure 7.1 The knowledge base of research		
Lay knowledge	Biomedical knowledge	Social science knowledge
Based on subjective personal experience or beliefs	Based on objective experiment and observation of the natural world through rigorous and repeated tests	Varied, but based on objective analysis or subjective observation of the social world

7.2.1 Lay knowledge

'Lay' knowledge, the knowledge that 'ordinary people' draw on to make sense of health and illness, as distinct from professional or academic understandings, has important characteristics that distinguish it in terms of its understanding of research. Some people would, of course, question whether the knowledge gathering undertaken in lay knowledge is research at all, because research is usually seen as a formal process of knowledge acquisition, whereas knowledge gathering in lay knowledge is largely informal and reliant on secondary sources. It is based mainly on experience – either one's own or the collective and historical experience of others – rather than on organised research practices, and is therefore inherently subjective rather than objective (although lay knowledge certainly draws on and assimilates over time accepted biomedical and social research). It is often claimed that lay knowledge is irrational, based on magic, religion, folklore and myth, rather than on scientific rationality or social scientific research; or that it is based on notions of 'common sense' that have no scientific or research basis. For this reason, lay knowledge is often accorded a relatively low status. However, increasingly public health practitioners (and many others) have argued that, in order to understand health and health actions, lay knowledge should be taken seriously as a valid 'truth' or explanation (Popay and Williams, 1996).

7.2.2 Biomedical knowledge

Biomedical knowledge has several characteristics that distinguish it from lay knowledge and most social scientific knowledge in terms of research (and which it tends to share with other 'natural' sciences). Biomedical research shares with other scientific research the understanding that it is dealing with universal laws that can be uncovered through experiment, observation and rigorous testing. Traditionally, natural science assumes that there is a measurable, material world which can be investigated through scientific methods which are logical and replicable. Although separate from lay and social science knowledge in important ways, biomedical knowledge is linked to both lay and social science understandings of health and illness, and drawn on by these.

Thinking point   what elements of biomedical knowledge inform your own lay understandings of health?

Michael Hardey points to the increasing use of the internet as a way for lay people to access biomedical knowledge and suggests that this will transform the relationship between health professionals and their clients (Hardey, 1999). He argues that this use of the internet is associated with a demystification of medicine and medical expertise and a consequent lay scepticism about health professionals. One way in which this increased access can be seen to be played out is in the popularity of NHS Direct, not just as a telephone helpline but as a web-based facility. This is just one example: there is a vast array of other health (and illness) information available on the internet.

One might argue that this increased availability of health knowledge must be empowering as it also challenges existing power relations between the knowledge-rich health professional and the knowledge-poor lay person. However, as Korp (2006) points out, there are also *dis*empowering aspects of health on the internet because it widens the gap between those who have access to this information and those who do not. There has also been a shift towards the control and evaluation, and therefore the legitimacy, of information by so-called 'experts' in health. Both these latter moves reinforce existing social and power divisions between what Korp (2006) calls the 'information-rich' and 'information-poor'.

7.2.3 Social science knowledge

Social science knowledge has at its heart the insistence on the primacy of 'the social' in researching and acting on the world. Social science research varies according to the theoretical understandings of the researcher, and their methodology (or the scientific or theoretical basis of the method). A researcher's methodological assumptions inform the choice of particular research methods. As discussed in previous chapters, some social scientists focus on health and illness as being socially caused. This view suggests, first, that illness is caused not simply by and within individual human beings, but is a result of social and human environmental causes such as poverty, industrialisation and urbanisation. Second, it suggests that a person's social position, and factors such as their class, gender, ethnicity, and so on, influence their health and illness and, indeed, the medical and social responses to these. In this view, research is a political act aimed at uncovering the causes of health inequality.

Other social scientists focus on health and illness as being socially constructed, in that both are cultural phenomena that people need to explain to themselves and to others. They therefore have meanings attached to them that are cultural rather than simply biological.

What health and illness mean will be different in different cultures and at different times in history, and research is aimed at understanding the relationship between the ways in which things are defined and the power that accrues to certain people and organisations as a result of those definitions. Yet other social science researchers focus on gathering objective data on the health of populations, while some focus on the personal experiences and feelings of the individual. As should be becoming obvious, social science research is complex and multifaceted.

Implications for researching health

What are the implications of these different bodies of knowledge for researching health, and how do the competing perspectives influence what and how research is carried out? Research is not value neutral and is supported and funded according to the political agenda of the time. Different researchers have competing priorities, but not everything gets researched. Small-scale research is often done without funding, whereas larger-scale research is often commissioned by the health or social care sectors, or is carried out in answer to calls for specific pieces of research by some of the large government-funded organisations such as the Medical Research Council (MRC) or the Economic and Social Research Council (ESRC). How these organisations decide on their research priorities is influenced by that same political agenda of the day.

Different bodies of knowledge are given credence depending on the perspective and epistemological assumptions of those commissioning, as well as those carrying out, research. Epistemology is the theory or the science of the methods or grounds of knowledge. It is concerned with how we know what we know and what we regard as valid knowledge. Different types of knowledge are considered valuable depending not only on the types of questions being asked, but also on the people both asking and answering those questions. The next section considers these links between knowledge and research in promoting public health.

7.3 Research and promoting public health

Bodies of knowledge about health and public health are not static; they develop and change. Mainly, they change through the gathering of new information and the development of different ways of interpreting that information. These alternative ways of information gathering and explaining the world are valued differently within a culture according to how dominant at the time is the body of knowledge within which they predominate.

Thinking point   is there one body of knowledge which is dominant in defining health in western societies today?

One might argue that the most dominant body of knowledge within health varies over time and is largely dependent on whose perspective is taken. As you saw in previous chapters, biomedical knowledge remains a powerful discourse or way of seeing and knowing about health; however, for those involved in promoting public health, a social model or approach to health may be more useful. For public health practitioners, it is important to understand the way in which these bodies of knowledge work and how they are linked to and influence research in health and illness, for two reasons:

1   to gain an understanding of where particular beliefs and understandings come from and how important they are in affecting public perception of health and therefore public health practice

2   in order to conduct research.

Public health practitioners will access in different ways the three broad types of research outlined in the three subsections below. Each and every person is implicated in lay knowledge and gathers information as a lay person, although practitioners or other health professionals may believe that their views are more rigorous and objective than many lay ideas. However, it is important not to dismiss lay knowledge since it clearly has an effect on individuals' responses to their health and on their health behaviours. At the same time, much of our understanding of illness is gained from biomedical research, and it is clear that the biomedical model is still dominant in many areas of interest to public health practitioners. Much of the research that underpins public health practice draws on social scientific methods. However, the broadening out of the public health field in recent years may well result in the use of an even wider range of research and research methods.

7.3.1 Lay information gathering

Much lay research or information gathering is based on a particular set of questions that focus on the nature of health and illness for the individual. It is distinct from the gathering of information *from* lay people, in that it is the lay person or persons themselves who are integral to the research process and the gathering of the information, rather than just providing that data as participants of a research study. Lay research often focuses on the answering of questions that are inherently personal. For example, rather than asking a general question such as 'What causes these symptoms?', the lay person will ask 'Why have *I* got these symptoms *now* and what *purpose* do they serve?' (Williams and Popay, 1994). Lay explanation is either characterised by a reliance on personal experience and experimentation, or based on a reliance on a set of principles or beliefs that explain a particular phenomenon. These explanations may contain elements of biomedical and social science knowledge, but this is likely to be given no more weight than information derived from friends, fellow sufferers, the media, or moral and spiritual beliefs of various kinds.

Lay information gathering has been a crucial part of the development of user group perspectives and self-help strategies. It has also been influential in underpinning the development of various political groupings based on self-advocacy (in this it has similarities to the critical perspective in social science knowledge outlined in Section 7.3.3 below). Many of these groups seek to confront biomedical knowledge, particularly by asserting the rights of people to define their health problems in their own ways, and to see labels such as 'disability' as prone to focus on the physical or mental impairments as the cause of the problem, rather than on the physical and social environment.

Lay information gathering at an individual level is not, of course, a formal process with a coherent set of techniques and methods. On the contrary, it is characterised by an informality that rarely questions the validity of the information other than in terms of whether it fits with a set of beliefs or chimes with personal experiences. However, this is not to say that lay information gathering has no value. First, biomedical and social science knowledge offer no convincing explanations for 'why me?' and 'why now?'; and, second, whether or not lay knowledge is 'right' or 'wrong' in biomedical or social scientific terms, the narratives created within it clearly have a role in supporting individuals in promoting their own health or in attempting to live with illness.

In recent years there has been a surge of interest in more formal lay involvement in research, often termed 'lay epidemiology'. Many people advocate participatory research, in which lay people are an integral part of the research process, designing and carrying out research. The greater acceptance of the idea that research is not value free but is influenced by the social and political agendas of the time, and that there is not only one 'scientific truth', opens up the possibility that the validity of lay ideas may also come to be accepted. In other words, if one no longer accepts the idea of complete objectivity and impartiality as the only true way of knowing about health, then the subjective experiences of those who are usually being researched (the research subjects) become equally valid as a way of knowing. Participatory research has its roots in the radical work of Paulo Freire, a Brazilian writing in the 1970s about oppressed groups in developing countries. Freire argued that, in order to be liberated from oppression, people need to acquire a critical awareness of the world in which they live and the structures that surround them. He called this critical awareness 'conscientisation', and described it as a process in which people, through a change in consciousness, are able to gain the knowledge needed to make a realistic appraisal of their position in the world in relation to others; this then enables them to act to transform their world (Freire, 1972). In research terms this involves having control over the setting of the agenda and the problem posing, as well as over the problem solving. Freire saw research and action as a seamless process. Decision making without what he called the 'stakeholder's' or the lay person's full participation is akin to what he referred to as 'cultural invasion', where the power of decision making is located outside rather than within the one who should decide, so that the latter has only the illusion of making decisions (Freire, 1972). For Freire, cultural synthesis is the only way in which human fulfilment can be achieved and people liberated from their oppression. This requires that: 'The actors who come from "another world" to the world of the people do so not as invaders. They do not come to teach or to transmit or to give anything, but rather to learn, with the people, about the people's world' (Freire, 1972, p. 155).

Thinking point   can lay involvement in research be consciousness building?

Current public health research often makes use of lay knowledge and expertise, but it is arguable whether this leads to 'conscientisation' or a critical awareness on the part of individuals in terms of their position in society. It could be argued, however, that it also leads to greater frustration and feelings of powerlessness. There is much rhetoric within the health service about listening to local voices and developing consumer-sensitive services (Handsley, 2007; Scriven, 2007), but there is much scepticism too. The claims made for empowerment and emancipation through participation have been questioned by Rissel (1994), who makes a distinction between psychological empowerment and political and economic empowerment. He argues that raising consciousness and confidence can be psychologically empowering, but political and economic empowerment requires a shift in power that is much harder to effect. Even if full emancipation from oppression is a remote dream, there are many achievable goals attached to participatory research which make it a worthwhile enterprise. Narrowing the gap between lay and expert knowledge, enabling people to take an active role in the structures that influence their lives, widening debates about health and creating people-sensitive services, must contribute in some way to a fairer and more just society than one based on a top-down approach.

One of the primary reasons for engaging in participatory research is to bridge the gap between lay and professional knowledge so that health and social care work can better reflect the needs of communities and those living within them. It therefore represents a two-way process of knowledge sharing, which is illustrated in Figure 7.2.

The attitude of outside experts is often characterised by the third quadrant in Figure 7.2, and lay people put themselves in quadrant II. The aim of

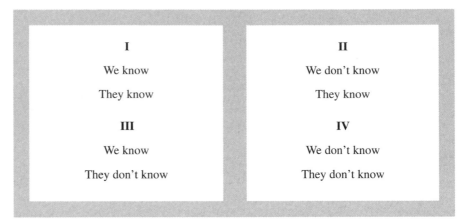

Figure 7.2   A two-way process of knowledge sharing (Source: Tolley and Bentley 1996, p. 51, Figure 5.1)

participatory research is to reach the first quadrant. The use of 'We' and 'They' is interchangeable in this context because, as de Koning and Martin put it:

> It is not only the poor, illiterate, and other categories of people classified as marginalized and deprived who need to think about how, in what ways and why they experience themselves and the world as they do. It is equally important for more privileged groups such as health professionals, researchers and activists to do the same.
>
> (de Koning and Martin, 1996, p. 10)

For researchers and professionals trained in conventional methods, the leap from telling people what to do, 'in their best interests', to finding out those people's own perspectives and ways of doing things, which may challenge that professional knowledge, can be a daring one. As Cornwall explains, the use of participatory methods:

> demands a style of interaction and a change in approach that in itself opens up transformational possibilities. By bringing health professionals into communities, to learn from rather than to teach people, participatory methods open up spaces for dialogue. This experience can be humbling for health workers. Realising that people are not only knowledgeable but also capable of generating their own solutions has, for many, been a revelation. Working together with local people, as counterparts, challenges deeply held prejudices about the poor.
>
> (Cornwall, 1996, p. 104)

The climate that has nurtured participatory research and the breaking down of barriers in terms of 'who knows' has also encouraged the breaking down of barriers between research methodologies. Different methodological approaches are considered later in this chapter, but it should be noted that this postmodernist view is one that has opened up the possibility of multiple views and realities of the world and which questions the idea that there is only one 'truth' to be researched. If there are multiple or competing 'truths' and ways of seeing the world, then research methodologies can be considered in terms of their fitness for purpose.

Participatory research is not without its difficulties, however, and its use in studies of community participation in health has sometimes been problematic (Handsley, 2007). Although the principles of community participation have long been operationalised in the developing world as part of the movement for social justice (El Ansari et al., 2002), in the UK the discrepancies between perceived levels of skill, knowledge or expertise between professional groups and lay members of the community can lead to difficulties in research (Bandesha and Litva, 2005). Community participation initiatives in the UK are still frequently led by professional researchers in health or social care, rather than utilising a broader, more egalitarian approach to research. You encounter examples of participatory research in Chapter 9.

7.3.2 Biomedical research

Whereas lay knowledge is rooted in the experience of health and illness, biomedical knowledge rests on the concept of disease and attempts to discover the causes and treatment of disease. It shares with most scientific research a reliance on the scientific method.

The scientific method is the process by which scientists, collectively and over time, endeavour to construct an accurate or objective (i.e. reliable, consistent and non-arbitrary) representation of the world. Recognising that personal and cultural beliefs influence people's perceptions and their interpretations of natural phenomena, this method aims to minimise those influences when developing a theory through the use of standard procedures and criteria. In summary, the scientific method attempts to reduce as far as possible the influence of bias or prejudice in the experimenter when testing a hypothesis or theory. The scientific method 'consists of a system of rules and processes on which research is based, following the principles of the hypothetico-deductive method, and against which it can be evaluated' (Bowling, 2002, p. 122).

The scientific method has four steps:

1   observation and description of a phenomenon or group of phenomena
2   formulation of a hypothesis to explain the phenomena
3   use of the hypothesis to predict the existence of other phenomena, or to predict quantitatively the results of new observations
4   performance of experimental tests of the predictions by several independent experimenters and 'properly performed' experiments.

Researchers are expected to conduct their research in such a way as to ensure that the methods of data collection, the analysis of data and the writing up and publication of the results are all carried out rigorously and systematically (Bowling, 2002).

The supporting or refuting of a hypothesis after rigorous testing is integral to the scientific method. However, not all research is carried out to test a specific theory, but may contribute to the development of a theory, during which time a hypothesis may or may not be modified. Sometimes a hypothesis might be partially supported by the data and will then be modified. The researcher will then again set out to test that hypothesis. A 'paradigm shift' can be said to have taken place if and when, after rigorous testing over time, a transformation of scientific beliefs occurs. A paradigm is a conceptual framework within which research is carried out. The concept of a paradigm shift was first described by Thomas Kuhn (1970). Bowling describes this phenomenon thus: 'over time evidence accumulates and challenges the dominant paradigm, leading to a crisis among scientists and the gradual realisation of the inadequacy of that paradigm; pressure for change eventually occurs, leading to a "scientific revolution", and the new paradigm becomes gradually accepted (until it, in turn, is challenged)' (Bowling, 2002, p. 124).

Although biomedical research shares the basic principles of the scientific method with the physical sciences, there are of course significant differences between what is appropriate in terms of experimentation when dealing with inanimate objects and human beings (and, arguably, the rest of the natural world). It is widely agreed that it is unethical to conduct medical experiments on human beings, and there are considerable ethical arguments against both blind trials (where one group of patients is given a drug and another not, to test its effectiveness) and animal experimentation.

Thinking point   what arguments might you put forward in favour of animal experiments?

As you read in Chapter 1, two central tenets of promoting public health are to do good and to avoid doing harm. These are core principles of utilitarianism, which states the greatest good should be secured for the greatest number of people (see Chapter 1). It might be argued that animal experimentation can be justified on the grounds of the greater good of the human race, in spite of doing harm to animals.

Because biomedical research relies on the scientific method, it attempts to maintain objectivity, although many critics would argue that, even though the method may be objective, the research itself is socially and politically embedded so that, for instance, decisions about which research gets funded and how the results of the research are used are deeply subjective. Apart from anything else, much biomedical research is often carried out by companies whose aim is to make a profit as well as to develop more effective treatments. It is also clear that not all the products of biomedical research have been wholly beneficial in their individual and social effects.

Biomedical research, of course, also has limits in terms of its reach. Clearly, the scientific method is not an appropriate way of understanding huge swathes of human experience and interaction, from the politics of healthcare to human emotions. For this it is necessary to turn to the social sciences.

7.3.3 Social science research

Social science is not a single, unified way of thinking – it contains many competing perspectives with radically different ways of understanding and researching the world. Some of the main perspectives are outlined below.

Positivism

The founders of the social sciences in the nineteenth century regarded social science as analogous to natural science. Emile Durkheim, one of the founders of sociology, claimed that 'our method is objective. It is dominated entirely by the idea that social facts are things and must be treated as such' (Durkheim, 1966 [1895], p. 143). According to this 'positivist' perspective, the social science endeavour is to describe the laws of society by deducing social facts. This makes it possible to explain how societies work and how they change.

Because positivism stresses the scientific nature of social facts, it shows a marked preference for measurement and quantification. Sociological notions that are not measurable are deemed meaningless, and much effort in this tradition is put into operationalising sociological concepts in order to subject them to research techniques leading to quantifiable conclusions. An allied tendency in positivism is towards social structural explanations as distinct from those that refer to human intentions and motives, which are not operationalisable. The research tools most commonly used within a positivist approach include surveys, standardised interview schedules, and experimental methods, with statistical techniques used to analyse the data.

In much contemporary sociological debate, positivism has become something of a term of abuse. The main criticism of positivism from within social science is that it ignores the importance of people's intentions and motives even though these are often fundamental in understanding social activity. What is the use, the argument goes, of counting how many people smoke cannabis, if you do not ask why they do so? Even if you record through an opinion survey the reasons people give for smoking cannabis, you cannot measure successfully people's hidden or underlying motives, or the deeper meanings and various interpretations attached to these.

Interpretivism

Radically different from positivism, interpretivism starts from the position that making sense of society involves understanding the thinking, meanings and intentions of those being researched. For interpretivists, quantifying social action is a limited way of understanding meanings. Positivists might record quantitative measures of social capital – for example, the number and frequency of social contacts people have, and even the satisfaction levels with regard to those social relationships – but they can tell us little about the lived experience of the individual, or the meanings that the person attaches to actual social encounters. (You can read more about social capital in Gibson, 2007.)

 Interpretivists tend also to ignore the structural determinants of human action, focusing instead on the ways in which individuals produce subjective frameworks of meaning in very local contexts. Although most interpretivists would not argue, for instance, with the suggestion that gender influences how individuals interpret the world about them, they would argue that a simplistic 'reading off' of an individual's actions from their gender is reductionist and ignores the complexity of each individual's response to their lived experience.

Interpretivists explore the social by examining the definitions and interpretations of individual 'actors'. To do this they examine the interpersonal construction of meanings in local contexts. The researcher seeks to understand experience by getting close to it, either by first-hand observation or by other techniques such as in-depth interviews that allow respondents to express their understandings, meanings and motivations.

Critical perspectives

Including a range of theoretical positions, from Marxism to feminism, critical perspectives see research as a way of changing society as well as understanding it: 'At the heart of critical research is the idea that knowledge is structured by existing sets of social relations. The aim of critical methodology is to provide knowledge which engages the prevailing social structures. These social structures are seen by critical social researchers ... as oppressive structures' (Harvey, 1990, p. 2). As Marx and Engels observe at the end of *The German Ideology*, 'The philosophers have only interpreted the world in various ways: the point is to change it' (Marx and Engels, 1998 [1932], p. 170).

Critical perspectives make three main points about research. First, research cannot ignore either the social context in which it is carried out, or the broad structures, such as capitalism or patriarchy, that control people's lives. For example, research on health that assumed that drug treatments are entirely progressive and ignored the influence of the large pharmaceutical companies would be meaningless.

Second, research must start from a position that acknowledges power relations and inequality. Most positivist and interpretivist accounts treat all social subjects as equal, disregarding social divisions and inequalities. Critical research, on the other hand, acknowledges power relations as determining factors in people's patterns of behaviour. For example, research on the causes of anorexia that ignored the unequal power relations between men and women would be fatally flawed. Campaigns against obesity that focus on the provision of information about healthy eating, but fail to recognise the importance of cost (and therefore poverty and access to resources) as a factor, will fail. (You consider research and obesity further in Chapter 12.)

Third, critical researchers raise questions about the impact of prevailing power structures on the research process itself. In whose interest is it, they would ask, for a particular piece of research to be commissioned, and who benefits from the research findings? The political and social context will always shape the knowledge that is generated from research, but it also shapes the frameworks of understanding used by researchers. Many feminist researchers, for instance, argue that, in a patriarchal society, men have power in social institutions; and male values, stereotypes of gender relations and male-dominated language and culture are significant in the production of knowledge, thus excluding women and subordinating them to male agendas (Stanley and Wise, 1993).

There are, of course, difficulties with critical research. If theory leads research, there is a danger that research findings simply confirm the theory. If a research project starts with the assumption that class is a primary structure in society, it is highly likely that the research findings will reflect that foundation. Research can become little more than an illustration of a theoretical argument, substantiating the researcher's theoretical predisposition. Clearly, also, the promotion of a particular political priority could be considered as rather a narrowly conceived research aim.

Cultural perspectives

Although the term 'culture' has many definitions, in social science it refers to the beliefs and practices of a society. The focus of cultural perspectives is on how meaning is constituted in particular societies at particular times through language and representation. The meaning of the word 'madness', for instance, has varied enormously across time, as have the beliefs and practices to which the word has been applied. Madness has been represented in various ways: as religious ecstasy, as moral laxity, as mental breakdown, as lovable eccentricity, and so on. It is also mediated by social divisions of class, race and gender; for example, 'madness' might be thought of as 'eccentricity' in people of higher social classes. Moreover, the construction of meaning is connected to power: the way in which people think about madness – the 'truth' about it – is regulated by the dominant medical discourse of the time.

Research on culture has generally focused on reading texts, by which is meant not simply the written word but any cultural artefact, such as images, clothing, and so on. By 'reading' is meant the exploring of the meanings carried by the artefact. So, for instance, a reading of the cultural significance of medical dressings might focus on their colour: the white of bandages symbolising purity and cleanliness; the pink of surgical plasters demonstrating dominant ideas about the most valued skin colour in some cultures.

Cultural perspectives are highly critical of other social science perspectives as reductionist (accounting for a range of phenomena in terms of a single determining factor, such as class or the meanings of participants). However, they are criticised in turn for their relativism and for the subjective nature of textual analysis.

A postmodernist approach

As should be apparent, there is a range of different perspectives or ways of seeing and knowing about the world and therefore about health: this is termed a postmodernist approach. Postmodernism holds that there is no single or overall 'truth'; rather, there are many 'truths' or ways of making sense of the world. A postmodernist view asserts that there is a multitude of alternative explanations and ways of seeing, and this opens up the possibility of alternative but equally valid explanations for health, or indeed for illhealth. This has implications for the relationship between lay and professional persons within the health environment; no longer is the doctor's perspective 'objective' and juxtaposed with the patient's 'subjective' experiences. It also has implications for the way research is carried out and especially for the methods used. If there is not only one truth, it follows that there might be more than one way of unearthing those truths. Different, but equally valid, methods might be used, depending on the subject of the research and the questions to be answered.

There are sceptics of the postmodernist position, however. Although some commentators (e.g. Morris 2001) see the potential for breaking down barriers between lay people and professionals, others argue that, by accepting the different discourses as merely different, this has taken the sting out of critical perspectives, with the power structure that governs people's lives left unchallenged (Kermode and Brown, 1996).

It has been important to describe some of the ways in which knowledge about health is generated, but there is no substitute for engaging with research in finding out the strengths and weaknesses of particular approaches. The remaining chapters in this part of the book concentrate on particular research techniques and settings. In the rest of this chapter you consider the first stages of research activity: the preparatory work that needs to be done before research can be effectively carried out.

7.4 Doing public health research

Although multidisciplinary public health research can take many forms (Baum, 2007), there are particular tasks that need to be carried out for all types of research. It can be thought of as a staged process, as demonstrated in Figure 7.3, which takes a social science perspective.

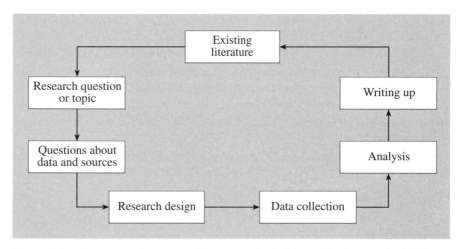

Figure 7.3   The research process (Source: adapted from Mackay et al., 2001, p. 47, Figure 3.3)

Imagine that you have been asked to help a school encourage its pupils not to smoke cigarettes and you want to conduct some research to help you decide on what action to take. Your first step is to gather information by looking at the existing literature about smoking in schools and any other relevant information you can find. At this stage any information from any source might be useful in scoping the issue. There are often vast sources of unpublished information, known as 'grey literature', which can be accessed via local authority departments, NHS hospital libraries, and so on, and which are valuable sources of knowledge. A list of sources of public health information is given in Box 7.1. This list, which focuses mainly on UK sources, is by no means comprehensive. At the time of going to press there are plans for the National Library for Health (NLH) to develop a National Library for Public Health which should provide a single initial access point to information.

Box 7.1 Sources of health information

Evidence-based resources

The Cochrane Library is an electronic publication designed to supply high-quality evidence to inform people providing and receiving care, and those responsible for research, teaching, funding and administration at all levels.

The Centre for Public Health Excellence at NICE (the National Institute for Health and Clinical Excellence) commissions research to support evidence on how to improve the public's health. Its evidence briefings provide a comprehensive, systematic and up-to-date map of the evidence base for public health and health improvement, with a particular focus on reductions in inequalities in health.

Journals

Key, peer reviewed, journals include:

Critical Public Health	*Health Promotion Practice*
Ethnicity and Health	*International Journal of Health Promotion Education*
European Journal of Public Health	*Journal of Epidemiology and Community Health*
Health Education Journal	*Journal of Mental Health Promotion*
Health Education Research	*Social Science and Medicine*

Databases

Although some of the key journals are listed above, public health research is published in a wide array of journals. The following databases should be used to trace relevant articles.

ASSIA	Global Health
British Nursing Index	HMIC (Health Management Information Consortium)
CINAHL	Medline

Statistics

National

National Statistics Online provides access to key statistics on population trends, mortality, health-related behaviour and indicators of the nation's health. The virtual bookshelf provides links to online versions of many statistical publications including *Social trends*,

Regional trends, Health and Personal Social Service Statistics and
Health Statistics Quarterly.

International

The World Health Organization provides statistics in both summary
format (e.g. World Health Statistics) and in more detail (e.g. levels of
mortality, deaths by cause).

The World Bank provides access to a range of health indicators for
countries and regions around the world. It includes summary
health data.

Local

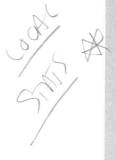

The Local Public Health Observatory is the main source of local
statistical information for public health. Links to these are available
from the website of the Association of Public Health.

The Neighbourhood Statistics part of National Statistics Online can
be searched by postcode and includes a section on health and social
care.

Policy

The Chief Medical Officer's section of the Department of Health
website has up-to-date information on key public health issues.

Other organisations' websites

The websites of many organisations provide information on public
health topics. The easiest way of tracing these is through gateways
that list only high-quality websites.

The Intute website (http://www.intute.ac.uk) has a 'Health & Life
Sciences' section which includes a range of information on public
health.

7.4.1 Searching for information

Although the internet has revolutionised how easily and quickly people can
gain access to vast quantities of information, finding the best research
evidence to inform your practice requires a systematic approach to
searching. This section takes you through a methodological process of
finding information (see Figure 7.4), although it is recognised that in
practice the steps may overlap and you may retrace them. To work through
the process, use the example mentioned above, and imagine that you have
been asked to help a school to encourage its pupils not to smoke cigarettes.
You need to find up-to-date information to support this work.

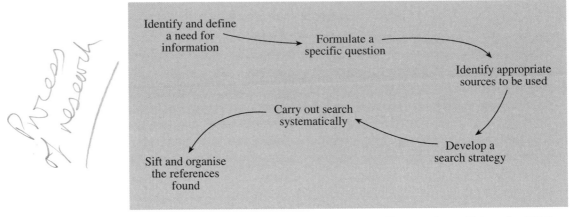

Figure 7.4   The information searching process (Source: Open University, 2004)

Step 1: identify and define a need for information

Before starting to search for information it is worth spending some time thinking about what you already know and what the gaps in your knowledge are. Two useful questions to ask when trying to identify a need for information are:

1   Why is the information needed?

2   What do you already know?

The answer to the first of these questions will usually help you scope your search. For example, you would have to be far more systematic in your search if you were planning to implement a regional or local health promotion campaign than if you just needed to find one or two references to support a course assignment. In this particular case the campaign is for one school and is something you are doing in your own time, so this may well limit the time for, and hence the comprehensiveness of, your search, although you will still be keen to make sure that it is based on the best evidence available.

Step 2: formulate a specific question

Once you have clarified why you need the information and what you know already you should be able to identify the key question(s) you need to address. Formulating clear and focused questions makes searching easier. It will help you to:

• identify relevant sources to search

• identify key concepts to search

• identify those parts of the information you retrieve that are most relevant.

The following questions could all be pertinent for your search and you can probably think of many more:

Q1 What is the prevalence of smoking in school-age children?

Q2 What statistics are available on mortality that is related to smoking?

Q3 What are the predictors of smoking in school-age children?

Q4 What reasons are given by children as being their main reasons for giving up smoking?

Q5 Are there examples of successful school-based programmes for preventing smoking in children?

Q6 What interventions have been successful in reducing or preventing smoking uptake in children?

Q7 What current national policies are there concerning children and smoking?

Q8 Are there any materials available which could be adapted for use with my school?

Step 3: identify appropriate sources to be used

As Box 7.1 demonstrates, there are many possible sources of public health information. The questions you have formulated should help you to identify the types of sources that are likely to contain the information you require. For example, Q1 and Q2, and possibly Q3 and Q4, would be answered with statistical resources; Q3, Q4, Q 5 and Q 6 with evidence-based resources or bibliographic databases to trace journal articles; Q7 with policy resources; and Q8 with organisations' websites.

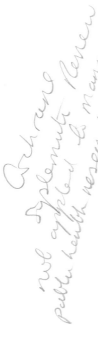

The evidence-based resources most frequently used as a starting point for searching for the effectiveness of clinical interventions – for example, Cochrane Systematic Reviews – are not the sources necessarily recommended for searching for the effectiveness of public health initiatives. Many health promotion interventions are not evaluated using the methods reported in these databases; for example, they do not use randomised controlled trials. Perkins et al. (1999) argue that this is because health promotion interventions are often too dynamic and complex to be evaluated in this way.

Step 4: developing a search strategy

Keywords   Once you have identified your key questions you can move on to identify the key terms you need for searching. The questions need to be broken down into the broad ideas or concepts that they cover. You will usually find that your question breaks down into two or more ideas or concepts.

Most of the questions identified in the example above involve the two concepts of 'smoking' and 'schoolchildren'. Other concepts which are question specific are 'prevalence' (Q1), 'mortality' (Q2), 'predictors' (Q3), 'prevention' (Q5), and 'school-based programmes' (Q5).

Synonyms   Because language varies and databases use their own thesauri or index of keywords, it is important to think of synonyms or alternative key words to use in your search. You need to consider:

- plurals (child, children)

- abbreviations (UK, United Kingdom)

- variations in spelling (colour, color [US spelling], specialised, specialized)

- variations in terminology used in different cultures and countries

- differences in terminology; for example, between the health and social care sectors.

Check to see whether any of the words you have used are vague or ambiguous and, if so, cut them out. You need to be as precise as possible to avoid retrieving irrelevant material. The following are examples of appropriate synonyms for some of your concepts:

smoking: no obvious synonyms

children: child; adolescent(s); young people

prevalence: frequency; incidence

mortality: death rate.

7.4.2 Combining terms

As well as listing all the possible terms, with many databases you also have to think about how you are going to combine them. There are three special words you can use for these: AND, OR and NOT. Combining terms in this way is called Boolean searching.

To use a very simple example, imagine a database has three sorts of documents: documents about children (represented by the oval shape, labelled children, in Figure 7.5), documents about smoking and documents about both children and smoking. The search terms would work in the way shown in Figure 7.5.

For questions 1 and 5, our search terms would be combined in the following ways:

Q1 (incidence OR frequency OR prevalence) AND smoking AND (children OR child OR adolescent OR adolescents OR young people)

Q5 school AND (programme OR programmes OR program OR programs) AND smoking.

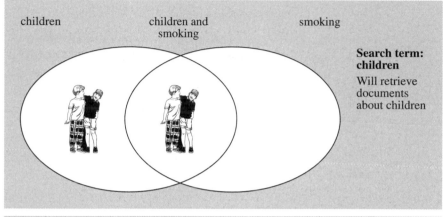

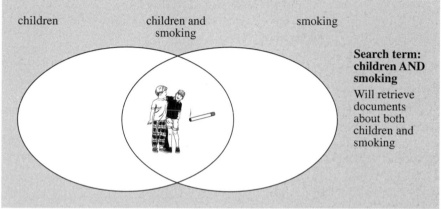

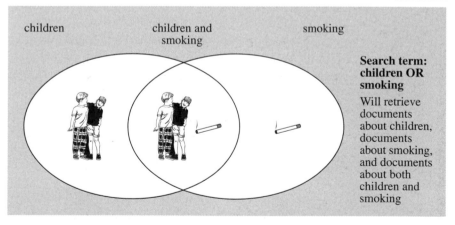

Figure 7.5 Combining search terms

7.4.3 Limits

You also need to consider ways of limiting the scope of the search. Some topics, for example, are time limited (e.g. only current policies), others may have geographical limits (e.g. you may only be interested in UK policy or intervention programmes), and yet others will have age limits (e.g. school-age children would not include those under four).

Step 5: carry out the search systematically

You are now ready to search the identified resources for information to answer your questions. The following are some general principles for any kind of searching.

- Although each source that you use may look quite different from the one you tried before, there are always features that are similar – a box in which to type your search terms, a clickable help button. Different databases refer to the same functions using different terminology, but the principles behind them are exactly the same. The trick is to check the clues given on the screen or in the 'help' of the individual database you are using.

- Before searching a resource for the first time check for the following:
  - Is there any online help?
  - Can I search for phrases? In our example, if you can search for 'school programmes' as a phrase your search will be a lot more specific than if you search for 'school' and 'programmes' as two separate words which could appear anywhere. It will depend on the resource you are using how phrase searching is entered. Check the search tips of the individual resources to find out how to do this.
  - Can I combine search terms and if so how?
  - Can I use truncation? Many databases allow you to use a symbol, often an asterisk (*), so that you can easily find all words with a common root; for example, program* will find program, programs, programme, programmes.
  - Can I use wildcards? Some databases let you use a symbol to search for variants of a word; for example, organi?ation would find organisation and organization.
  - Can I do an advanced search?
  - How can I get a list of what I've found?

- Be prepared to change your search strategy if you are finding too much or too little.

 - Be systematic and keep a record of your progress.

7.5 Assessing research findings

As you search the various information sources you will retrieve a lot of material. There is a skill in deciding what to include and what to exclude, and this is the focus of the next step.

Step 6: sift and organise the references found

Various criteria exist to help you evaluate the information retrieved. Some of those you should consider are:

- **Provenance**   What are the author's credentials? Which organisation do they work for and who funds them? Has the material been reviewed by others?

- **Relevance**   Is the information retrieved from the right geographical area? Is it at the right level? Does the information have the correct emphasis?

- **Objectivity**   Do the authors state clearly the viewpoint they are taking? Be particularly careful about opinion expressed as fact.

- **Method**   If some kind of research or data collection is involved, is it clear how the research was carried out? Were the methods appropriate?

- **Timeliness**   Is it clear when the information was produced? Is it obsolete?

During your searching you will probably gather information from a wide variety of sources, and you will need to keep track of what you have got, where you found it and what it is about. Keeping a record of your information sources will ensure that you don't have to retrace your steps. It will also enable you to cite references and provide an accurate bibliography when you are writing up your work.

7.6 The research process: next steps

Once you have done your information gathering and reviewed the existing evidence, and you are convinced that there are still new things to learn and research that has not been done, you should have some idea of the sorts of questions you want to find answers to. It may be that you will choose to replicate research that has already been done somewhere else, to find out whether it applies in your specific situation; it may be that you will choose simply to work with the existing information and to apply it to your situation. However, it may be that there is a gap in your knowledge that can only be filled by doing some primary research of your own. (Primary research involves gathering new data; secondary research involves using data that has already been gathered by other researchers.) The important thing about your research question is that it must be answerable; that is, you must be able to conduct the research that will answer your question within the resources you have and using appropriate methods.

7.6.1 Questions about data and sources

In order to refine your research question still further, and to ask whether it is answerable, as well as to help with research design, you now need to scope the actual research process. This involves answering such questions as

'How will I gain access to the people whose views I want to research?', and 'How will I deal with analysing the data that I collect?', as well as such basic questions as 'What sort of data will best suit my purpose?'. It is at this stage that various ethical questions will need to be addressed.

There are six key principles of ethical research that the Economic and Social Research Council expects to be addressed, whenever applicable:

- Research should be designed, reviewed and undertaken to ensure integrity and quality

- Research staff and subjects must be informed fully about the purpose, methods and intended possible uses of the research, what their participation in the research entails and what risks, if any, are involved. Some variation is allowed in very specific and exceptional research contexts for which detailed guidance is provided in the policy Guidelines

- The confidentiality of information supplied by research subjects and the anonymity of respondents must be respected

- Research participants must participate in a voluntary way, free from any coercion

- Harm to research participants must be avoided

- The independence of research must be clear, and any conflicts of interest or partiality must be explicit

(ESRC, 2005, p. 1)

In addition, any research carried out in schools, hospitals and many other settings will need to be submitted to the ethics committee of the relevant institution.

7.6.2 Research design: choosing methods – the quantitative/qualitative debate

Perhaps one of the most important choices to be made when planning to gather data is that between quantitative or qualitative methods. Methods themselves (i.e. the particular techniques used in research) are the subject of the next two chapters, but it is worth setting up the distinction between quantitative and qualitative data collection strategies at this stage to highlight the vast range of approaches to research that can be taken.

Quantitative research uses methods adopted from the physical sciences that are designed to ensure objectivity, generalizability and reliability. These techniques cover the ways research participants are selected randomly from the study population in an unbiased manner, the standardized questionnaire or intervention they receive and the statistical methods used to test predetermined hypotheses regarding the relationships between specific variables. The researcher is considered external to the actual research, and results are expected to be replicable no matter who conducts the research.

The strengths of the quantitative paradigm are that its methods produce quantifiable, reliable data that are usually generalizable to some larger population. Quantitative measures are often most appropriate for conducting needs assessments or for evaluations comparing outcomes with baseline data. This paradigm breaks down when the phenomenon under study is difficult to measure or quantify. The greatest weakness of the quantitative approach is that it decontextualises human behavior in a way that removes the event from its real world setting and ignores the effects of variables that have not been included in the model.

Qualitative research methodologies are designed to provide the researcher with the perspective of target audience members through immersion in a culture or situation and direct interaction with the people under study. Qualitative methods used ... include observations, in-depth interviews and focus groups. These methods are designed to help researchers understand the meanings people assign to social phenomena and to elucidate the mental processes underlying behaviors. Hypotheses are generated during data collection and analysis, and measurement tends to be subjective. In the qualitative paradigm, the researcher becomes the instrument of data collection, and results may vary greatly depending upon who conducts the research.

The advantage of using qualitative methods is that they generate rich, detailed data that leave the participants' perspectives intact and provide a context for health behavior. The focus upon processes and 'reasons why' differs from that of quantitative research, which addresses correlations between variables. A disadvantage is that data collection and analysis may be labor intensive and time-consuming. In addition, these methods are not yet totally accepted by the mainstream public health community and qualitative researchers may find their results challenged as invalid by those outside the field ...

(Weinreich, 1996)

Thinking point   do you agree with Weinreich's comments?

Although some would take issue with some of the terminology in the above extract, and others would take issue with the point about the lack of acceptance of qualitative research methods, many public health researchers would support Weinreich's assertions. Many researchers, including

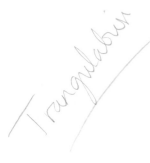

Weinreich, would argue for an integration of quantitative and qualitative methods, for a process of 'triangulation'. Triangulation involves using more than one method to produce different forms of data (or the same method to gather data from different sources). The data can be compared, and similar findings from different methods may support the validity and comprehensiveness of the research findings. In practice, many researchers commonly deploy a variety of methods.

Selecting a method and the balance between methods is often influenced by the researcher's methodological predispositions (their choice of perspective or their political and theoretical views), although it will also be influenced by the resources and time available. Once a decision has been reached, and ethical approval has been received, the process of data collection and analysis can commence. Chapters 8 and 9 examine this more closely, but before you move on it is necessary to go into a little detail about what makes research findings useful and what makes them open to criticism. Section 7.6.3 offers some criteria by which research findings may be judged.

7.6.3 Criteria for assessing research findings

Whenever information is gathered and findings are produced, it is important to ask how useful this information is. Some of the criteria that might be used to assess the usefulness of information gathering and research are outlined below.

- **Validity**   This is based on the degree to which data actually measure what they say they do. For example, to test the hypothesis that a ban on smoking in public places will reduce lung cancer rates, a direct relationship between the two needs to be established for research to be valid. It is not enough to demonstrate a fall in lung cancer rates and to demonstrate that levels of smoking in public have also fallen and then to assume that the two are connected, when the fall in lung cancer rates might be due to some other significant change, such as a drop in the number of young people taking up smoking. An important part of the researcher's quest for validity is making sure the concepts being used are clear and operationalisable.

- **Reliability**   This is about the extent to which repeated measurements using the same research technique in the same conditions produce the same results. Reliability is tested by repetition, so that the most reliable results are those that can be repeated on several occasions using a similar but different sample. Biomedical research is often said to be more reliable than social science research: social science research is difficult to repeat because the contexts, settings and actors are dynamic and ever-changing.

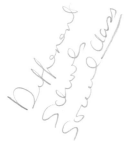

- **Comprehensiveness**   This is based on the extent to which a piece of research is applicable to all the different contexts and cases to which it is claimed to apply. For instance, in order to be comprehensive, research that showed that 75 per cent of restaurant customers in Manchester in October 2003 wanted to ban smoking in restaurants would need to show that the respondents' views were the same irrespective of their gender, class, age, ethnicity, and so on, as well as their geographical location and the type and size of restaurant in which they were interviewed. The more general a claim made about a research finding is, the more comprehensive the research that underpins it needs to be.

- **Generalisability**   This refers to the idea that the findings of a piece of research in one setting or section of a population can be applied to other settings or populations. For example, if 75 per cent of young people aged 16–25 responded negatively to a survey question asking whether or not smoking should be banned from all public places, this would be observed in older people too if the findings could be said to be generalised to all adults.

- **Coherence**   This is based on the extent to which a piece of research is logical and consistent in its argument and use of concepts and theory. Tests for coherence explore the logic of the argument being put forward. In order to test for coherence, in many cases the hidden assumptions behind research must be teased out and checked for plausibility and clarity of reasoning.

Conclusion

This chapter has explored the different bodies of knowledge that inform and impact on the gathering of information for public health research. Researchers and public health practitioners do not start from an objective position outside society and culture. The questions that are asked and the ways in which people ask them, the interpretation of findings and the ways in which they are used in practice, are all influenced by people's perspectives and the different bodies of knowledge that pre-exist any information gathering. Public health research methods of data collection can take a vast range of forms, some quantitative, some qualitative and some that contain a mix of the two. In Chapters 8 and 9 you consider first quantitative and then qualitative methods, before applying these, in Chapters 10 and 11, to the planning and evaluation of public health practice.

References

Bandesha, G. and Litva, A. (2005) 'Perceptions of community participation and health gain in a community project for the South Asian population: a qualitative study', *Journal of Public Health*, vol. 27, pp. 241–5.

Baum, F. (2007) 'Dilemmas in public health research: methodologies and ethical practice' in Douglas et al. (eds) (2007a).

Bleier, R. (1984) *Science and Gender: A Critique of Biology and its Theories on Women*, Elmsford, NY, Pergamon Press.

Bowling, A. (2002) *Research Methods in Health: Investigating Health and Health Services*, Buckingham, Open University Press.

Cornwall, A. (1996) 'Towards participatory practice: participatory rural appraisal (PRA) and the participatory process' in de Koning and Martin (eds) (1996).

de Koning, K. and Martin, M. (eds) (1996) *Participatory Research in Health: Issues and Experiences*, London, Zed Books/Johannesburg, NPPHCN.

Durkheim, E. (1966 [1895]) *The Rules of Sociological Method*, London, Free Press.

Economic and Social Research Council (ESRC) (2005) *Research Ethics Framework*, London, Economic and Social Research Council; also available online at: http://www.esrcsocietytoday.ac.uk/ESRCInfoCentre/Images/ ESRC_Re_Ethics_Frame_tcm6-11291.pdf (Accessed 7 October 2006).

El Ansari, W., Philips, C.J. and Zwi, A.B. (2002) 'Narrowing the gap between academic professional wisdom and community lay knowledge: perceptions from partnerships', *Public Health*, vol. 116, pp. 151–9.

Freire, P. (1972) *Pedagogy of the Oppressed*, London, Sheed and Ward.

Gibson, A. (2007) 'Does social capital have a role to play in the health of communities?' in Douglas et al. (eds) (2007a).

Handsley, S. (2007) 'Community involvement in public health promotion' in Handsley et al. (eds) (2007b).

Handsley, S., Lloyd, C.E., Douglas, J., Earle, S. and Spurr, S. (eds) (2007a) *A Reader in Promoting Public Health: Challenge and Controversy*, London, Sage/Milton Keynes, The Open University.

Hardey, M. (1999) 'Doctor in the house: the internet as a source of lay knowledge and the challenge to expertise', *Sociology of Health and Illness*, vol. 21, pp. 820–35.

Harvey, D. (1990) *The Condition of Postmodernity*, Oxford, Blackwell.

Kermode, S. and Brown, C. (1996) 'The postmodernist hoax and its effect on nursing', *International Journal of Nursing Studies*, vol. 33, pp. 375–84.

Korp, P. (2006) 'Health on the internet: implications for health promotion', *Health Education Research*, vol. 21, pp. 78–86.

Kuhn, T.S. (1970) *The Structure of Scientific Revolutions* (2nd expanded edn), Chicago, IL, University of Chicago Press.

Lloyd, C.E., Handsley, S., Douglas, J., Earle, S. and Spurr, S. (eds) (2007b) *Policy and Practice in Promoting Public Health*, London, Sage/Milton Keynes, The Open University.

Mackay, H., Maples, W. and Reynolds, P. (2001) *Investigating the Information Society*, London, Routledge.

Marx, K. and Engels, F. (1998 [1932]) *The German Ideology*, London, Elecbook.

Morris, D. (2001) 'Postmodern illness' in Heller, T., Muston, R., Sidell, M. and Lloyd, C. (eds) *Working for Health*, London, Sage/Milton Keynes, The Open University.

Open University (2004) K223 *Knowledge, Information and Care*, CD-ROM 2 'The evidence base', Section 3, Topic 4, Milton Keynes, The Open University.

Perkins, E.R., Simnett, I. and Wright, L. (1999) *Evidence-Based Health Promotion*, Chichester, Wiley.

Popay, J. and Williams, G. (1996) 'Public health research and lay knowledge', *Social Science and Medicine*, vol. 42, pp. 759–68.

Rissel, C. (1994) 'Empowerment: the holy grail of health promotion?', *Health Promotion International*, vol. 9, no. 1, pp. 39–47.

Scriven, A. (2007) 'Developing healthy alliances through partnership and collaboration' in Lloyd et al. (eds) (2007b).

Stanley, L. and Wise, S. (1993) *Breaking Out Again: Feminist Ontology and Epistemology*, London, Routledge.

Tolley, E.E. and Bentley, M.E. (1996) 'Training issues for the use of participating research methods in health' in de Koning and Martin (eds) (1996).

Weinreich, N.K. (1996) *Integrating Quantitative and Qualitative Methods in Social Marketing Research* [online], http://www.social-marketing.com/research.html (Accessed 2 November 2005).

Williams, G. and Popay, J. (1994) 'Lay knowledge and the privilege of experience' in Gabe, J., Kelleher, D. and Williams, G. (1994) *Challenging Medicine*, London, Routledge.

Done
7/5/10

Chapter 8

Studying the population's health

Moyra Sidell and Cathy Lloyd, incorporating previously published material from Jeanne Katz (2000)

Introduction

There is, in the UK, a 60 per cent rise in chlamydia infection. Syphilis and gonorrhoea are on the increase, while HIV infection is not diminishing. Heart disease kills more people than cancer, and more women are surviving breast cancer. This information appeared in the media at the time of writing (in 2006). Where does this type of information, which is the stuff of public health, actually come from? How is it generated and what purpose does it serve? More importantly, is it credible? This chapter is devoted to exploring these questions in relation to the type of evidence that informs public health policy and practice. Chapter 7 introduced you to the idea of different bodies of knowledge relating to health and illness. These different bodies of knowledge are, in effect, producers of knowledge and information about health and, therefore, as Chapter 7 pointed out, have a profound effect on health policy and practice. This chapter focuses on the production of knowledge about the health of populations, using quantitative methods of inquiry from a biomedical and positivistic social scientific perspective. It starts by considering the major disciplines involved in collecting information about the public's health, those of *demography* (the study of human populations, focusing in particular on numbers of people) and *epidemiology* (the study of the occurrence and spread of illhealth and disease and its relationship to other phenomena). The chapter then moves on in the last section to examine attempts, using positivistic social scientific methods such as surveys, to explore wider aspects of the public's health, including wellbeing, lifestyles and quality of life.

8.1 Demography

Demography provides a framework for studying different aspects of a population, for instance, education and crime, as well as health. Since 1801 a census has been conducted to determine the number of people of different types, groups or categories residing in the UK. Demographers count people according to certain social characteristics such as age, gender, marital status, housing conditions and, more recently, ethnicity. Demography can identify how many people live and/or work in a particular geographical area, what kind of work they do, and the age and gender distribution of that population. It is concerned with change resulting from births, deaths, movement of people and alterations in population characteristics. Demography can also provide statistics on unemployment, indicating the numbers of long-term unemployed people as well as the temporarily unemployed, such as school leavers. Demographic data can be divided into two discrete forms:

1   data gathered through population *censuses*

2   data collected through *registration systems*.

8.1.1 The UK national census

The UK national census gives a snapshot view of individuals at a particular moment in time. The information it yields is about the size and structure of a particular population as it was on census night. Some of the questions in a census relate to people's health directly or indirectly and therefore are of interest to public health. The first modern periodic, direct and complete census took place in the USA in 1790. The first UK census followed shortly after in 1801 and has been repeated decennially on a regular basis, except in 1941 during the Second World War. The 1840 Population Act appointed a Registrar General responsible for a complete census of the population.

Questions asked in censuses have changed over time, reflecting contemporary concerns, and increasingly since 1891 data providing information about aspects of health and lifestyles has been collected. In the 1891 census, questions were asked about the types of dwelling and the number of rooms each household occupied, reflecting concern about overcrowding. From 1911, details were asked about family size, to be considered alongside mortality and morbidity data. The 1921 census contained questions about place of work and methods of transport to work, reflecting growing concern with traffic density. By this time, questions were included about educational level as well as about the ages and numbers of children in the population (for educational planning purposes). Between the 1991 and 2001 census the changes in the nature of the UK population prompted questions about ethnicity. However, issues have been raised concerning the use of ethnicity data in relation to health (Bhopal, 2001; Gunaratnam, 2007).

Social class, on the other hand, has been identified as a major indicator of health (Townsend and Davidson, 1982). The 1921 census redefined occupational classification and introduced five socio-economic groups. This Registrar-General's social classification has been the subject of much debate and controversy, culminating in a reclassification known as the National Statistics Socioeconomic Classification (NS-SEC). This classification was used in the census of 2001 and, although welcomed, this change could cause some problems in comparing the 2001 census with previous ones. The system adopted by the 2001 census is set out in Figure 8.1.

Figure 8.1   Descriptive definitions of NS-SEC categories

Combined NS-SEC category description	NS-SEC category	NS-SEC category description
Managerial and professional occupations	L1, L2	Large employers and higher managerial occupations
	L3	Higher professional occupations
	L4, L5, L6	Lower managerial and professional occupations
Intermediate occupations	L7	Intermediate occupations
	L8, L9	Small employers and own account workers
Routine and manual occupations	L10, L11	Lower supervisory and technical occupations
	L12	Semi-routine occupations
	L13	Routine occupations
Excluded when the classification is collapsed into its analytical classes	L14	Never worked and long-term unemployed
	L15	Full-time students
	L16	Occupation not stated or inadequately described
	L17	Not classifiable for other reasons

(Source: Babb et al., 2004, pp. 107–8)

Since 1911, census data has been analysed mechanically. Initially, data was entered on punch cards and sorted by electrical machines; computers were used for the first time in 1961. The Data Protection Act 1998 ensures that personal and identifiable census information stored on computer files remains confidential. Census data forms the basis of a great deal of statistical information at the national, regional and district level. Indeed, since contemporary censuses extend over some 100,000 separate districts, accurate statistical information about each and every one of them is available. This facilitates accessing information about, for example, lone parents, employment, housing, education and other health-related issues for small areas of the country. The topics covered by the 2001 census are presented in

Box 8.1. The censuses of 1971 and 1981 saw the introduction of a 'cohort study' on a sample section of the population. This is known as the OPCS (Office for Population Censuses and Surveys) longitudinal study, which also links to a wide range of health and social indicators. Babies born on four days in 1971 were identified and followed up in subsequent censuses. This data is used for medical research as well as demographic purposes.

Box 8.1 The 2001 census requested the following information from residents

1 Name
2 Sex
3 Date of birth
4 Marital status
5 Relationship to others in household
6 Student status
7 Term time address of students and school children
8 Usual address one year ago
9 Country of birth
10 Knowledge of Gaelic (Scotland), Welsh (Wales)
11 Ethnic group
12 Religion (not Scotland)
13 General health
14 Long-term illness

15 Provision of unpaid personal care
16 Educational and vocational qualifications
17 Economic activity in the week before the Census
18 Time since last employment
19 Employment status
20 Job title and description of occupation
21 Size of workforce of employing organisation at place of work
22 Nature of employer's business at place of work (industry)
23 Hours worked per week
24 Name of employer (if self-employed give the name and nature of the person's business)
25 Address of place of work
26 Means of travel to work

Questions for households

1 Tenure of accommodation

2 Whether rented
   accommodation
   is furnished or
   unfurnished
   (Scotland only)

3 Type of landlord (for
   households
   in rented
   accommodation)

4 Number of rooms

5 Amenities (bathroom, WC, etc.)

6 Lowest floor level of
   accommodation

7 Number of floor levels in
   the accommodation
   (N. Ireland only)

8 Availability of central
   heating

9 Type of accommodation,
   including whether or not
   it is self-contained

10 Cars and vans (available
   for use)

(Stationery Office, 1999, pp. 9–10)

The census of 2001 included, for the first time, a question specifically on general health in addition to the question on long-term illness. Respondents were asked to assess their own health over the past twelve months as either 'good', 'fairly good', or 'not good', providing subjective quantitative data on general health which is valuable data for public health practitioners. It allows for the comparison of regional variations in self-reported health as shown in the maps of the UK given in Figure 8.2.

8.1.2 Registration systems: counting births and deaths

Demographers count and compare birth and death rates in different places and at different times. These rates are calculated on the basis of returns to the registrar following a birth or death. Since 1836, registration of births and deaths has been compulsory. Prompt registration was encouraged by instituting a fee payable if the birth was not registered within six weeks. Local registrars were responsible for registering deaths and births. This, combined with other kinds of local registration, has facilitated recording movement within different localities and computations of local populations.

Through compulsory recording of deaths (without a death certificate, for example, it is illegal to dispose of a body) the Office for National Statistics (ONS) is able to publish detailed mortality statistics. In addition, using population data from the census, information about mortality in relation to cause of death and occupation is obtained, and this is published every ten years. The combination of mortality and census data facilitates the study of trends and changes in mortality over time. Mortality statistics, then, are based on death certificates which list the name, age and sex of the deceased, the date and place of death and the cause of death.

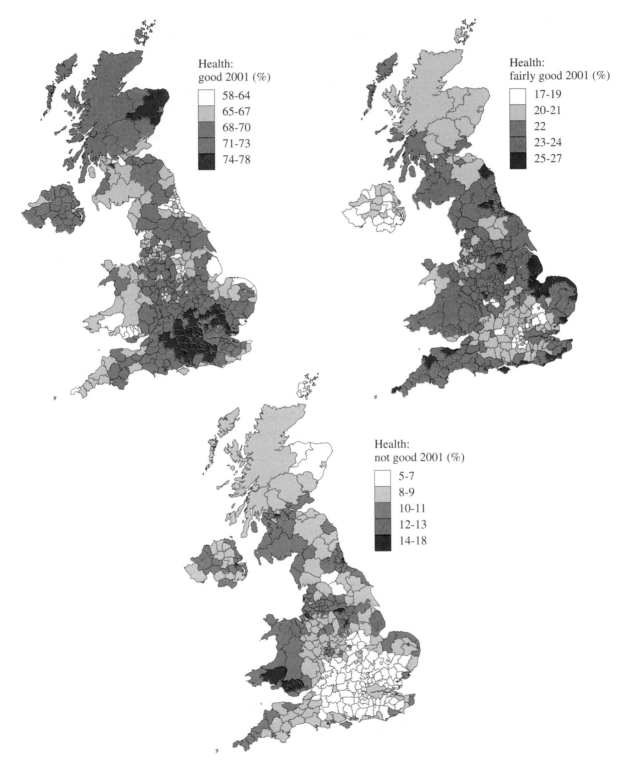

Figure 8.2   Mapping of good and poor health in the UK (Source: Dorling and Thomas, 2004, pp. 134–5)

Thinking point   which aspects of the death certificate might present problems in recording a death?

The accurate assessment of the cause of death is recognised as being problematic. In fact the original death registration bill of 1836 did not include provision for cause of death and it was not until the Births and Deaths Registration Act of 1874 that it became a requirement that the cause of death be recorded by the medical practitioner who last attended the deceased unless there was to be an inquest or post-mortem. This aspect of the death certificate has provided vital epidemiological information for decades, but its usefulness depends on the accuracy with which death certificates are completed. The procedure is that, if the deceased has been seen by a doctor within fourteen days before the death and the circumstances of the death are not suspicious, then the doctor fills in the 'cause of death' box. The death certificate asks the certifier to record direct causes of death as well as contributory causes. But it is the 'underlying' cause of death which is most important and that should appear in the lowest completed line of Part 1 of the death certificate. It is this information on the underlying cause of death which is transformed at the ONS by codifiers into a number which is given to a particular cause of death on a list called the International Classification of Diseases, Injuries and Causes of Death (ICD). For example, cancer of the lung is numbered C34. Routine mortality statistics are based on this classification of the recorded 'underlying' cause of death, but the ONS now also codes additional causes mentioned on a death certificate.

The validity of mortality statistics is dependent on the accuracy and veracity of the certifier. Even when the cause of death is straightforward there is a wide range of factors that can result in reporting differences. For instance, there are variations in diagnostic decisions between countries, between physicians and over time that can influence mortality statistics. In addition, the cause of death mentioned on the death certificate might mask a serious disease problem which is not identified either because the person completing the certificate is unaware of it, or because the dying person or their family put pressure on the doctor certifying the cause to withhold this information.

Thinking point   can you think of such a cause?

Stigmatised causes such as AIDS or suicide, the latter of which is unacceptable for some religions, can be under-reported. Figure 8.3 shows marked international differences in suicide rates.

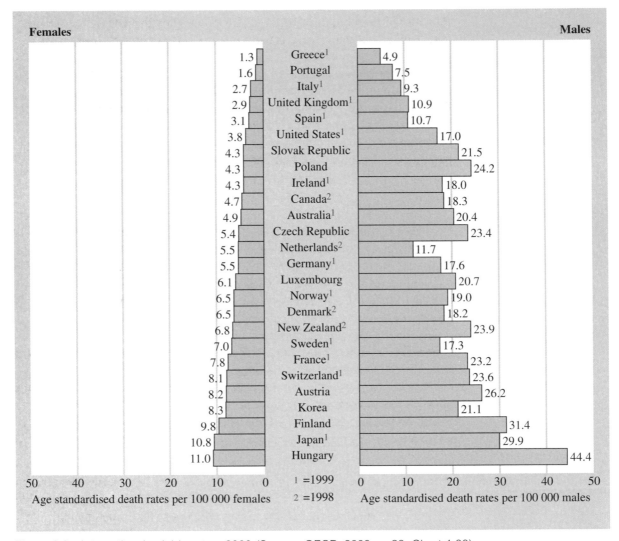

Figure 8.3   International suicide rates, 2000 (Source: OECD, 2003, p. 29, Chart 1.30)

The Organisation for Economic Co-operation and Development (OECD) admits that:

> The international comparability of death rates from suicide can be affected by reporting differences across countries. A stigma is associated with suicide in many countries, and those recording causes of death may come under pressure to record deaths from suicide as 'unknown' or due to other causes. Caution is required therefore in interpreting variations across countries.

(OECD, 2003, p. 28)

Pneumonia might appear on the death certificates of many older people when the actual underlying cause of death was senile dementia, with pneumonia a co-pathology. In fact, there has been much controversy in the past about 'old age' as an acceptable cause of death. Peto (1994) estimated that there may be inaccuracies in 30–50 per cent of cases and that this is likely to be more common in older people where multiple pathologies are likely. Nevertheless, death certificates are, potentially, a rich source of evidence for epidemiology which helps to provide valuable data on the patterns of disease within and between countries.

8.2 Epidemiology

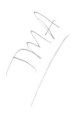

Epidemiology has been defined as 'the study of how often diseases occur in different groups of people and why' (Coggon et al., 2003, p. 1). It is concerned not only with the distribution of disease within a particular group or population, but also with the causes of disease. Epidemiologists are in many ways disease detectives (Bailey et al., 2005), tracking down disease to discover why it occurs as well as when and where it occurs. Although the term 'epidemiology' literally means the 'science of epidemics', it actually has a much broader remit and explains why and how diseases occur and spread, what causes them and how they can be contained. The types of events that are of interest to epidemiology include morbidity (disease), disability, mortality (death), recovery and the use of health services. There is also a whole area known as 'psychiatric epidemiology' where the distribution of, and risk factors for, mental illness are studied.

Epidemiology focuses on populations or communities. These can be very large, such as a nation or continent, or groups within larger populations. So a population such as that of the UK might be broken down into the four nations, or specified health districts. But epidemiology is concerned not just with geographical groupings: often it focuses on such diverse groups as different occupations or residents in nursing homes. The key feature is that it investigates a 'population at risk': 'The population at risk is the group of people, healthy or sick, who would be counted as cases if they had the disease being studied' (Coggon et al., 2003, p. 1). It is therefore important to ensure that the population under study is capable of having the disease or condition.

Thinking point   why might an epidemiologist study pregnant women only?

A reason for studying pregnant women might be to investigate morning sickness or gestational diabetes or the use of antenatal facilities. Studies of prostate cancer, on the other hand, would exclude women.

Epidemiology is the scientific foundation for public health in that it assists in identifying the health problems in particular communities, can assess the relevance of prevention and evaluate the effectiveness of preventive interventions (Tannahill, 1994, p. 97). Public health practitioners rely, to a large extent, on epidemiological data to provide valuable information about the health of their population. It is therefore important to understand the principles behind epidemiological methods and techniques.

Methodologically, epidemiology adheres to the principles of the 'scientific method'. You will recall from Chapter 7 that this is the way of knowing that is considered to be acceptable within biomedicine. The research method embedded in this paradigm falls under the umbrella of quantitative research methods; that is, it emphasises the collection of objective quantifiable data which can then be subjected to statistical procedures. Before exploring some of the methods and procedures used in epidemiology, the origins of modern epidemiology are briefly examined.

8.2.1 Early studies in epidemiology

The following three examples serve to illustrate, albeit very briefly, the origins of modern epidemiology.

In the mid-nineteenth century, Dr John Snow suspected that drinking water might have caused the spread of cholera in Soho, London. He plotted all the cholera cases in Soho on a local map and noted that they clustered around Broad Street, which had a water pump. He found that people who had drunk water provided by a particular water company were more likely to have developed cholera than those who had not. Snow's interest was not so much in treating the individuals with cholera as in the *patterns* of where the victims lived and where they obtained their water supply, so that he could prevent further spread of the disease. Thus, the link between the water and cholera was established before it was understood precisely what was in the water that caused the illness. Hence, the epidemiological explanation preceded the biological explanation and was able to halt the rapid spread of the disease.

There are two twentieth-century parallels to this nineteenth-century example: the link between smoking and increased incidence of lung cancer (Doll and Hill, 1950) and AIDS, for which understanding of the biology of the disease is far behind epidemiological explanations of how the infection spreads. Epidemiology can, thus, help identify populations or certain groups with an above-average death rate, or high disease rates, and that information is essential to all those involved in working towards equality in health.

There are two broad types of epidemiological inquiry: one is descriptive, the other analytic. Although they are interdependent, they use different methods. Before exploring the scope of these two types of epidemiology, the basic levels of measurement are explained. These are measures of deaths in a population (mortality) and measures of disease in a population (morbidity).

8.2.2 Measures of mortality and morbidity

Mortality statistics

Mortality data from death certificates and from census and population registers are routinely collected; from these the death rate in a population can be calculated. To calculate a death rate the number of deaths recorded is divided by the number of people in the population, and then multiplied by 100, 1,000 or another convenient figure.

The *crude death rate* shows the number of deaths in the total population and, for the sake of manageability, is usually calculated per 1,000. It is calculated as follows:

The annual *crude death rate* per 1,000 population $= \dfrac{\text{Total number of deaths in a calendar year}}{\text{Estimated mid-year population that year}} \times 1{,}000$

Crude death rates do not show the burden of deaths in particular groups in the population. For example, one might assume that a town such as Bournemouth is an unhealthy place because it has a high crude death rate, but on closer examination this is found to be due to the fact that it is a popular place to retire to and so has a high proportion of older people. To counter this problem, *age-specific* rates can be calculated as follows:

The annual *age-specific death rate* for the age group 25–50 years per 1,000 population $= \dfrac{\text{Total number of deaths among people aged 25–50 years during a calendar year}}{\text{Estimated mid-year population aged 25–50 that year}} \times 1{,}000$

As well as straightforward age-specific rates, certain special age rates can be calculated which are of particular importance in public health. The infant mortality rate (IMR) is used as an indicator of the overall health of a nation or community because this rate correlates well with young adult mortality, but is more sensitive to socio-economic and environmental improvements as well as to improvements in healthcare. The IMR is calculated as follows:

The annual *infant mortality rate* per 1,000 live births $=$ Total number of deaths under the age of one year during a calendar year/total number of $\times$ 1,000 live births in that year

Other special rates of deaths in infants under one year of age include the annual stillbirth rate, late foetal deaths after 24 weeks of gestation and the annual perinatal mortality rate (stillbirths plus deaths in the first week of life), and are calculated in the same way as infant mortality. Figure 8.4 shows these rates for the UK in 2003.

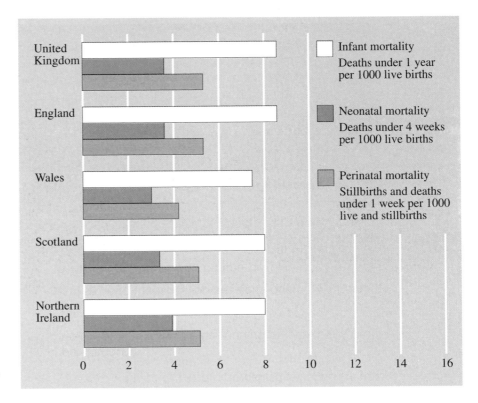

Figure 8.4   Infant neonatal and perinatal mortality rates, 2003 (Source: Glickman et al., 2006, p. 33, Figure 2.3)

The death rates discussed above are based on all causes of death. The cause-specific death rate is used to calculate how many deaths occurred from specific diseases such as cancer or heart disease. This would be calculated as follows:

$$\text{The annual } \textit{cause-specific death rate} \text{ per 1,000 population} = \frac{\text{Total number of deaths from a particular cause during a calendar year}}{\text{Estimated mid-year population in that year}} \times 1,000$$

The calculations made so far can provide the overall crude death rate for a population, the death rate for different age groups and deaths from different causes, but do not allow for a comparison to be made between one part of the country and another. For instance, as we noted above, south coast resorts such as Bournemouth have a preponderance of older people and consequently a high death rate, whereas a population with a high proportion of young people, as in a new town, is likely to have a low death rate. A direct comparison of crude mortality rates for the two localities would obviously produce a distorted picture. So the death rate for a specific condition in a particular area may be higher than the national average simply because the area contains relatively more residents in a susceptible age group than the national population. *Standardised Mortality Ratios* (SMR) can compare mortality rates between different geographical areas, taking age differences into account. (How an SMR is calculated in given in Box 8.2.) So despite the very different age structures of the populations involved, regional comparisons can be made, as Figure 8.5 demonstrates for cities in Wales.

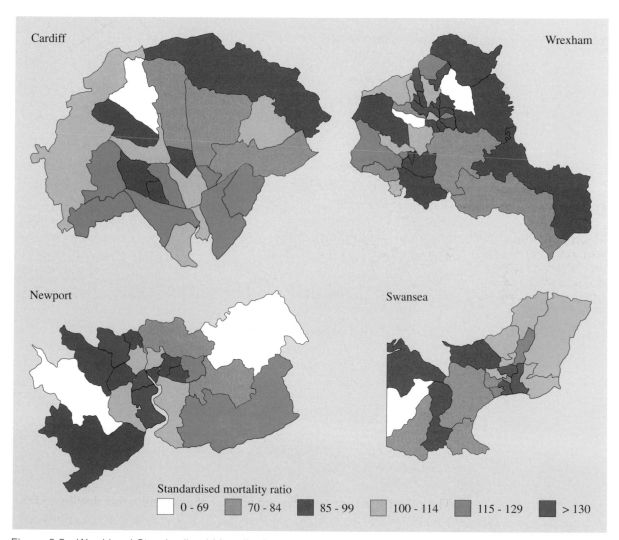

Figure 8.5   Ward-level Standardised Mortality Ratios for four major cities, 1990–92 (all causes; ages 0–74) (Source: Williams et al., 1994, Figure 4.4)

Box 8.2 Calculating a Standardised Mortality Ratio

Death rates for age groups (or other groups) in the standard [national] population are multiplied by the population of the same groups in the study population. This produces an 'expected' number of deaths representing what the number of deaths in the study population would have been, if that population had the same death rates as the standard population. The observed (or actual) number of deaths in the study population is then divided by the total expected number and multiplied by 100. This produces an *SMR*. The standard population always has an SMR of 100, with which the SMR of the study population can be compared. The SMR figure is actually a percentage. This means that if the study population's SMR is 130, its death rate is 30% higher than that of the standard population. If the study population's SMR is 86, then its death rate is 14% lower than that of the standard population.

(Stewart, 2002, p. 80)

As well as comparing death rates for different regions the SMR can be used to compare the death rates in other groupings of the population; for instance, between different occupational groups. The SMR for male bus drivers between the ages of 25 and 65 in the UK in 2000 would be calculated as:

$$\frac{\text{Observed deaths in male bus drivers in the UK aged 25--65 years}}{\text{Expected deaths of male bus drivers based on male death rates in UK, aged 25--65}} \times 100$$

A somewhat tongue-in-cheek study reported in the *British Medical Journal* (Crayford et al., 1997) used SMRs to study the death rates of characters in soap operas on British television. They found that being a character in *EastEnders* was the most dangerous job in Britain, as Figure 8.6 shows.

Figure 8.6   Standardised Mortality Ratios for various high-risk groups in comparison with the general population

	SMR
EastEnders characters	771
Formula One drivers	581
Coronation Street characters	353
Oil rig divers	235
Bomb disposal experts	196
Steeplejacks	148
General population	100

(Source: Crayford et al., 1997, p. 27)

So far we have been focusing on mortality data, but how is the distribution of morbidity measured?

Morbidity statistics

Epidemiology also involves estimating the frequency and distribution of diseases in populations. Measures of disease frequency are tools with which to describe how common an illness is in relation to the size of the population (the population at risk). These measures count the number of cases in a population and a measure in time. The two main types of measure of disease frequency are incidence and prevalence.

1   **Incidence**   This is the number of new cases of a disease or disorder that arises in a defined population over a defined period of time.

Incidence rates are calculated as follows:

$$\text{The } \textit{incidence rate} \text{ per 1,000 population} = \frac{\text{The number of new cases of a disease occurring in a population during a specified time period}}{\text{The population at risk during that period of time}} \times 1{,}000$$

(Source: Royal Free Medical School, 2001, p. 83)

The specified time period is usually a calendar year. Therefore, to calculate the incidence of ovarian cancer in women in Wales in 2002 per 1,000 of the population, you would need to divide the number of new cases of ovarian cancer in women in Wales by the number of women resident in Wales in 2002 and then multiply by 1,000.

Figure 8.7 shows the number of newly diagnosed cases of chlamydia infection in the UK in 2002. It gives new cases of chlamydia diagnosed in genito-urinary medicine (GUM) clinics in England, Wales and Scotland.

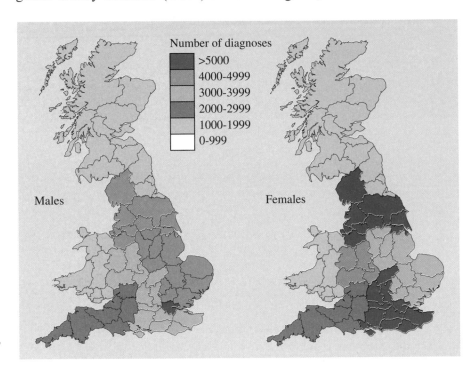

Figure 8.7   Map of new cases of chlamydia in 2002 (Source: Health Protection Agency, 2003, p. 28, Figure 7a)

Thinking point   what additional information would you need in order to calculate the incidence of chlamydia in a given area: for example, Scotland?

You would need the actual numbers of men and women in Scotland. If you wanted to calculate the age-specific incidence rate for men and women, because chlamydia infection is higher in younger adults, then you would need the new cases of chlamydia broken down by age as well as by sex. You would then need the numbers of men and women in different age groups in Scotland. Incidence, of course, only applies to reported and diagnosed cases of chlamydia. The actual size of the problem is likely to be higher. The same applies to prevalence rates.

2   **Prevalence**   This is the total number of people suffering from a specific disease at a certain point in time. Prevalence studies are commonly used to survey characteristics such as smoking habits or alcohol use.

Prevalence rates are calculated as follows:

$$\begin{array}{l}\text{The } \textit{point} \\ \textit{prevalence} \\ \textit{rate} \text{ per 1,000} \\ \text{population}\end{array} = \frac{\text{The number of existing cases of the disease in the population at a specified moment in time}}{\text{The population at risk at that specified time; for example, June 2000}} \times 1{,}000$$

$$\begin{array}{l}\textit{The period} \\ \textit{prevalence} \\ \textit{rate} \text{ per 1,000} \\ \text{population}\end{array} = \frac{\text{The number of existing cases of the disease present in the population during a specified time period}}{\text{The population at risk during that specified period of time; for example, June 1990 to June 1995}} \times 1{,}000$$

(Source: Royal Free Medical School, 2001, p. 83)

Incidence and prevalence rates can be calculated separately for men and women. Figure 8.8 shows the period prevalence rates of chlamydia, gonorrhoea and genital herpes simplex for Scotland between 1992 and 2002.

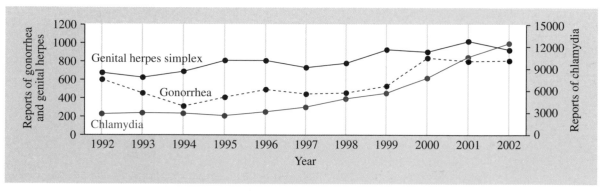

Figure 8.8   Laboratory reports for chlamydia, gonorrhoea and genital herpes simplex for Scotland, 1992–2002 (Source: Health Protection Agency, 2003, p. 29, Figure 7b)

These measures of morbidity, as well as those of mortality, are the raw data used in both descriptive and analytic epidemiology.

8.2.3 Descriptive epidemiology

A large part of the epidemiological task is concerned with surveillance. Public Health Departments and agencies such as the Health Protection Agency quite literally keep watch on the incidence and prevalence of disease in the population. Data on these is collected regularly and routinely from a range of sources throughout the UK. Sources of morbidity data in the community include those listed in Box 8.3 (all of which can be found on the ONS website, http://www.statistics.gov.uk).

Box 8.3 Sources of morbidity data in the community

1 **Cancer registers** These are a national record of newly diagnosed cases of cancer in England and Wales. The following information is recorded: site of the primary tumour and type of growth; place of birth; usual place of residence of patient; age; sex; occupation; social class; initial treatment date; duration of survival and date of death.

2 **Hospital episode statistics** These comprise an annual report based on a 25 per cent sample of finished consultant episodes in all NHS hospitals. Data on the principal diagnosis and operative procedure are provided by age, sex and region of the patients.

3 **Psychiatric morbidity** Since 1993 a series of surveys on the mental health of the population of Great Britain has been commissioned by the Department of Health, the Scottish Executive and the National Assembly for Wales (or their predecessors). The series began with a survey of the adult population aged between sixteen and sixty-four, living in private households in Great Britain. Since then, additional surveys have covered children aged five to fifteen, living in private households; prisoners in England and Wales; and five of the main minority ethnic groups in England (Bangladeshi, Black Caribbean, Indian, Irish and Pakistani people), together with a general population White group to provide a point of comparison.

4 **Key health statistics for general practice** The report *Key Health Statistics from General Practice* (Office for National Statistics, 1998) was the third in a series of morbidity and treatment data derived from the General Practice Research Database which holds anonymised, patient-based clinical records submitted regularly by general practices.

Other sources of data include:

- notifiable industrial diseases
- notification of congenital malformations
- Royal College Confidential Inquiries, including suicides and maternal mortality.

(Adapted from Royal Free Medical School, 2001, pp. 84, 85)

Notifiable diseases

The diseases listed opposite are notifiable and should be reported to the Office of National Statistics.

Anthrax	Malaria	Acute poliomyelitis paralytic non-paralytic	Tuberculosis (all forms)
Cholera	Measles	Rabies	Typhoid fever
Diphtheria	Meningitis	Relapsing fever	Typhus fever
Dysentery	Meningococcal septicaemia (without meningitis)	Rubella	Viral haemorrhagic fever
Acute encephalitis infective post-infectious	Mumps	Scarlet fever	Viral hepatitis
Food poisoning	Ophthalmia neonatorum	Smallpox	Whooping cough
Leptospirosis	Paratyphoid fever Plague	Tetanus	Yellow fever

(Adapted from Royal Free Medical School, 2001, p. 87)

As well as the basic data on incidence and prevalence of disease, epidemiology is particularly interested in the patterns of disease distribution in human populations. In particular, it aims to discover who develops health problems, when they contract illness and in which locations a problem is particularly prevalent. Thus disease is studied in relation to *persons*, *place* and *time*. Each of these is considered in turn below.

Persons: which groups in the population have health problems?

In order to discover the patterns of disease distribution, data is needed on the personal characteristics of the population: the age groups, proportions of men and women, and occupational groups. Other population variables that are important are the social circumstances and conditions in which people live, as well as their religion, culture and ethnic origin. This is important since there are associations between these variables and the health status of individuals.

Thinking point   look at Figure 8.9 which illustrates the prevalence of hazardous drinking by age and sex. Which age groups do you think are most at risk?

You will see that, for women, the greatest prevalence is between 16 and 19, after which it declines steadily. For men, it peaks around 20–24, but has always been higher than for women. However, women are at particular risk because physiologically they are less tolerant of alcohol than men.

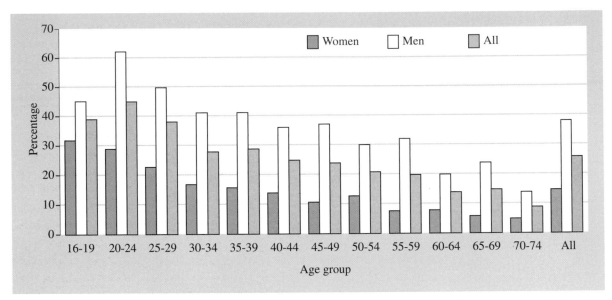

Figure 8.9   Prevalence of hazardous drinking by age and sex, UK, 2000 (Source: Singleton et al., 2001, p. 28, Figure 2.6)

Place: where do the problems occur?

The cholera epidemic of the 1850s, mentioned in Section 8.2.1, demonstrates the influence of geographical and environmental factors on the occurrence of disease. Disease patterns also vary internationally; for example, the global pandemic of HIV infection is not geographically uniformly distributed (United Nations, 1998), as Figure 8.10 shows.

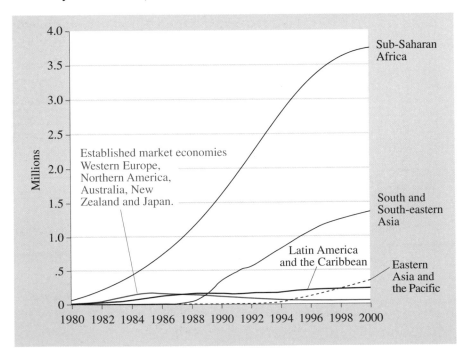

Figure 8.10   Annual number of new HIV infections, selected world regions (Source: United Nations, 1998, p. 25, Figure V)

Within countries, regional variations in the occurrence of diseases are not uncommon. In addition, differences in disease patterns between urban and rural communities are frequently observed. Even within one health district, mortality rates due to particular diseases may vary from one electoral ward to another.

Studies of immigrant populations focus on separate groups within geographical areas. One such population was that which migrated from Japan to the USA between 1890 and 1924. It was found that heart disease in Japan was only one-quarter the rate of that in the USA, whereas stroke and cerebral haemorrhage were two or three times more common (Marmot et al., 1975). Stomach cancer was five times more common in Japan, but cancer of the breast and prostate were very uncommon; cancer of the cervix was twice as common in Japan as in the USA. As the Japanese population settled in the USA, some of their disease patterns changed, and conditions such as stroke, cerebral haemorrhage and cancer of the cervix approached the rates of the community to which they had migrated. This suggests that environmental factors played a considerable part in the causation of these particular diseases. Cancer of the stomach also declined, but not to a very great extent (Hirayama et al., 1980). Cancer of the breast, however, did not alter significantly when the population had settled in the USA.

Caution must be exercised when making international comparisons of illhealth. In developing countries, access to biomedical treatment and the availability of facilities for investigation can be restricted. This means that there may be problems with the accuracy and completeness of diagnosis. The age structure of the population in developing countries, with a greater proportion of young people than in the industrialised world, also makes comparisons of disease frequency difficult.

Time: when do health problems occur?

The question of when (in time) diseases occur or peak is of considerable interest in epidemiology. For example, it is well established that a range of well-known infectious diseases (e.g. measles, influenza and whooping cough) show cyclical variations in occurrence, which result in epidemics every few years.

Thinking point   look at Figure 8.11 and identify in which years notifications about pertussis (whooping cough) cases peaked.

You will note that, in 1978, over 60,000 cases were reported and this fell dramatically in 1981, only to rise again in 1982. The rises may be explained by media coverage of the dangers of the vaccine in the mid-1970s and then again in the early 1980s.

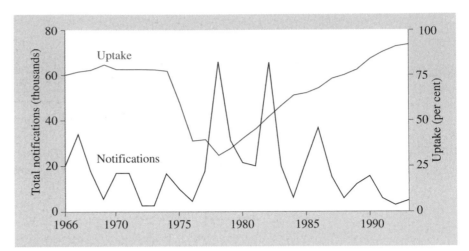

Figure 8.11   Pertussis notifications and immunisation uptake, 1966 to 1993 (England and Wales) (Source: Katz et al., 2000, p. 235, Figure 13.4)

When considering time in relation to the occurrence of diseases, it has to be noted that time can be measured in a variety of ways: as secular time (referring to centuries), as cyclical time or time intervals such as five yearly, as seasonal time (i.e. summer, autumn, winter and spring), or by specifying particular times of the week or times of the day. In relation to 'secular time' in the UK and elsewhere, infectious diseases constituted a major health problem throughout the nineteenth century. Fortunately, most of these diseases have declined and some, such as smallpox, have almost been eliminated. By the end of the twentieth century, however, heart disease and cancer had become the major health problems.

Seasonal variations in the incidence of disease are most common for respiratory tract infections (during winter months). Salmonella food poisoning also frequently shows seasonal variations, with peaks during the summer and in the Christmas period. Hay fever and other allergies occur primarily in the early summer.

Outbreaks of diseases can also be related to specific points in time, locations or events. For example, the sudden occurrence of infection such as typhoid or salmonella food poisoning is usually due to the simultaneous (or near simultaneous) exposure of groups of susceptible people to a certain micro-organism, as might happen at a wedding reception or in a hotel.

Despite considerable evidence about the influence various factors have on people's health, epidemiologists cannot infer that the link between a factor and illhealth is a causal one. However, descriptive studies give an indication of the cause of a disease, but special studies in epidemiology can explore causation further.

8.2.4 Analytic epidemiology

Causation of illhealth is difficult to determine. Apart from infectious diseases, most evidence relates to the risk associated with particular factors, rather than the direct causes of illhealth. Even in the case of infectious diseases, it is not known why certain people succumb to them when other seemingly similar people do not. Only certain types of causative mechanism are amenable to investigation by epidemiological methods and few diseases can be said to have a single cause. Epidemiological evidence regarding disease causation is mainly circumstantial. So how can the information on persons, place and time help in the understanding of the causes of disease? An important model, originally developed for use with infectious diseases, but which has been adapted for much broader use in recent years, is the *epidemiological triad.*

The epidemiological triad

The epidemiological triad is best represented diagrammatically (see Figure 8.12). This represents the interaction between an agent, host or persons and environment or place within a specific time dimension. The epidemiological triad can be applied to non-infectious diseases where the agent could be 'unhealthy behaviours, unsafe practices, or unintended exposures to hazardous substances' (Miller, 2002, p. 64).

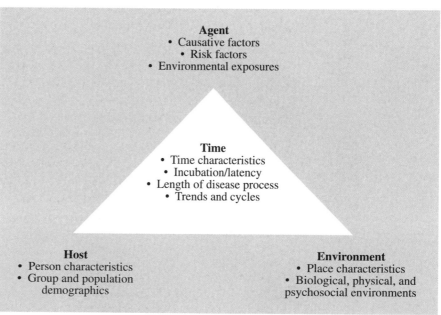

Figure 8.12   The epidemiological triad (Miller, 2002, p. 63, Figure 3.1)

Within the epidemiological triad the agent is known as a 'necessary' factor. It has to be present for morbidity, although it may not inevitably lead to disease. For the disease to occur it needs the combination of what have been called 'sufficient' factors. These would include a host, which might be an individual or group of individuals who are susceptible to the agent. Susceptibility might be on the basis of age, sex, ethnic group or occupation. Environmental factors can also be sufficient factors that combine with the agent.

With reference to the case of chlamydia as the agent in Figure 8.7, there is some very limited information on the hosts and their environment within a particular timescale (i.e. 2002). The map in Figure 8.7 shows the geographical distribution of male and female cases of chlamydia reported in genito-urinary medicine clinics. The source of that data – the statistical returns made from GUM clinics (the KC60 form) – records age as well as sex. This indicates that the highest rates of diagnoses were among women aged between aged 16 and 19 and men aged between 20 and 24, and that the rate for women begins to fall dramatically after the age of 24 (Health Protection Agency, 2003). In order to contribute to causal understanding, Bhopal suggests that three main questions need to be asked:

1   How does the pattern of disease vary over time in this population?

2   How does the place in which the population lives affect the disease pattern?

3   How do the personal characteristics of the people in the population affect the disease pattern?

(Bhopal, 2002, p. 18)

Thinking point   which of the three questions do you think would be the most fruitful line of investigation in the case of a sexually transmitted disease?

The third question about personal characteristics would seem most useful because the risk factor is behavioural in that the practice of safe sex seems to be important.

However, identifying causal variables is far from straightforward. Aggleton (1990) cites three conditions identified by Armstrong (1983) which must be met before two variables can be said to be causally related. These are outlined below:

1   The variable must be in the correct temporal sequence. The variable which is thought to be the cause must precede the one that it is predicted to affect.

2   There must be a correlation between the variables that are believed to be related. As one varies, so should the other. Correlations can be positive; that is, when one variable increases, so does the other. They can also be negative; that is, as one increases, the other decreases.

3   There must be no hidden or confounding variable (i.e. a variable that could also be a causative factor) causing both of the variables to change.

(Adapted from Aggleton, 1990, pp. 77–8)

8.2.5 Types of epidemiological studies

Epidemiological studies generally fall into four broad categories:

1   cross-sectional studies
2   case-control studies
3   cohort studies
4   intervention studies.

Each of these is addressed in turn below.

Cross-sectional studies

Cross-sectional studies measure the prevalence of conditions or characteristics of people in a population at a point in time or over a short period. Although they are essentially descriptive studies, their results can often suggest causative or risk factors associated with particular illness or behaviour; for instance, the causal relationship between cataracts and vitamin status was originally investigated through a cross-sectional study (Coggon et al., 2003). They may also be used to ascertain the prevalence of a health-related behaviour, such as the wearing of seat belts or participation in exercise. In cross-sectional studies, it is not always necessary to investigate the whole population: a sample is usually sufficient, provided that the individuals in the sample are representative of the total group under consideration. Cross-sectional studies are useful in planning public health interventions, something you will consider in Chapter 10.

A population or group can be studied in a variety of ways: by questionnaire, by taking measurements (such as blood pressure), by analysing blood specimens (e.g. for blood cholesterol levels), or by examining healthcare records.

Case-control studies

These focus on determining disease causation. The 'case' is a person who has a particular symptom or medical condition. Thus, the focus is on a group of cases which is then compared with a 'control group' consisting of persons not having the symptom or the medical condition. Investigations are then carried out into the previous exposure of the two groups to particular factors that are suspected of causing the symptom or condition. If the two groups differ regarding their exposure to such factors, a causal link between the symptom/condition and the factor is inferred.

A classic example of a case-control study was the important study reported by Herbst et al. (1971) and Herbst and Scully (1980), in which a clinician noticed a cluster of unusual cancers in adolescent girls. On investigation, it was found that the mothers of these girls had been treated with a hormone during pregnancy, while the mothers of the adolescent girls in the control group had not. (The particular hormone had been prescribed to prevent miscarriages in the girls' mothers, but no one had suspected that their children might develop cancer.)

Cohort studies

These focus on groups of people who show certain attributes or characteristics (e.g. with respect to their health behaviour). The groups are then observed over a period of time in order to discover what happens to their individual members and to check whether there are any associations between behaviour and the development of disease. In this way the famous epidemiologist, Sir Richard Doll, and colleagues investigated doctors' smoking habits and *prospectively* followed the sample over forty years, by which time two-thirds of the sample had died. The finding obtained during the first twenty years was that doctors who were heavy cigarette smokers were thirty-two times more likely to die of lung cancer than doctors who were non-smokers (Doll and Peto, 1976). Mortality associated with smoking doubled during the second half of the study (Doll et al., 1994). Examples of cohort studies include the National Study of Health and Growth of School Children, started in 1974 (Stamatakis et al., 2005), and the Millennium baby study (Millennium Cohort Study, 2006).

Longitudinal studies are a form of cohort studies, which study groups of people over time; they can be retrospective as well as prospective. Longitudinal studies can be very costly in time and money and require the following up of subjects, which may prove difficult. However, they have the advantage of being able to accumulate very useful information for the determination of the long-term effects of biological, environmental and social factors on health. For example, comparing cohorts born every twelve years – say, in 1946, 1958 and 1970 – could throw light on the effects of changes in social and health policy and education on beliefs about diet, smoking, exercise and other issues of interest to those engaged in promoting public health.

Intervention studies

Whereas the types of study described so far, including case-control studies, are purely observational in nature (i.e. they only observe what is happening), intervention studies involve intervening with a group of people, and include an equivalent group which acts as a 'control'. The most popular study of this kind is the *randomised controlled trial* (RCT). RCTs divide the population to be studied into groups on a random basis; one group is then subjected to a treatment, procedure or intervention, the other not. If the two groups are matched in terms of their characteristics, then any measurable differences between them should be due to the intervention. Ideally, the RCT should be carried out using a double-blind method: that is, neither the researcher nor the subject knows who is in the intervention or control arm of the study.

Intervention studies are conducted in the following way. Initially, observations (or measurements) are made on a population which is then divided (by random sampling) into two equivalent groups. Of these, one is subjected to the intervention. After some predetermined period following the intervention, the observations are repeated and the results for the two groups compared to establish whether or not the intervention had any effect.

Drug trials are by far the most common type of intervention studies. Their purpose is to discover the effects and effectiveness of new drugs developed by the pharmaceutical industry. Objections to trials such as these are often on ethical grounds. If a study is investigating the effects of a particular treatment on cancer sufferers, for instance, then it could be seen as unethical to withhold the potentially beneficial treatment from the control group who would also need to be cancer sufferers. However, conventionally, the control group would be receiving the current best treatment. Other ethical problems relate to whether the participants are fully informed about the potential effects of participating. The 1964 Declaration of Helsinki on medical ethics (see World Medical Organisation, 1996) makes it clear that RCT participants must receive adequate information about the aims, methods, expected benefits and possible hazards involved in the intervention. Participants must feel free to withdraw without putting at risk their previous treatment.

Thinking point   can you think of any groups in the population who may be vulnerable to exploitation in RCTs?

Older people have traditionally been highly deferential to the medical profession and may feel that they cannot refuse to take part for fear of losing the goodwill of their doctor. Also, great care needs to be taken with people for whom English is not their first language to ensure that they fully understand what is involved. To safeguard the rights of vulnerable groups, all trials must gain ethical approval from local ethical committees before they are allowed to recruit people to their study.

Randomised controlled trials use an experimental approach which is largely restricted to single-factor interventions and interventions in closed systems such as schools or health clinics, because these are the contexts in which it is possible to exercise more control and to have more knowledge about the various factors that may influence the outcomes. The experimental approach assumes a greater degree of control over extraneous factors than is usually possible or desirable in most social settings.

Thinking point   what might be the main problems with trying to use an experimental approach in public health settings?

The random assignment of people in a community to intervention and control groups can be problematic given that people are social and cultural beings whose lives cannot become separated from one another. Many interventions are meant to influence whole communities and in these situations the problem of trying to create experimental conditions is great.

Quasi-experimental design

One response to some of these difficulties has been to use a modified or quasi-experimental design. Instead of using a control group formed by random assignment, the investigator may choose a highly comparable but not randomly selected comparison group.

An alternative method is to identify the control group as those individuals who will be exposed to the intervention eventually but are on a 'waiting list', and are thus termed a 'waiting-list control group'. Even so, the question remains as to how useful experimental and quasi-experimental designs are in public health. Here is one view relating to health education that reflects the gap between experimental design and the demands of normal practice settings:

> In practical terms it can be difficult to plan and implement fully controlled experimental studies of health education activities. The use of laboratory type conditions can be both artificial and inappropriate and where interventions have been tested in such artificial situations we have to ask questions about the generalizability of findings to the real world. Even when experimental studies in health education have taken place in normal practice settings the outcomes which result from the extra efforts which typically go into an evaluated study may be an unrealistic guide to what can be achieved in routine practice. Finally, while experiments can establish statistical significance, it may be more important to focus on practical significance.
>
> (Tones and Tilford, 1994, p. 59)

Some of these tensions are explored further in Chapters 10 and 11, where the practical use of all the measurements are examined. However, so far this chapter has focused on studying illhealth and disease. How can the health of a population in a more positive sense be studied? The next section looks at surveys which address a broad range of factors in relation to health.

8.3 Health surveys

A range of health-related surveys has been carried out regularly by the Office for National Statistics (ONS) since the Second World War when the Social Survey Division monitored population morale as well as diet during food rationing and sickness absences from work. In addition, in contrast to the census, government agencies commission other studies to elicit opinion or attitude; for example, those undertaken by the Social and Community Planning Research Organisation. The General Household Survey: Living in Britain (undertaken by the ONS) collects information annually from 12,500 households on five topics: population and family, housing, employment, education, and health. The Health Survey for England is carried out annually for the Department of Health, and there is comparative data available for Wales and Scotland. The annual National Food Survey reports on expenditure on food and dietary patterns for a representative sample of the population. Since very close links exist between diet and health, this is a particularly useful source of information about the types of food that make up a typical British diet; and, additionally, it looks at the relationship between income and diet. As well as these annual national surveys there is a plethora of surveys which focus on the health of different groups in the population; for instance, the Health Survey for England 1999, which focused on the health of minority ethnic groups (Erens et al., 2001); the ONS Disability Surveys; the labour force surveys covering the population eligible for work, which ask about health problems that affect work; and dental health surveys. In addition, many surveys are carried out at the local level. For example, Mid Devon County Council regularly surveys its citizens' panel, asking questions about transport and housing that are relevant to health.

8.3.1 What is a survey?

It is hard to escape surveys. They come in all shapes and sizes and, although they relate to vastly different subjects, they do all have some things in common. The survey is a method of researching a population or a sample of that population. As Aldridge and Levine (2001, p. 5) put it, a survey is strategic: 'The strategy involved in a survey is that *we collect the same information about all the cases in a sample*'. The items of information gathered are known as variables.

Surveys can focus on factual variables such as age, sex, socio-economic circumstances and, in the case of health surveys, measurements of health status. They frequently explore attitudes, beliefs and opinions and they can gather information on behaviours, all of which can inform public health.

Scope of health-related surveys

It was noted in Section 8.1.1 that the 2001 census included, for the first time, a question on general health, asking people to rate their health as 'good', 'fairly good' or 'not good', as well as a question about long-standing illness or disability. Before that the only other national large-scale regular survey to ask those two questions was the General Household Survey (GHS). This is an annual survey of around 17,000 people which has been conducted by the ONS since 1971. As well as the two core questions about general health it asks a wide range of questions about socio-economic conditions. Every alternate year it asks about health-related behaviours such as smoking and drinking. In 1994 it asked questions on the causes of long-standing illness. In 1998 and 2001 data was collected on the use of the internet, mobile phones and other consumer durables. Its 2002 edition, 'Living in Britain', investigated the notion of social capital, to which you were introduced in Chapter 3. This range of variables enables researchers to link health to a much broader social model, and so can throw light on and monitor the determinants of health and inequalities in health. Researchers can access the findings and carry out further statistical analysis on variables that interest them. For instance, they may want to draw out the links between those who rate their general health as 'good' with measures of social capital.

The Health Survey for England (HSFE) is, as its title suggests, a dedicated health survey. It was started in 1991 and has been carried out annually since then. It combines a health interview with a physical examination carried out by a qualified nurse. It now interviews similar numbers to the GHS. As well as core questions asked annually, it takes a different focus each year. In 2002, it focused on the health of children and young people and on maternal health.

However, although covering some behaviours, neither the GHS nor the HSFE are concerned with attitudes and opinions. Other surveys do cover these aspects. At the national level, the British Social Attitudes (BSA) survey is carried out annually and monitors the nation's attitudes to a whole range of issues, from religious affiliation to membership of community organisations and participation in voluntary activities, to the impact of transport policies on car use. The BSA survey covers England, Wales and Scotland.

The King's Fund, an independent foundation which undertakes research and health policy analysis, carried out a survey in 2004 into *Public Attitudes to Public Health Policy* which was mentioned in Chapter 1. They interviewed 1,002 members of the public about their 'health expectations', their views on 'individual responsibility and control', the 'role of government' and the 'role of the NHS' (Kings Fund, 2004, pp. 4, 5). They found a great deal of support for a public smoking ban. With regard to diet and nutrition, they found that government action to ensure that schools provide only healthy meals was very popular. Eighty-two per cent would support laws to limit levels of salt, fat and sugar in foods and 73 per cent would support government action to stop junk foods and sweets being advertised to children. The bar diagram in Figure 8.13 shows the percentage of people who agreed with statements about the role of government. This provides useful information on public health (for the full report see Kings Fund, 2004).

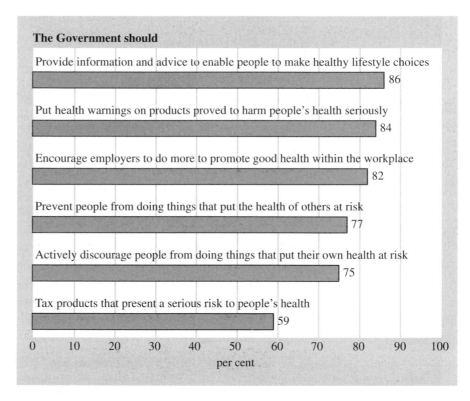

Figure 8.13   Percentage of people who agreed with statements about the role of government (Source: Kings Fund, 2004, p. 13. Figure 3)

Another important area of health surveying is the often quite difficult and contentious attempt to measure quality of life. It has been argued that 'social, lifestyle, and psychological factors account for 50 per cent of preventable morbidity and mortality' (McHorney, 2000, p. 352). There is little national data on quality of life, although much information is collected on what might be considered to be 'indicators' of quality of life; for example, lifestyle, social exclusion, poverty, mental health or transport. Smaller scale but still large surveys of quality of life are frequently carried out, often using well-known instruments such as the General Health Questionnaire (with its mental health focus) or the SF-36 questionnaire, which takes a multidimensional approach to measuring life quality (including physical, mental and emotional wellbeing). (Further information about these can be found at http://www.workhealth.org/UCLA%20OHP%20class%202004/GHQ%20and%20scoring.pdf and http://www.sf-36.org [accessed 24 November 2006].)

Health-related quality of life has increasingly come to be recognised as an important factor in the measurement of health status. But it is notoriously difficult to measure, as Bowling points out: 'Quality of life and health related quality of life are multi-level and amorphous concepts, and both are increasingly popular as end points in the evaluation of public policy ... But the wider research community has accepted no common definition or definitive theoretical framework of quality of life' (Bowling, 2005, p. 7)

Arguments abound about what makes up quality of life and therefore what should and could be measured. Bowling (2005) goes into the complexity of the concept of health-related quality of life, which she describes as an interaction of subjective and objective dimensions, and reviews a plethora of multidimensional measurements of quality of life which are used in surveys. However, as she points out, breaking down the concept into many parts and measuring them separately defeats the object because simply summing the parts does not allow for the dynamic interaction of the parts. Others have argued for a unidimensional quality of life rating (Beckie and Hayduk, 1997, cited in Bowling, 2005), simply asking 'How do you feel about your life as a whole?' As McHorney (2000) argues, this type of question in a cross-sectional survey only indicates the way the person was feeling at the time of the survey and could certainly change over time and in different circumstances. This problem of trying to measure such a subjective concept using quantitative measures applies, of course, to many of the variables measured in health surveys, and it is one of the criticisms to which we will return at the end of this section.

8.3.2 Characteristics of surveys

Surveys fall mainly within the quantitative research paradigm in that they aim to quantify the information collected in such a way that the data can be subjected to statistical analysis and that generalisations can be made from it. The quality of surveys is judged in terms of five interrelated criteria (May, 1997):

1   **Standardisation**   Each respondent should be asked exactly the same question in exactly the same way so that any difference in their reply is not due to the way the question is asked.

2   **Replicability**   The survey should be able to be carried out with different but matched respondents and different researchers, and produce the same findings.

3   **Reliability**   It should be possible to obtain the same results using the same questions with the same respondents at different times and with different interviewers.

4   **Validity**   The survey should measure what it intended to measure.

5   **Representativeness**   It should be possible to generalise from the survey to the whole population.

Criteria 1, 2 and 3 are closely linked. Standardisation is in many ways an attempt to ensure replicability and reliability. If more than one interviewer is involved in a survey, and in large surveys this is inevitably the case, then they must all be trained in asking the questions. Many surveys give elaborate instructions to the interviewers. Nevertheless, different interviewers can illicit different reactions from respondents merely on the basis of factors such as age or gender.

Thinking point   why might it be difficult to achieve reliability in obtaining the same results from respondents at different times?

Certain questions might be more difficult in terms of reliability than others. For instance, the question on self-assessment of health begs the question 'What is health?', which was discussed in Chapter 2. It might also depend on how a person feels that day or that morning which might be different from how they feel on another day. Nevertheless self-assessment of health has been found to be a reliable indicator of future health.

Criterion 4, on validity, is very much dependent on the question asked, which needs to be clear and unambiguous. Criterion 5 is dependent on the sampling procedures. Sampling procedures and the use of questions are addressed next in relation to the characteristics of surveys.

8.3.3 Sampling

The census is the only form of data collection from the population which targets the whole population of the UK. All the other surveys discussed above have, of necessity, to focus on a sample of the population. A 'sample' in research is a technical term for a smaller subset of a larger group which is the 'population'. This may or may not be the whole population; that is, all UK residents. It may be all students currently at UK universities or any other defined group. Practicalities and issues of manageability govern the need for sampling, but the important issue is that the sample should represent the population from which it is drawn. There are a number of ways to ensure this, depending on the purpose of the survey.

Random sampling

Random samples are also known as probability samples because they enable a statistical generalisation to be made from the sample to the population. Random sampling is a technique whereby each member of the target population has an equal chance of being selected. The usual way to select a random sample is to use a sampling frame; this is a list of those in the target population. Sampling frames frequently used in large health surveys include the electoral register (EL), the postcode address file (PAF) and lists from primary care trusts (PCTs). From the chosen list a system, such as selecting every tenth person on the list, is used to create the sample. Stratified random sampling means that the population is divided into subgroups according to particular characteristics – perhaps age, sex or social class – which are then subjected to random sampling. This is not to be confused with quota sampling in which a proportion of a particular group in the population is required to be included because the research has a particular interest in that group. For instance, a random sample of people in London may fail to include many older women from minority ethnic groups, so the researcher will set a quota of such women to include in the sample in order to be able to elicit their views. A quota sample is actually therefore a non-random sample.

Non-random sampling

A *purposive* sample is one where people, or organisations, exhibiting particular characteristics are chosen for study; for example, pregnant women over the age of forty with diabetes. A *snowball* sample is sometimes used for groups that are hard to reach: for instance, homeless people. One interviewee is asked to suggest others who may be willing to be interviewed; each of these others will in turn be asked to suggest further people, and so on. These two types of sample are typical of small-scale surveys which, although producing quantitative data, do not claim to be representative. Another type of sample which is becoming increasingly familiar on our streets is a 'next available person' sample, where interviewers try to engage the next available member of the public who passes by.

8.3.4 Asking questions

All surveys ask questions of their respondents in some form or another. This might be in the form of a questionnaire or an interview schedule. Technically, a questionnaire is designed to be filled in by the respondent, whereas an interview schedule is designed to be administered by an interviewer. (This is the way we use the terms in this chapter, but the term 'questionnaire' is often used for both ways of asking questions.) In some circumstances questionnaires and interview schedules are now completed by or with a third party, such as a relative or health/social care assistant or an interpreter; for example, when the population being studied has a high rate of illiteracy in English (Lloyd, 2007).

Questionnaires are part of everyday life, but you may have noticed how some questionnaires are easier to complete than others. In fact, they are quite difficult to design. Some general principles exist for the production of good questionnaires. Punch (2003, p. 61) suggests the following:

- keeping questions and items short and as simply worded as possible;

- ensuring that each item and question carries only one idea;

- avoiding negatives and double negatives;

- using language that is clear, unambiguous, relevant and appropriate, and unbiased.

(Punch, 2003, p. 61)

In questionnaires it is probably better to use mainly closed questions which are easier to codify. It has been argued that open questions are more difficult to answer in self-filled questionnaires because respondents have to reflect on their answer and this may take time and effort which they do not want to invest. Open questions have a higher non-response rate than closed questions (Aldridge and Levine, 2001).

Thinking point   do you agree that open questions can be problematic in questionnaires?

There is an argument for saying that open questions allow more attention to be paid to the respondent's point of view, and certainly more use can be made of them in an interview schedule where the interviewer records the response. Brevity is a virtue in questionnaires which should not take more than 20–30 minutes of a respondent's time. If there is a need for complex questions then the questionnaire format is probably not appropriate.

Some common pitfalls in questionnaires are:

- the use of insensitive language or language that is class, race or region specific; for instance, it is better to use the term 'midday meal' than 'lunch' which might have class connotations

- overlapping categories; for instance, when asking about age it is usual to provide age groups such as 30–40, 40–50, but where does a 40-year-old woman place herself? It is better to use the format 30–39, then 40–49, and so on. And when asking about age, always be specific and say 'at your last birthday'.

- double-barrelled questions such as 'Do you swim and walk regularly?' with the option to tick just 'yes' or 'no'. This would need to be formulated as two questions with a 'yes' and 'no' reply for each.

(Adapted from Aldridge and Levine, 2001)

Many questionnaires deal with sensitive subjects, and often the anonymity of a questionnaire is useful in gaining information in these circumstances as it avoids the embarrassment of responding to an interviewer (Kelly et al., 1994). Questionnaires can be sent through the post, but this often results in a low response rate. The response rate can be improved if they can be given out; for example, at a clinic, with a box for the receipt of the completed ones.

Many of the issues relating to asking questions on a questionnaire also apply to interview schedules, but because they are administered by a trained interviewer they can be much more complex. Large-scale surveys employ teams of researchers to carry out the interviews and they are usually trained together. But if the requirements of reliability and replicability are to be satisfied, they need to contain full instructions for the interviewer in order to try to ensure consistency in the way in which different interviewers carry out the interview. In effect, they are rather like stage directions in a play when the author wants to make sure that, whichever actor plays the part, the lines will be delivered in the way the author intended. The fact that interview schedules can include many more open questions makes them more attractive for use in any survey which is attempting more than some simple and specific measurements.

Health surveys can provide a wealth of information on a population – some of it descriptive, some of it analytic – and it should be possible to make generalisations from the survey about the whole population on a wide range of health-related topics. For this to be the case, they have to have followed specific sampling procedures and to ask questions which are meaningful, relevant and unambiguous to the respondent. Surveys have attracted a good deal of criticism, some of which is attributable to poor design, but some criticisms are more fundamental.

8.3.5 Critical views of surveys

Surveys have been criticised for lack of scientific rigour by those who see randomised controlled trials as the only viable form of health research (Aldridge and Levine, 2001). It is claimed that surveys cannot make causal inferences from correlations between variables: to say that there is a correlation between age and poor health does not mean that age causes illhealth (May, 1997, p. 104). What surveys do well is to identify correlations between a large number of variables which can then be tested through an experimental design.

However, most criticism of surveys is made from a humanistic perspective on the basis that surveys are atomistic: 'they treat society and culture as no more than the sum of the individuals within it' (Aldridge and Levine, 2001, p. 12). In fact, surveys do not pretend to be focusing on individuals per se, but on the aggregate of individuals who make up a population. They describe and analyse populations rather than individual people; that is their strength as well as a limitation. In this way they can identify a great deal about which people adopt a particular health behaviour, but they cannot provide an understanding of the processes involved in *why* people adopt such behaviour. The next chapter looks in detail at the potential of qualitative research in understanding people's behaviour.

A further major criticism of surveys is that they reflect the concerns and presuppositions of the researcher. The questions they ask restrict the respondent's options in answering them. This is particularly the case with closed questions, but even open questions are inviting the respondent to respond to a question which the *researcher* deems to be important. In addition, in order to ensure replicability and reliability surveys go to great lengths to ensure that questions are asked in a standardised way, but as May (1997, p. 104) points out: 'By using the concept of standardization, people do not have the opportunity to challenge ideas on their own terms. Furthermore, the myriad of differences in people's attitudes and the *meanings* which they confer on events can hardly be accommodated by compartmentalizing them into fixed categories ...'.

This problem is compounded by what Aldridge and Levine term the problem of social desirability:

> Respondents' answers are influenced by their desire to be helpful and to live up to their own self-image or to an ideal which they think will look good to the researcher ... They will also try to appear consistent, with the result that their opinions and beliefs will seem more coherent than they really are.
>
> (Aldridge and Levine, 2001, p. 13)

Others have objected to the mythical power of quantitative research:

> Quantification has acquired a bogus value – if something can be measured or counted it gains a scientific credibility often not afforded to the unmeasured or unmeasurable. Because of this, a finding or result is more likely to be accepted as a fact if it has been quantified than if it has not. On occasions, our love affair with numbers goes even further: sometimes we may suspect our critical faculties when faced with quantitative information, whether derived from routine or ad hoc sources. As a result, many well known, widely accepted 'facts' of doubtful accuracy have become entrenched in our supposed knowledge of health, disease and health care.
>
> (Black, 1994, p. 425)

Black is not suggesting here that quantitative methods do not have their strengths in describing many aspects of our world. Indeed, he believes that quantifying information is so essential that we need constantly to monitor and improve the way it is collected and analysed. He proposes three ways to improve health research: by developing more sophisticated statistical methods to handle this kind of data, by using quantitative methods in combination with qualitative methods, and by acknowledging that some areas of inquiry are simply not amenable to quantitative inquiry, but could be investigated using qualitative methods (Black, 1994, p. 426).

The next chapter is devoted to qualitative research methods and discusses further the potential for combining quantitative and qualitative methods in the pursuit of public health promotion. Using qualitative methods in combination with quantitative methods can help prevent the problem of ensuring that the questions asked in surveys do not reflect just the concerns of the researcher or those commissioning the research. In-depth qualitative methods used with a small but purposive sample of people can help to define and refine the research questions and give them salience to the respondents in a large-scale survey. Qualitative methods can also be useful as a follow-up to a survey and can contribute to the development of understanding of, for example, certain behaviours or attitudes expressed in the survey.

Conclusion

Quantitative methods have their limitations, but they make a vital contribution to finding out about the population's health. Without such data the extent and nature of inequalities in health would not be exposed. Demography, epidemiology and survey research are powerful and essential tools in efforts to promote public health. Without information on the levels of mortality and morbidity in the population it is inconceivable that policies and practices to prevent and combat disease could prevail. And without a greater understanding of the distribution of disease within a population it is difficult to see how policies and practices could be targeted at the appropriate groups in that population. Health surveys can provide much needed information on numerous aspects of a population's health in a much broader sense than disease and death statistics, and they can identify attitudes and behaviours as well as social factors that contribute to the way in which health and illhealth is distributed in the population. Nevertheless, the quantitative data that is generated can never be taken at face value and should always be open to critical review and, where appropriate, it should be informed and enhanced by qualitative methods.

References

Aggleton, P. (1990) *Health*, London, Routledge.

Aldridge, A. and Levine, K. (2001) *Surveying the Social World: Principles and Practice in Survey Research*, Buckingham, Open University Press.

Armstrong, D. (1983) *An Outline of Sociology as Applied to Medicine,* Bristol, John Wright.

Babb, P., Martin, J. and Haezewindt, P. (eds) (2004) *Focus on Social Inequalities*, London, The Stationery Office.

Bailey, L., Vardulaki, K., Langhan, J. and Chandramoha, D. (2005) *Introduction to Epidemiology*, Maidenhead, Open University Press.

Beckie, T.M. and Hayduk, L.A (1997) 'Measuring quality of life', *Social Indicators Research*, vol. 42, no. 21, p. 39.

Bhopal, R. (2001) 'Is research into ethnicity and health racist, unsound, or important science?' in Heller, T., Muston, R., Sidell, M. and Lloyd, C. (eds) *Working for Health*, London, Sage/Milton Keynes, The Open University.

Bhopal, R. (2002) *Concepts of Epidemiology: An Integrated Introduction to the Ideas, Theories, Principles and Methods of Epidemiology*, Oxford, Oxford University Press.

Black, N. (1994) 'Why we need qualitative research', *Journal of Epidemiology and Community Health*, vol. 48, no. 5, pp. 425–6.

Bowling, A. (2005) *Measuring Health: A Review of Quality of Life Measurement Scales* (3rd edn), Maidenhead, Open University Press.

Coggon, D., Rose, G. and Barker, D.J.P. (2003) *Epidemiology for the Uninitiated*, London, British Medical Journal Books.

Crayford, T., Hooper, R. and Evans, S. (1997) 'Death rates of characters in soap operas on British television: is a government health warning required?', *British Medical Journal*, vol. 315, pp. 20–7.

Doll, R. and Hill, A.B. (1950) 'Smoking and carcinoma of the lung', Preliminary Report, *British Medical Journal*, vol. 2, pp. 739–48.

Doll, R. and Peto, R. (1976) 'Mortality in relation to smoking: 20 years' observations on male British doctors', *British Medical Journal*, vol. 2, pp. 1525–36.

Doll, R., Peto, R., Wheatley, K., Gray, R. and Sutherland, I. (1994) 'Mortality in relation to smoking: 40 years' observations on male British doctors', *British Medical Journal*, vol. 309, pp. 901–11.

Dorling, D. and Thomas, B. (2004) *People and Places: A 2001 Census Atlas of the UK*, Bristol, Policy Press.

Douglas, J., Earle, S., Handsley, S., Lloyd, C.E. and Spurr, S. (eds) (2007) *A Reader in Promoting Public Health: Challenge and Controversy*, London, Sage/Milton Keynes, The Open University.

Erens, B., Primatesta, P. and Prior, G. (eds) (2001) *Health Survey for England 1999: The Health of Minority Ethnic Groups '99*, London, The Stationery Office.

Glickman, M., Corbin, T., Tortoriello, M. and Devis, T. (2006) *United Kingdom Health Statistics*, Newport, Office for National Statistics.

Gunaratnam, Y. (2007) 'Complexity and complicity in researching ethnicity and health' in Douglas et al. (eds) (2007).

Health Protection Agency (2003) *Renewing the Focus: HIV and other Sexually Transmitted Infections in the United Kingdom in 2002*, London, Health Protection Agency.

Herbst, A.L. and Scully, R.E. (1980) 'Adenocarcinoma of the vagina in adolescence: a report of seven cases including six clear-cell carcinomas (so-called mesonephromas)', *Cancer*, vol. 25, pp. 754–7.

Herbst, A.L., Ulfelder, H. and Poskaner, D.C. (1971) 'Adenocarcinoma of the vagina associated with maternal stilboestrol therapy with tumor appearance in young women', *New England Journal of Medicine*, vol. 284, pp. 878–81.

Hirayama, T., Waterhouse, J.H. and Fraumeni, J.F. (1980) *Cancer Risk by Site*, UICC Technical Report Series No. 41, Geneva, Union Internationale Contra Le Cancer.

Katz, J. (2000) 'Studying populations' in Katz et al. (eds) (2000).

Katz, J., Peberdy, A. and Douglas, J. (eds) (2000) *Promoting Health: Knowledge and Practice* (2nd edn), Basingstoke, Palgrave Macmillan/Milton Keynes, The Open University.

Kelly, L., Burton, S. and Regan, L. (1994) 'Researching women's lives or studying women's oppression?' in Maynard, M. and Purvis, J. (eds) *Researching Women's Lives from a Feminist Perspective*, London, Taylor & Francis.

King's Fund (2004) *Public Attitudes to Public Health Policy*, London, King's Fund; also available on line at http://www.kingsfund.org.uk/free (Accessed 29 May 2006).

Lloyd, C.E. (2007) 'Researching the views of diabetes service users from South Asian backgrounds: a reflection on some of the issues' in Douglas et al. (eds) (2007).

Marmot, M.G., Syme, S.L., Kagen, A., Kato, H., Cohen, J.B. and Belsky, J. (1975) 'Epidemiologic studies of coronary heart disease and stroke in Japanese men living in Japan, Hawaii and California: prevalence of coronary and hypertensive heart disease and associated risk factors', *American Journal of Epidemiology*, vol. 102, pp. 514–25.

May, T. (1997) *Social Research: Issues, Methods and Process*, Buckingham, Open University Press.

McHorney, C.A. (2000) 'Concepts and measurement of health status and health-related quality of life' in Albrecht, G.L., Fitzpatrick, R. and Scrimshaw, S.C. (eds) *The Handbook of Social Studies in Health and Medicine*, London, Sage.

Millennium Cohort Study (2006) *Millennium Cohort Study: First Survey, 2001–2003* (5th edn) [online], http://nesstar.esds.ac.uk/ (Accessed 31 October 2006).

Miller, R.E. (2002) *Epidemiology for Health Promotion and Disease Prevention Professionals*, New York, The Haworth Press.

Office for National Statistics (1998) *Key Health Statistics for General Practice: Analyses of Morbidity and Treatment Data Including Time Trends, England and Wales*, Series MB6, No. 2, London, Office for National Statistics.

Organisation for Economic Co-operation and Development (OECD) (2003) *Health at a Glance: OECD Indicators 2003*, Paris, Organisation for Economic Co-operation and Development.

Peto, R. (1994) 'Smoking and death: the past 40 years and the next 40', *British Medical Journal*, vol. 309, pp. 937–9.

Punch, K.F. (2003) *Survey Research: The Basics*, London, Sage.

Royal Free Medical School (2001) Lecture Notes (Personal Communication).

Singleton, N., Bumpstead, R., O'Brien, M., Lee, A. and Meltzer, H. (2001) *Psychiatric Morbidity Among Adults Living in Private Households, 2000*, London, The Stationery Office.

Stamatakis, E., Primatesta, P., Chinn, S., Rona, R. and Falaschetic, E. (2005) 'Overweight and obesity trends from 1974 to 2005 in English children: what is the role of socio-economic factors?', *Archive of Disease in Childhood*, vol. 90, no. 10, pp. 999–1004.

Stationery Office (1999) *The 2001 Census of Population*, Cm 4253, London, HMSO.

Stewart, A. (2002) *Basic Statistics and Epidemiology: A Practical Guide*, Oxford, Radcliffe Medical Press.

Tannahill, A. (1994) *Health Education and Health Promotion: From Priorities to Programmes*, World Health Organization Regional Office for Europe/Health Education Board for Scotland.

Tones, K. and Tilford, S. (1994) *Health Education: Effectiveness, Efficiency and Equity*, London, Chapman and Hall.

Townsend, P. and Davidson, N. (eds) (1982) *Inequalities in Health: The Black Report*, Harmondsworth, Penguin.

United Nations (1998) *Health and Mortality: A Concise Report*, New York, United Nations, Department of Economic and Social Affairs, Population Division.

Williams, H., Dodge, M., Higgs, G., Senior, M. and Moss, N. (1994) *Mortality and Deprivation in Wales,* Cardiff, University of Wales, Department of City and Regional Planning.

World Medical Organisation (1996) 'Declaration of Helsinki', *British Medical Journal*, vol. 313, pp. 1448–9.

Chapter 9

Qualitative research towards public health

Linda Finlay

Introduction

Qualitative research aims to explore, describe and/or interpret personal and social experiences, taking into account particular cultural contexts. Qualitative approaches are inductive, exploratory, hypothesis generating and focused on understanding meanings. This is in contrast to quantitative research which is deductive and hypothesis-testing, and aims to predict or explain behaviour.

The vast majority of official or statutory public health research projects are based on quantitative methods and approaches. Occasionally, as you discovered in the previous chapter, these studies offer a qualitative component: for instance, in a survey, a few people may be interviewed in greater depth, adding richness and texture to the quantitative statistics. However, there is a growing call for qualitative research to be undertaken in its own right (Green and Thorogood, 2004). There is increasing recognition of the value of such research, with its sharper focus on both the individual's lived experience and the social context of health/illness. Exciting projects are being developed and new opportunities are opening up for understanding people's health and health needs.

The process of carrying out qualitative research, and the challenges this involves, are the focus of this chapter. It explores different routes open to those seeking to use qualitative methods to promote public health. Section 9.1 begins by examining the contribution of qualitative research to public health. Section 9.2 explains how qualitative research is characterised by an array of methodologies. It examines three concrete exemplars of qualitative health research to indicate the scope and diversity of research methodology and practice. Section 9.3 focuses on 'doing' research. Some of the issues, methods and procedures that make up the data collection and analysis phases of research are examined – again, in reference to the exemplar studies. In the final section, modes of evaluating qualitative research are examined, with the point being made that such modes draw on different criteria from those used in conventional quantitative research.

9.1 The contribution of qualitative approaches to public health

Doing qualitative research is like going exploring or, as Willig (2001) suggests, going on an 'adventure'. People doing qualitative research commonly begin their research journey with a reasonably open mind about their destination and how they are going to get there. They know that any qualitative process is likely to throw up many challenges and potentially false or misleading trails. On route, they recognise they may well get 'bogged down' and have to negotiate a 'swamp' of interpretive analysis. At the same time, they expect to be excited and surprised (Finlay, 2006a).

Denzin and Lincoln (1994, p. 2) state that: 'Qualitative researchers study things in their natural settings, attempting to make sense of, or interpret, phenomena in terms of the meanings people bring to them.' They start with open research questions rather than having a hypothesis to test. Rich, textured description is valued, with a focus on the 'hows', 'whys' and 'whats' rather than on questions of 'whether' or 'how many'. In qualitative research the researcher's role and the research context are viewed with a critical eye. Where possible, the aim is to promote collaborative, empowering, participatory and/or egalitarian relationships.

In the case of public health, qualitative research focuses on individuals' everyday meanings, motivations and behaviours related to health. It aims to locate lifestyle risk behaviours within individuals' broader life and cultural contexts to examine how social factors (relational, institutional and ideological) impact on health. In general, qualitative research in the field of public health aims to help both practitioners and policy makers ensure that health education and provision are relevant to the needs of service users (see Box 9.1). Some qualitative research will also specifically focus on giving a 'voice' to marginalised, vulnerable or disempowered individuals and groups, with a view to empowering them to take control of their own health. For instance, Choudhry et al. (2002) used a method called participatory action research to examine health issues for a group of South Asian immigrant women. In addition to exploring the women's health needs and understandings, the researchers offered various workshops over a three-year period designed to help the women develop knowledge about their own health.

Box 9.1 Summary of qualitative research aims in public health

1   To explore individuals' everyday meanings, motivations and behaviours related to health.

2   To locate lifestyle risk behaviours within individuals' broader life and social context.

3   To examine how social factors (relational, institutional and ideological) impact on health.

 4   To empower individuals to take control of their own health towards engaging in health-enhancing behaviours.

5   To give voice to marginalised, vulnerable or disempowered individuals and groups.

6   To better inform service providers and policy makers of users' needs and interests.

Thinking point   which of the six aims in Box 9.1 would you be most interested in pursuing if you were going to undertake qualitative research?

These different aims are illustrated in action by three examples from research on public health issues, given in Box 9.2.

Box 9.2 Exemplar studies: aims and rationale of public health research

Flowers et al. (1997) aimed to understand unprotected sex in relationships between gay men. Specifically, they sought to discover what individual gay men thought and felt about the connection between unprotected anal sex and their relationships. They argue that previous (largely quantitative) research did not pay sufficient attention to the quality of gay men's specific relationships and tended to lump all relationships together. Significantly, their research findings showed that, within romantic relationships, men often place more importance on the expression of commitment, trust and love than on their own health.

Fazil et al. (2004) examined how concepts of empowerment and advocacy impinge on power relationships for service providers working with Pakistani and Bangladeshi families who have children with disabilities. Specifically, they investigated the processes and challenges involved in running an advocacy programme for this group. They argue that there are important cultural and gender factors which need to be taken into account if services for this vulnerable and relatively powerless group are to make a positive impact.

Pavis and Cunningham-Burley (1999) explored male youth street culture with the aim of understanding the context of health-related behaviours. In particular, they examined the motivations, meanings and behaviours of the young men in terms of their vandalism, under-age drinking and drug use. They argue that there is a need to see such behaviour in the context of the particular subculture concerned. Public health policies cannot hope to be effective if they fail to take into account the ways in which these risk behaviours link to broader life circumstances.

In recent years the qualitative research movement has gained growing acceptance in the health and social science arenas. However, in the field of public health the legitimacy of qualitative methods is still challenged (Green and Thorogood, 2004). Researchers face questions about the validity and generalisability of their findings and are challenged about whether or not their interpretive methods are 'scientific'. Critics claim that qualitative findings are too anecdotal, subjective, vague, 'soft' and 'airy fairy' (Zyzanski et al., 1992; Labuschagne, 2003). They argue that, because qualitative research often involves small numbers of participants, its findings cannot be generalised and are therefore of little value. The critical backlash against some Department of Health funded qualitative research on the use of complementary and alternative medicine is a case in point. For example, Walton (2006) calls instead for more scientific, quantitative research: 'While those projects already supported are likely to generate results of considerable interest ... they constitute, in my view, no more than preliminary and explorative projects that need to be followed by others, with well-defined concrete objects and firmly established endpoints.'

In response, qualitative researchers argue that such criticisms display ignorance about the nature of their work (Mason, 2002). Critics, they say, fail to grasp the central aim of qualitative research: to capture and contextualise complex meanings. Further, qualitative research has the potential to be 'a more powerful persuader than scientific publication in changing clinical practice' (Britten and Green, 1998, p. 1230).

In pursuit of these aims, qualitative research employs methods that are systematic and rigorous. While its findings cannot necessarily be statistically extrapolated to wider populations, concepts and theories can certainly be applied to other groups and settings. And rather than regarding the subjective, often ambiguous aspects of the findings as a problem, qualitative research embraces them, seeing these as bringing richness and depth to the research undertaking.

Green and Thorogood (2004) offer three key arguments about the contribution of qualitative research in public health. First, qualitative research fills some gaps which quantitative approaches cannot reach. It has a distinctive role in its search for understanding and context: qualitative methods can therefore address questions about the meaning and purpose of health and interventions, from the perspective of both users and providers.

Second, qualitative approaches are better able to capture complex attitudes and behaviours as they recognise that these are based on people's multiple, ambivalent, ambiguous meanings. Traditional survey research, such as asking people about their health concerns, can result in simplistic, unnuanced answers. In qualitative research it is acknowledged that respondents will be influenced by the context; for example, their relationship with the researcher. If the research is carried out at different times by different people, different 'stories' will be told.

Finally, qualitative research is useful in terms of application at both the practice and policy levels. At the level of practice, qualitative research can sensitise service providers not only to users' views, but also to how such views might affect health behaviours. Similarly, practitioners' values, beliefs and reactions can be studied to better understand, and so improve, service provision. At the policy level, qualitative studies can provide evidence of population needs. This can inform the implementation of appropriate policies.

With these arguments in mind, advocates of qualitative research are seeking wider acceptance for its specialised research methodologies. When qualitative research is done as a minor adjunct to quantitative research, there can be a tendency for the qualitative component to be limited to a few superficial, descriptive quotes from participants. For many qualitative researchers this hardly merits the status of 'qualitative research'; in reality, it amounts to little more than the qualitative presentation of quantitative findings. What is needed is a growing commitment to genuine, thoroughgoing qualitative research geared to generating deeper and more informative results. Such results can only enhance the findings of quantitative research.

A good example of how qualitative work can enhance quantitative studies is offered by Winch (1999, cited in Green and Thorogood, 2004), who uses a multidisciplinary approach to evaluate an intervention to promote insecticide-treated bed nets in Africa. Significantly, qualitative methods were utilised initially to access local views (and myths) about malaria. This knowledge was fed into various health-promotion interventions, including the use of street theatre emphasising the importance of using nets all year round. To evaluate these interventions, a survey of bed net use was undertaken. When it was discovered that there was still resistance to its use, interviews were used in a further study to investigate the barriers. The results indicated that villagers were concerned about both the cost and the possible toxic effects of the insecticide nets.

In this example, qualitative research was used at the beginning and end of the project to answer the 'what' and 'why' questions relating to people's beliefs about malaria and net use. In contrast, the quantitative survey research addressed the question of whether or not the nets were used. The choice of methodology thus follows logically from the research question being asked.

9.2 Choosing between multiple qualitative approaches

One of the biggest differences between quantitative and qualitative research is that qualitative research spans many more quite distinct and specialised approaches. This section describes some of these before discussing further the value – and potential problems – of mixing quantitative and qualitative methodologies.

9.2.1 Competing methodologies?

Methodology is the overarching approach to research that encompasses both the underpinning philosophy or perspective and the methods used in the research (see Figure 9.1). Unlike quantitative research stemming from the positivist tradition where the choice is largely between survey or experimental methods, qualitative research offers an extensive range of choices about how to approach research and which methodology to adopt (Finlay, 2006b). Phenomenology, action research and ethnography are just the tip of the iceberg of options available for qualitative researchers. To name a few more, there are ethnomethodology, grounded theory, discourse analysis, conversation analysis, narrative analysis, biographical and historical approaches, co-operative enquiry, case studies, repertory grid technique, and so on. Cresswell goes as far as to describe this spread of options as 'baffling' (Cresswell, 1998, p. 4). Each of these methodologies has its own aims and implies particular research designs. Although a researcher embarking on public health research cannot be expected to understand all these options, they need to be conscious that, at the very outset, they will be making some critical choices.

Underpinning the different methodologies are particular philosophical assumptions or perspectives. In Chapter 7 you were introduced to the significance of the role played by interpretivist, critical or cultural perspectives. Returning to the exemplars introduced in Box 9.2, the examples in Box 9.3 demonstrate how the three different groups of researchers have conducted their public health research in different ways – ways that depend fundamentally on which perspective they have adopted.

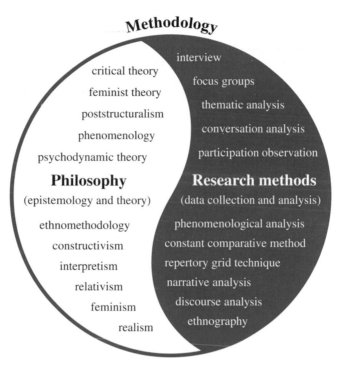

Figure 9.1   Methodology spanning philosophy and research methods (Source: Finlay, 2006b, p. 10, Figure 2.1)

Box 9.3 Exemplar studies: varied methodologies incorporating perspectives and methods

The interpretive phenomenological analysis (IPA) research by Flowers et al. (1997) is underpinned by interpretivist understandings. Here the researchers focus on the meanings, intentions and thinking of the gay men being researched. In-depth, relatively unstructured interviews are their method of choice to access these subjective 'insider' meanings. Taking an idiographic (individual/particularly focused) approach, the researchers value and celebrate the individuals' different voices.

Fazil et al. (2004) engage in an action research project arising from the critical perspective to evaluate the effectiveness of an advocacy programme offered to Asian families who had children with a disability. (The role of the advocates here was to befriend the families, link them into relevant services and aid communication with services.) They interview the families on four separate occasions to monitor the progress of the advocacy service. The findings of the research are then fed back to the local service providers and advocates so that they can take on board the issues and problems identified.

Pavis and Cunningham-Burley's (1999) ethnography of youth street culture is an example of research arising from a cultural perspective. Although – like Flowers et al. – they are concerned with individuals' meanings and health behaviours, their attention is focused on local cultural practices. They use participant observation to gain first-hand understandings about this culture. In addition to this fieldwork, the researchers conduct semi-structured interviews with community workers, and employ documentary analysis of the town's history, together with structured (quantitative) questionnaires.

Each of these research projects, then, has distinct research objectives underpinned by distinct perspectives and values which influenced how the researchers set about collecting and then analysing data. The researchers tended to have single research questions which they chose to explore under the umbrella of a single research methodology. In practice, however, it is rarely as simple as this. The use of multiple methods of inquiry is becoming quite common in public health research (Green and Thorogood, 2004) and is increasingly encouraged by the large funding bodies such as the Department of Health (DoH), the Economic and Social Research Council (ESRC) and the Medical Research Council (MRC). Often, public health research is multidimensional where different aspects of a health intervention project are investigated (such as the research by Winch, 1999, mentioned earlier). In such cases, it may well be desirable to combine quantitative with qualitative methodologies.

9.2.2 Combining qualitative and quantitative methods

Qualitative research may be used in tandem with quantitative methods when the researchers aim to address different aspects of the research topic. For example, participant observation may be used alongside survey type research (as in the Pavis and Cunningham-Burley exemplar) (participant observation is explored in greater depth in Section 9.3.2). Here, the qualitative data can add colour, texture and richness to any demographic data and statistical results. Qualitative data can also help clarify quantitative findings, particularly where there seems to be a puzzle or contradictions in the findings (as the research by Winch, 1999, illustrated).

The Health Impact Assessment (HIA) study carried out by Hirschfield et al. (2001), as part of their 'Stepping Out' project, is one example of mixing methods in public health research. The Stepping Out programme aimed to empower vulnerable young women in the Liverpool area of the UK by encouraging them to participate in social, educational and cultural facilities. The interventions included the use of groups and one-to-one work to offer support, training and practical skills development. For example, a team of youth workers joined the women on the streets two evenings a week rather than in more formal, centre-based venues.

The researchers describe a fairly complicated and wide-ranging research design which utilises many different methods, including documentary evidence, interviews, surveys, focus groups and fieldwork observation (see Box 9.4 for a sense of the range of what they evaluated) (interviews and focus groups are looked at in more detail in Section 9.3.2). In a way, such a large-scale project can be seen as a collection of different research studies, each using a different research design.

Box 9.4 Multiple methods for a Health Impact Assessment project

The research was designed so that each stage in the process informed the next. The logical place to start was a review of the documentary evidence already in existence. This included: monitoring and evaluation reports of the project, the Crime and Disorder Audit for the Borough of Sefton ... a full geodemographic profile of the two wards that the project serves and the score on the Index of Local Deprivation. This information enabled the researchers to develop a good understanding of the demographic, social and policy context in which the project works and knowledge of the type of work that it undertakes.

It was then considered appropriate to interview the project manager and a number of the workers in order to ascertain their views about the nature of the intervention, the needs and issues of the client group and the geographical area in which the project operates. Following one of the interviews, one of the researchers was invited to accompany two of the detached youth workers in their street work ... This exercise was extremely useful since it enabled the researcher to talk informally with the workers and to observe their interactions with the groups of young women that they went up to or who were approached by them.

Having gathered the youth workers' perceptions of the service Stepping Out provides and the impact it has on the young women that they work with, the sensible next step was to find out the views of the users. In the first instance, this was done through a series of face-to-face interviews carried out by the One-to-One workers with their clients using a semi-structured questionnaire ... The research team also had access to the results of a survey (the Self Assessment Questionnaire – SAQ) designed by the research director for another purpose and filled out by over twenty of Stepping Out's users. Finally, one of the researchers carried out two focus groups at Venus, the centre in which the Stepping Out Partnership is based.

The last stage of the research entailed speaking to other key informants and stakeholders who are not directly associated with the project as either employees or users.

(Hirschfield et al., 2001, pp. 17–18)

Sometimes researchers use multiple methods to offset the weaknesses of one method over another. This triangulation (a commonly used metaphor indicating the use of different points to navigate, to which you were introduced in Chapter 7) is used to enhance or confirm the validity of findings. For instance, the evidence base could be seen as strengthened if people report similar things when they are being both surveyed and interviewed.

However, there is some debate about how easily qualitative and quantitative methods can and should be combined. Problems can arise when methods are combined in the same single study. Research by Steward (2006) is a case in point. She studied the nature and impact of teleworking (i.e. remote or homeworking), using a survey to identify teleworkers' views of their work and then in-depth qualitative interviews with the same group to follow up the survey and explore how health, illness and sickness were defined and experienced. She found that, far from providing complementary accounts, the positivist and interpretive perspectives of the two methodologies clashed. Significantly, she discovered that the survey data was often refuted by participants in follow-up interviews and that participants responded differently depending on whether they were writing down their responses or giving them verbally. For instance, Steward found that asking about days 'off sick' produced different answers because the meanings teleworkers ascribed to the terms 'off' and 'sick' varied. She concludes that neither approach can be seen as 'right' (although she gained more information and understanding from the qualitative data): 'A mixed methodological approach', she says, 'served to highlight the complexity and ambivalence [of teleworking] ... It showed how individuals generate information about themselves ... in many ... often irreconcilable ways' (Steward, 2006, p. 105).

For Steward, the point is that it is impossible to produce a consistent version of the object of study. This is because 'truths' are relative; they vary from one person to another and one person's views may vary depending on the context. The object needs to be seen as socially constructed rather than as a fixed reality. As Denzin explains:

> each method implies a different line of action toward reality – and hence each will reveal different aspects of it, much as a kaleidoscope, depending on the angle at which it is held, will reveal different colours and configurations of objects to the viewer. Methods are like the kaleidoscope: depending on how they are approached, held, and acted toward, different observations will be revealed.
>
> (Denzin, 1989, cited in Green and Thorogood, 2004, p. 208)

Thinking point   given that different methods can produce different results, is this an argument for or against mixing methods?

Care needs to be taken when combining methods as their aims can vary considerably (Yardley and Marks, 2004). Much depends on whether researchers are taking a 'realist' or 'relativist' approach (i.e. whether they believe there is one reality out there that they are studying, or whether it is only possible to capture relative meanings). Studies that seek to combine methods that are compatible, in that they draw meaningfully on their different potentials, tend to yield more fruitful results. The practice of combining qualitative and quantitative methods is probably most useful if different questions are being asked or if this helps the researcher to unpack complex meanings. But, more importantly, qualitative methods used in the planning stage of a quantitative survey can help to generate survey questions which do resonate with people's understandings and meanings and might help avoid the problem identified by Steward (2006), and mentioned above.

The next section explores the potential of different qualitative methods and how they might be used in practice to unpack meanings.

9.3 Doing qualitative research

The actual 'doing' of research poses many challenges in qualitative research. Three particular stages of the research are discussed here: early planning, collecting data and data analysis. Across all these stages, the challenge lies in conducting the research appropriately, ethically, systematically and rigorously.

9.3.1 Early planning

In the early stages of planning research, researchers have much to decide. What, precisely, is the research focus and question? Who will constitute the participants and how will they be recruited? (In the case of documentary research that doesn't use participants, how will documents be obtained and how much will be sampled?) Are there particular 'gatekeepers' who need to be approached first (i.e. people who control access to participants: for instance, parents and teachers in the case of research with young people)? What methods of data collection and analysis will be used? What kind of roles will the researcher and participants play? To what extent will participants be involved in the formulation or validation of findings? How will the participants be briefed in order to give their 'informed consent' and how will they be 'de-briefed'? How will the participants' rights and safety be protected?

Given this special relationship between the researcher and what is studied, what exactly should the researcher's role be? Beyond seeking to do no harm, qualitative researchers often aim to empower and 'give voice' to their participants. They need to be mindful that their research – which encourages participants to reflect on themselves and the social world around them – has the potential to be transformative, changing both themselves and their participants. In short, there is a power dimension at play – demanding recognition and management. Two key questions here are: 'Whose interests are served by our research?' and 'What wider impact might this research have?' (Finlay, 2006a). Answers to all the questions mentioned here are needed prior to beginning data collection.

After this early planning stage, the research project is likely to need formal approval; for instance, by the local research ethics committee following the Research Governance Framework (DoH, 2001). The committee's remit includes adjudicating on issues such as informed consent, confidentiality/ anonymity, rights and safety of the participants, risk to research participants, the legal liability of the researcher and the degree of independent monitoring of the research (e.g. by a supervisor) (Ballinger and Wiles, 2006).

Space does not permit a full exploration of all these issues. However, the three exemplars provide some insights into the issue of recruiting participants ethically (see Box 9.5).

Box 9.5 Exemplar studies: recruiting participants ethically

In the research conducted by Flowers et al. (1997), participants were being asked to speak about a deeply personal and intimate topic. Interestingly, however, the researchers had no trouble recruiting the participants. It seems they actively welcomed a chance to share experiences about this normally taboo subject. Initial contact was made through the first author's involvement in the local gay community. Subsequent contacts, from these initial informants, traced gay men's sexual networks. During the interviews, the researchers strove to be sensitive and they were concerned to develop trust. Without this care, the participants would have been less likely to disclose personal information.

In the research by Fazil et al. (2004), developing trust during the interviews was also a priority. When the researchers asked the participants whether the interviews could be tape-recorded, some participants refused. The researchers therefore recorded the interviews by hand. After each interview, the researcher carefully went through the text with each participant to ensure that they were happy with the recorded information. In addition, throughout the action research process, the advocates and researchers found themselves confronted by a number of sensitive ethical issues. These related to conflicts over ethnicity and gender; for instance, advocates working with just the women in the family found that their interventions had the potential to create family tensions.

The Pavis and Cunningham-Burley (1999) research raised the issue of the role of the fieldworker when making initial contact with young people. Simply approaching groups of young people 'cold' was going to be problematic. The young people would be unlikely to trust such an advance, while the researcher was likely to feel quite intimidated and would possibly be at physical risk (for this reason, local police and youth workers were informed of the research). The researcher eventually spent a great deal of time initially observing at a distance. Eventually, out of curiosity, it was the youths themselves who approached him. The young people were then told that the researcher was 'from the university and wanted to understand what it was like for them on the streets'. While such a strategy may have secured their trust, it raises questions about the extent to which the participants in this particular study gave their informed consent. Inevitably, there were some young people who remained in ignorance that they were being researched.

Thinking point   in the three exemplar studies, what 'risks' did the researcher need to be alert to?

Qualitative research often deals with sensitive, difficult topic areas where risk and safety are germane. However, research risk assessment involves further debate. At what point is a participant deemed to be in danger of harm? For instance, if a participant gets upset during an interview, is that 'harm'? Does this mean that researchers should avoid tackling potentially emotive topics? Some participants welcome the opportunity to talk at a deep and personal level; participants getting upset may therefore not necessarily be a 'problem'. Similarly, precautions taken to minimise risk for the researcher (e.g. interviewing in pairs or avoiding going into 'risky' environments) may well be interpreted negatively by participants and be counter-productive. In short, there may be trade-offs between 'safety' and being effective or productive as a researcher. According to Green and Thorogood, 'Ethical research practice requires a consideration of responsibilities to research participants, professional and academic colleagues, research sponsors and the wider public. Although ethical guidelines exist for most disciplines, qualitative health research often generates ethical dilemmas, which are not easily solved by reference to codes of practice' (Green and Thorogood, 2004, p. 51).

In these cases, probably the best a qualitative researcher can do is to be sensitive to, and critically aware of, the ethical implications of each stage of the research. Attempts should be made to handle these as conscientiously as possible. Care needs to be taken during data collection to regularly review the terms of the research agreement and to check with the participant that they are prepared to continue. The participant may value the opportunity to say something 'off the record' and this needs to be respected.

9.3.2 Collecting data

There are natural affinities between methodology and methods or procedures used to collect and analyse data. The choice of methods generally follows from the choice of methodology (Finlay, 2006b). A phenomenological researcher, for instance, usually draws on interviews or on personal written accounts (as in the case of the research by Flowers et al., 1997). Action research, such as that by Fazil et al. (2004), tends to rely on focus groups or interview data, perhaps in combination with surveys. In ethnography, as Pavis and Cunningham-Burley's (1999) research shows, researchers do fieldwork which requires them to engage in varying degrees of 'participation' and 'observation' (perhaps in combination with formal interviews and the reading of documents). Other research methodologies also have their particular methods. For instance, a discourse analytic study requires a 'text' to analyse linguistically (some analysts are content to use interviews while others prefer naturally occurring texts culled from conversations, media resources or published documents).

Whichever of the many data collection methods are chosen, the challenge lies in being able to carry the procedures off skilfully, rigorously and sensitively. To illustrate some of the issues and challenges involved, the examples of interviews, focus groups, participant observation and participatory action research – the most frequently employed qualitative methods – are now examined in more detail.

Researchers choosing interview (whether structured or unstructured) as a method need to take much care to build a relationship with the participant such that the participant feels listened to, safe and respected. Having enabled the participant to share something of themselves, the researcher then needs to ensure that the participant isn't being forced to disclose information beyond the point where they are comfortable. Henry and Finlay offer some advice to novice interviewers:

> Talking about thoughts, feelings or one's own present or future plans, can be a threatening and moving experience as well as an enjoyable one. Anyone engaged in a depth interview needs to be aware that new personal understandings might sometimes be disclosed without the participant recognising that this is the case.

> Your participant needs to be fully informed at the outset, and both of you need to recognize the extent to which personal revelations can be unsettling.
>
> (Henry and Finlay, 2001, p. 6)

Focus groups involve similar challenges, given that they are, in effect, group interviews. The role of the facilitator (who may or may not be the researcher) is vital as they need to try to promote a relaxed atmosphere initially to enable people to feel comfortable talking in the group. Facilitators might, for example, hand out refreshments as they greet participants or provide some initial warm-up interaction games. Great care needs to be taken when running groups on sensitive topics – particularly if participants have to live or work together after the research.

Green and Thorogood (2004, p. 128) suggest that the key to analysing group interviews is to remember that the researcher 'must be aware of the context of the data production ... Utterances ... cannot be presented as the essential "views" of the participants'. Group members may say things simply because they are part of the group. For example, perhaps they are feeling some peer pressure and wish to be seen to be going along with what others are saying. Also, sometimes individual members can dominate and influence others in groups. In other words, group dynamics will play a part and need to be taken into account.

In participant observation studies, the challenges are somewhat different. Negotiating access to the research 'field' can prove problematic as often there are gatekeepers who need to be satisfied. Studies attempting to explore service users' views and experiences of their treatment, for example, could be derailed by a gatekeeper manager who is defensively reluctant to have user 'complaints' researched by a stranger.

Having gained access, the next challenge is how to observe without unduly changing what is being studied. Care needs to be taken to minimise any intrusions to ensure observations are naturalistic. For instance, the use of video is gaining popularity as a means of recording details of interactions, such as those between healthcare providers and users. Here, having the camera in place before recording can help participants get used to its presence.

A third challenge for those doing fieldwork relates to the degree of researcher participation. This challenge comes to the fore in 'covert' field studies where researchers run the risk of participating rather than simply observing. One researcher, who wishes to remain anonymous, was studying drug use in the clubbing culture. He admits that he took drugs in order to be accepted in the group he was researching. Although most health research will not involve decisions of such an extreme nature, negotiating the extent and manner of the participant observation always involves choices and both practical and ethical questions.

Thinking point   should covert research always be avoided in order to preserve 'informed consent'?

Ethical dilemmas such as those related to 'informed consent' challenge every researcher. Although researchers tend to view covert practice in different ways, they would probably all agree that harm (emotional as well as physical) to participants must be avoided.

With participatory action research (also known as PAR) all the issues raised above with regard to the other methods discussed are relevant, but additional considerations need to be taken into account. PAR is action research with the emphasis on collaborating *with* community members. The overall goal of PAR is to work with community members to implement and research an intervention or social change needed to improve a health problem (Kelly, 2005).

As the requirement is to work with community members, PAR poses many challenges. It can be incredibly time consuming. Projects can often take several years from the initial discussion stage through to the 'action' being conceived, implemented and evaluated. A second challenge is the need to consult and work with community partners at all stages of the research, including the last stage of making public the results of the research. Even the first stage of discussing an idea can be problematic as communities may not have the people, energy or time resources to focus on less-than-pressing health promotion. Kelly explains the difficulties:

> To achieve meaningful results, participants must retain a sense of involvement, while the program is simultaneously moving toward its goals. Community members' voices must be heard continuously ... Keeping a diverse group of people together is challenging, and sustaining enthusiasm can be even more difficult, especially as competing needs arise and the group experiences setbacks.
>
> (Kelly, 2005, p. 70)

9.3.3 Data analysis

Most qualitative researchers would agree that difficulties encountered during the early stages of research pale into insignificance compared with the challenge of analysing the huge amount of descriptive data invariably generated by qualitative procedures. It is all too easy for researchers to feel overwhelmed as they work through the minutiae of the data. In Box 9.6, Flowers et al. describe their thematic analysis method. While their procedure refers to the particular method of analysing using interpretive phenomenological analysis, the process is similar in other qualitative methods which call for rigorous *thematic analysis*.

Box 9.6 Exemplar study: an IPA example of analysing data

The transcripts were analysed for recurrent themes. Themes emerged within the individual interviews and across different interviews. The process of identifying themes involved several steps. Throughout, the analyst attempted to acknowledge and suspend any existing knowledge of the field, and indeed, personal experiences within it. This was done in an attempt to 'see' the world as it is experienced by the respondent. Bearing this in mind, each transcript was repeatedly read. Following this, the analysis of each transcript began, in which both semantic content and language use were examined; key words, phrases or explanations which the respondent used were highlighted. These were then coded with a key word or phrase which captured the essence of the content. These represented emergent themes. The process was repeated with each transcript. Following this, repetitions of these emergent themes (between each individual transcript) were taken as indicative of their status as recurrent themes which reflect shared understandings. In this manner, for each theme, a file of transcript extracts was created. While an emphasis is placed here on themes emerging from the data, inevitably this selection process requires interpretation on the part of the analyst. One is attempting to capture the meaning of the phenomenon to the participant but this necessarily involves interpretative engagement with the respondent's text.

(Flowers et al., 1997, p. 76)

Having applied their thematic analysis method, Flowers et al. came up with such themes as 'Casual sex and detachment', 'Penetrative sex, relationships and self-involvement' and 'Unprotected anal penetration and the romantic rationality'. In their extended analysis and discussion they note how, in the men's accounts of sexual decision making, there seems to be a 'consistent awareness of sexual acts as being communicative ... capturing very powerful expressions ... Semen exchange within a relationship highlights sharing bodies, whilst condom use ... exemplifies keeping bodies separate and isolated' (Flowers et al., 1997, p. 82).

Having analysed their data, qualitative researchers often engage in further analysis to examine the ethics of their research and the central role they have played in the construction and production of the findings. Here, researchers utilise reflective diaries and engage in a process known as reflexivity (Finlay and Gough, 2003). This requires them to critically self-reflect on the ways in which their social background, assumptions, positioning, behaviour, presence and power relations impact on the research process. Reflexivity involves a continuing self-awareness of the research dynamics and claims being made. How this is achieved varies. The reflexive analysis offered by Gunaratnam (2007), on methodological and ethical dilemmas faced when researching ethnicity, provides one good example. Another example is the participatory action research project undertaken by McFadden and McCamley (2003) who investigated young people's sexual health. The authors used reflexivity to explore issues of identity and disempowerment throughout the research project. They tell of their struggle to relinquish their authority as university researchers so that they could share responsibility for the research with younger peer researchers who were taking on the responsibility of interviewing young people:

> At the end of the first phase the peer researchers felt sufficiently equipped to comment critically on the data obtained ... even questioning the supposed expertise of the university researchers ('they should have done it better') and imagining how they (the peer researchers) might improve the study. Listening to such feedback produced initial feelings of annoyance for us – we considered the young people's comments to be overly critical, and quite cheeky! ...
>
> However, such instances were invaluable in challenging our thinking around what constitutes collaborative research. Despite our aim to diminish the power differentials which dog traditional research approaches, we realised that we had overlooked some central issues within the wider research matrix involving young people as users of power.
>
> (McFadden and McCamley, 2003, pp. 206–7)

Reflexivity is one of the key ways in which qualitative researchers evaluate the value, integrity and trustworthiness of their research. Subjective elements which are so much a part of the qualitative research journey are identified and highlighted in the process of reflexive analysis. Indeed, they are actively celebrated (Finlay, 2003). This contrasts with the efforts made in quantitative research to minimise the element of subjectivity in the conduct of the research.

In the following passage, Peter Reason reflects on the need of researchers to examine the impact of their inquiry. Although he is referring to action research specifically, his points apply equally to qualitative research in general:

> our sense of quality must reach wider than simply 'does it work?' It must include whether we have helped the development of an effective community of inquiry among participants; whether questions of power have been addressed; whether the inquiry has been emancipatory and deepened the experiential basis of

understanding; and so on. In this way we can avoid being trapped in a heroic, agentic vision of action research: it is not just about solving the immediate problem but of articulating the subtle ways in which the inquiry is affecting our world.

(Reason, 2006)

In these ways, the use of reflexivity merges with evaluating the research as a whole – the subject of the next section.

9.4 Evaluating qualitative research

The examples of research offered throughout this chapter show something of the potential richness, complexity, depth and power of qualitative work. It is also important to remember that qualitative findings are always limited, partial and emergent. If you accept that qualitative work involves interpretation of meanings, it follows that analyses can only be presented as 'tentative statements opening upon a limitless field of possible interpretations' (Churchill, 2000, p. 164).

Unlike quantitative research, qualitative research is less concerned with positivist conceptions of reliability and validity as criteria for judging the quality of research. Reliability (i.e. repeatability and the inner consistency of the means of data collection) is largely irrelevant in the case of qualitative research which, by definition, does not seek to repeat the research; rather, it seeks to elicit a participant's responses within a specific and interpersonal context. Such a situation can never be replicated. As for validity, quantitative research with its goal of generalisability is concerned that the research measures what it is intended to measure. De Vaus (1991, pp. 54–5) takes the example of using educational level to measure social status, saying that: 'the issue is not whether we have measured education properly but whether this is a suitable measure for social status'. Qualitative research is less concerned with generalisability and more concerned to look at underlying meanings and explore the uniqueness of people's accounts. Validity, then, has a different meaning which should reflect the 'shifting nature of our realities' (Johnson, 2000, p. 82).

Thinking point   if qualitative researchers reject traditional quantitative criteria for evaluation, how can the quality of their research be judged?

New and different criteria, responsive to qualitative research ideals, are necessary to ensure the integrity and value of the research (Finlay, 2006c). Guba and Lincoln (1994) argue for at least two sets of criteria to judge the quality of investigation: trustworthiness and authenticity. Good research also has the power to convince. As Kvale (1996, p. 252) puts it, 'Ideally, the quality of the craftsmanship results in products with knowledge claims that are so powerful and convincing in their own right that they, so to say, carry the validation with them, like a strong piece of art.'

In the light of such criteria, it is suggested that evaluating a given piece of qualitative research is done in terms of five dimensions, called the '5 Cs' (Finlay, 2006c):

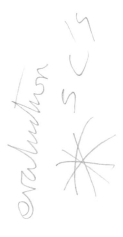

1. *Clarity*: Does the research make sense? To what extent is the research systematically worked through, coherent and clearly described?

2. *Credibility*: To what extent do the findings match the evidence and are they convincing? ... Are the researcher's interpretations plausible and justified? ...

3. *Contribution*: To what extent does the research add to debate and knowledge of an issue or aspect of human social life? ... Is it empowering and/or growth-enhancing? ... Does it offer guidance for future action or for changing the social world for the better? ...

4. *Communicative resonance*: Are the findings sufficiently vivid or powerful to draw readers in? Do the findings resonate with readers' own experience or understandings? Alternatively, do the findings unsettle or disturb challenging unthinking complacency? ...

5. *Caring*: Has the researcher shown respect and sensitivity to participants' safety and needs? To what extent is the researcher reflexive about the way in which meanings are elicited in an interpersonal [and cultural] context? Does the research demonstrate ethical integrity and does the researcher show concern for the impact of the research?

(Finlay, 2006c, p. 322)

The three exemplar studies were selected for this chapter in part because they represent good, clear, trustworthy and convincing examples of research. All three have much to offer in terms of being 'caring' as well as making a 'contribution' to knowledge and understanding towards better practice/policy. For instance, the research by Fazil et al. (2004) makes an important contribution to the understanding of empowerment and of the cultural and gender issues raised when setting up an ethnically sensitive advocacy service. For example, the authors found that empowering individual mothers to negotiate their own lives through advocacy can interfere with family dynamics. Mothers would make decisions which were later overturned by husbands. The authors concluded that: 'any process of empowerment will need to demonstrate a high level of cultural sensitivity ... [Further] an advocacy service needs to be very much family orientated to succeed' (Fazil et al., 2004, p. 396).

The IPA study by Flowers et al. (1997) also achieves an impressive communicative resonance. There is a richness, power, authenticity and poignancy in the quotations from the study's gay participants. For instance, one participant talked of not holding himself back once he fell in love:

PE: It took me a long time to love John ... for us to have anal sex it kind of, put the icing on the cake [pause] a sense the relationship was complete because sexually we were ... embarrassed to approach anal sex and then when we did do it, it got that obstacle out of the way ... I've always held a bit of myself back, relationship-wise, because I've been dumped so many times ... once we'd had anal sex, then I knew I'd given myself completely over, there was nothing else really I was holding back.

P: And you did it without condoms?

PE: Yeah. Yeah.

(Flowers et al., 1997, p. 78)

The research by Pavis and Cunningham-Burley (1999) achieves extra credibility by offering many descriptive examples of the behaviours observed. The 'street-life' is brought to life, and this serves as a powerful demonstration of the authors' central finding: the need to locate lifestyle risk behaviours within the broader cultural situation. Through their research examples and discussion, the authors manage to offer readers a different way of seeing the youths' problematic health behaviours. To pick up one theme from their discussion:

> Our young men's street culture arguably provided a group of relatively alienated and marginalized young people with a source of interest and excitement. The streets were 'colonized' space that was 'adult-free'. It provided a place where they could meet with friends and, using very limited resources, 'have a laugh'. The streets also provided a social context in which the young men could experiment with their sexuality and/or develop a certain type of masculinity. It was somewhere that they could achieve peer status and recognition through conspicuous consumption, e.g. of designer labelled clothes, and/or via the less overt mechanisms of knowledge about and use of illicit drugs, and/or involvement in small-scale gang violence.

(Pavis and Cunningham-Burley, 1999, pp. 593–4)

When applying qualitative research methods to public health, researchers are concerned that their research has both value and impact. The hope is that the research will increase understanding of individuals' health behaviours, or change society in some way: be it in terms of informing or changing health practice or policy. Ultimately, the value of qualitative research – whether on its own or as an adjunct to quantitative research – rests on this.

Conclusion

This chapter has looked at qualitative research in the field of public health. It has explored the processes involved and some of the challenges that qualitative research raises. The diversity of qualitative research practice has been illustrated through three exemplar studies.

Qualitative researchers often enter uncharted territory that is seemingly beyond the reach of conventional quantitative research. There are challenges at every stage, from planning a project to analysing and evaluating its findings. The extra demands placed on the qualitative researcher – for example, establishing sound, ethical relationships with participants and being reflexive about their role – should not be underestimated. At journey's end, the research may well yield findings that extend – or perhaps run counter to – those of conventional quantitative research. What is certain is that much can be learned about people's health-related meanings and motivations by placing them in their broader social context. For the purposes of effective health promotion and a higher profile for public health, such understanding is vital.

The diversity and richness of qualitative research, and its ability to go beneath the surface, are beyond dispute. Public health practitioners and policy makers need to emulate professionals in other fields by embracing qualitative research in its own right.

References

Ballinger, C. and Wiles, R. (2006) 'Ethical and governance issues in qualitative research' in Finlay and Ballinger (eds) (2006).

Britten, N. and Green, J. (1998) 'Qualitative research and evidence based medicine', *British Medical Journal*, vol. 316, pp. 1230–2.

Choudhry, U.K., Jandu, S., Mahal, J., Singh, R., Sohi-Pabla, H. and Mutta, B. (2002) 'Health promotion and participatory action research with South Asian women', *Journal of Nursing Scholarship*, vol. 34, no. 1, pp. 75–81.

Churchill, S.D. (2000) 'Phenomenological psychology' in Kazdin, A.D. (ed.) *Encyclopedia of Psychology*, Oxford, Oxford University Press.

Cresswell, J.W. (1998) *Qualitative Inquiry and Research Design: Choosing Among Five Traditions*, Thousand Oaks, CA, Sage.

de Vaus, D (1991) *Surveys in Social Research*, London, UCL Press.

Denzin, N.K. (1989) 'Strategies of multiple triangulation' in Denzin, N.K. *The Research Act: A Theoretical Introduction to Sociological Methods* (3rd edn), Englewood Cliffs, NJ, Prentice Hall.

Denzin, N.K. and Lincoln, Y. (eds) (1994) *Handbook of Qualitative Research*, Thousand Oaks, CA, Sage.

Denzin, N.K. and Lincoln, Y. (1994) 'Introduction: entering the field of qualitative research' in Denzin and Lincoln (eds) (1994).

Department of Health (DoH) (2001) *Research Governance Framework for England*, London, Department of Health.

Fazil, Q., Wallace, L.M., Singh, G., Ali, Z. and Bywaters, P. (2004) 'Empowerment and advocacy: reflections on action research with Bangladeshi and Pakistani families who have children with severe disabilities', *Health and Social Care in the Community*, vol. 12, no. 5, pp. 389–97.

Finlay, L. (2003) 'The reflexive journey: mapping multiple routes' in Finlay and Gough (eds) (2003).

Finlay, L. (2006a) 'Going exploring: the nature of qualitative research' in Finlay and Ballinger (eds) (2006).

Finlay, L. (2006b) 'Mapping methodology' in Finlay and Ballinger (eds) (2006).

Finlay, L. (2006c) '"Rigour", "ethical integrity" or "artistry"? Reflexively reviewing criteria for evaluating qualitative research', *British Journal of Occupational Therapy*, vol. 69, no. 7, pp. 319–26.

Finlay, L. and Ballinger, C. (eds) (2006) *Qualitative Research for Allied Health Professionals: Challenging Choices*, Chichester, Wiley.

Finlay, L. and Gough, B. (eds) (2003) *Reflexivity: A Practical Guide for Researchers in Health and Social Sciences*, Oxford, Blackwell Science.

Flowers, P., Smith, J.A., Sheeran, P. and Beail, N. (1997) 'Health and romance: understanding unprotected sex in relationships between gay men', *British Journal of Health Psychology*, vol. 2, no. 1, pp. 73–8.

Green, J. and Thorogood, N. (2004) *Qualitative Methods for Health Research*, London, Sage.

Guba, G.G. and Lincoln, Y.S. (1994) 'Competing paradigms in qualitative research' in Denzin and Lincoln (eds) (1994).

Gunaratnam, Y. (2007) 'Complexity and complicity in researching ethnicity and health' in Douglas, J., Earle, S., Handsley, S., Lloyd, C.E., and Spurr, S. (eds) *A Reader in Promoting Public Health: Challenge and Controversy*, London, Sage/Milton Keynes, The Open University.

Henry, J. with Finlay, L. (2001) 'The interview project: capturing experience and meaning' in D317 *Social Psychology: Personal Lives, Social Worlds*, Milton Keynes, The Open University.

Hirschfield, A., Barnes, R., Hendley, J. and Scott-Samuel, A. (2001) *Health Impact Assessment Case study: The Stepping Out Project* [online], http://www.phel.nice.org.uk/hiadocs/measuring_the_effect_SteppingOut.pdf (Accessed 2 May 2006).

Johnson, K. (2000) 'Interpreting meanings' in Gomm, R. and Davies, C. (eds) *Using Evidence in Health and Social Care*, London, Sage.

Kelly, P.J. (2005) 'Practical suggestions for community interventions using participatory action research', *Public Health Nursing*, vol. 22, no. 1, pp. 65–73.

Kvale, S. (1996) *Interviews: An Introduction to Qualitative Research Interviewing*, Thousand Oaks, CA, Sage.

Labuschagne, A. (2003) 'Qualitative research – airy fairy or fundamental?', *The Qualitative Report*, vol. 8, no. 1 [online], http://www.nova.edu/ssss/QR/QR8-1/index.html (Accessed 6 May 2006).

Mason, J. (2002) *Qualitative Researching* (2nd edn), London, Sage.

McFadden, M. and McCamley, F.A. (2003) 'Using reflexivity to loosen theoretical and organisational knots within participatory action research' in Finlay and Gough (eds) (2003).

Pavis, S. and Cunningham-Burley, S. (1999) 'Male youth street culture: understanding the context of health-related behaviours', *Health Education Research*, vol. 14, no. 5, pp. 583–96.

Reason, P. (2006) 'Choice and quality in action research practice', *Journal of Management Inquiry*, vol. 15, no. 2, pp. 187–203.

Steward, B. (2006) 'Investigating invisible groups using mixed methodologies' in Finlay and Ballinger (eds) (2006).

Walton, J. (2006) 'Invited response' [online], http://journals.medicinescomplete.com/journals/fact/current/fact0804a06d01.htm (Accessed 1 May 2006).

Willig, C. (2001) *Introducing Qualitative Research in Psychology: Adventures in Theory and Method*, Buckingham, Open University Press.

Winch, P. (1999) 'The role of anthropological methods in a community-based mosquito net intervention in Bagamoyo District, Tanzania' in Hahn, R. (ed.) *Anthropology in Public Health: Bridging Differences in Culture and Society*, Oxford, Oxford University Press.

Yardley, L. and Marks, D.F. (eds) (2004) *Research Methods for Clinical and Health Psychology*, London, Sage.

Zyzanski, S.J., McWhinney, I.R., Blake, R., Crabtree, B.F. and Miller, W.L. (1992) 'Qualitative research: perspectives on the future' in Crabtree, B.F. and Miller, W.L. (eds) *Doing Qualitative Research*, Research Methods for Primary Care Series, vol. 3, Newbury Park, CA, Sage.

Chapter 10

Using research to plan multidisciplinary public health interventions

Revised by Jenny Douglas, Cathy Lloyd and Moyra Sidell[1]

Introduction

Public health action has been termed 'eclectic' (McQueen, 2007) and can incorporate a range of different activities, from the development of policies and strategies, to service and programme development and delivery, and the implementation of interventions aimed at reducing inequalities in health and improving health and wellbeing. One of the challenges for public health practitioners is to develop effective and appropriate programmes and interventions which meet the needs of the population and improve health. In planning these, public health practitioners often need to make decisions about which interventions to choose. In a review of public health, Wanless (2004) proposed that public health interventions should be evidence based. In describing the history of public health reports, he stated that, since the 1970s, the same public health problems had been described, but effective implementation of solutions remained a challenge (Wanless, 2004).

Effective planning and implementation requires information about which public health interventions are likely to work, in what circumstances and with whom, thereby utilising existing evidence of the effectiveness of public health practice. In the White Paper *Choosing Health* (2004), the English Department of Health, responding to the call for evidence from the Wanless review, developed measures to strengthen the evidence for effective public health interventions. It announced a major new public health research and development initiative, for which up to £3.5 million was to be made available over five years. This was referred to in *Choosing Health:* 'Early in 2005, we will launch a public health research consortium, bringing together national policy makers and researchers from a wide range

[1] from an original chapter by Linda Jones, Jeanne Katz and Moyra Sidell (2000), with contributions from Gayle Letherby, Geraldine Brown and Geraldine Brady

of disciplines relevant to public health, to focus effort on strengthening the evidence for effective health interventions to support White Paper delivery' (DoH, 2004, p. 189, Annex B, paragraph 11). It was recognised by the public health research consortium that there was a need to involve a multidisciplinary research team utilising a wide range of research methodologies and applying these methodologies to public health practice.

Thinking point   how can research help in the planning of public health interventions?

Researching health can provide a wealth of information about factors that influence health and health behaviour, as well as ways in which the health of the population can be improved. However, the choice of research methodologies poses challenges for practitioners making decisions about planning public health interventions. Research can inform public health in a number of ways, including determining priorities for interventions which promote and improve the public's health, and assessing health needs to determine which public health problem should be addressed. Evaluative research can shed light on the acceptability or effectiveness of specific interventions, and an audit can assess the resources or systems available in participating organisations (Naidoo and Wills, 2005). Inherent in all these activities is the development of theory and knowledge about factors that influence and improve the health of the population.

This chapter will examine the application of research to multidisciplinary public health practice by exploring the ways in which different research methodologies contribute to planning and implementing effective interventions. This will take further some of the debates about the nature of knowledge and the meaning of evidence in public health which you have encountered in earlier chapters in this part of the book. Section 10.1 starts with a consideration of the term 'planning', and Section 10.2 moves on to think about the use of theory and models in planning public health interventions. A case-study of a project in Coventry in the West Midlands, on using research to plan and evaluate specialist services for pregnant teenagers and young parents (Letherby et al., 2006), is then used in the subsequent sections of this chapter in order to illustrate the different stages of planning.

In the preceding chapters you explored the nature of 'knowledge' and the types of knowledge and information that can be provided by adopting particular research methodologies. Planning and implementing public health interventions can be fraught with difficulties, tensions and complexities. Public health practitioners can experience these complexities as fundamentally baffling, but the challenges they present are inescapable and go right to the heart of the knowledge base that needs to be acquired in order to become competent public health practitioners.

10.1 What is planning?

The term 'planning' is used in a variety of ways. However, other terms are often used to describe aspects of planning, and the terminology can be ambiguous. Box 10.1 sets out some of the terms used and their different meanings.

Box 10.1 Some planning terminology

Plan: how to get from your starting point to your end point and what you want to achieve.

Policy: guidelines for practice which set broad goals and the framework for action.

Programme: overall outline of action; a package of services, or information, in planned sequence that is intended to produce a particular result.

Strategy: the methods to be used in achieving goals.

Priority: the first claim for consideration.

Aim: broad goal.

Objective: specific goal to be achieved.

(Adapted from Dignan and Carr, 1992; Naidoo and Wills, 2000)

10.1.1 Why plan?

Multidisciplinary public health activity takes place at many levels. Careful and systematic planning of public health interventions can help to ensure that resources are used well and most effectively. It also ensures effective evaluation of public health interventions. Without planning, interventions run the risk of being marginalised and of not being given priority in resource distribution. Perhaps most important of all, planning is a reflective activity: it focuses the mind on the job in hand and forces people to prioritise and justify their activities. Plans can be made for small-scale activities, such as giving a talk to a parent and toddler group, as well as for large events, such as a national no smoking day or public health intervention to reduce teenage pregnancy and develop appropriate sexual health services. Whatever the scale of the initiative, the planning process is fairly similar. Ewles and Simnett (2003) suggest that all plans should provide answers to three basic questions:

- What am I trying to achieve?

- What am I going to do?

- How will I know whether I have been successful?

However, before starting to plan a public health intervention the key question that should be asked is:

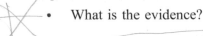

- What is the evidence?

10.1.2 What counts as evidence in planning?

Since the mid-1990s, there has been an increasing emphasis on the importance of evidence in health and social care generally and, more specifically, in multidisciplinary public health. In 1998, the Fifty-first World Health Assembly urged all member states to: 'adopt an evidence-based approach to health promotion policy and practice, using the full range of quantitative and qualitative methodologies' (WHO, 1998). In the UK, since the 1990s the accepted orthodoxy has been to base public health practice on the available evidence (McQueen, 2007). Evidence is obtained not only from major pieces of research: Davies et al. (2000) observe that critical evidence is held by practitioners and users in a range of public sector organisations and that this evidence is also important in any decision-making process. But what is meant by 'evidence-based practice'? Does it mean having an open and critical mind, and the ability to consider competing claims of knowledge, as Naidoo and Wills have argued?

Naidoo and Wills (2005) describe particular stages in adopting an evidence-based approach as:

- identifying an answerable problem

- searching for potential evidence

- data extraction

- critical appraisal and synthesis.

In order to plan and implement public health interventions, practitioners need to have some idea of the nature of the specific public health problem and a critical approach to research and evidence. This requires the knowledge, skill and ability to find out, access, critically appraise, synthesise and apply evidence from different disciplines and diverse sources.

Thinking point   what might be some of the sources of evidence that you could use in planning a public health intervention?

You considered some sources of evidence in Chapter 7. In particular, vital sources include published and unpublished papers. Published papers may be peer reviewed – where a paper is subject to scrutiny by experienced researchers and academics who are experts in the field – prior to its publication. Unpublished reports, conference papers and presentations, and independently published reports are also all vital sources of information (Naidoo and Wills, 2005).

Before looking at the process of planning, it is important to consider where information is obtained from and what counts as evidence in planning public health interventions. There are now many centres aimed at disseminating 'evidence' – for example, the NHS Centre for Reviews and Dissemination and the UK Cochrane Centre (dedicated to providing clinicians with up-to-date information on randomised clinical trials) – as well as national and local initiatives to help make healthcare research based. The Evidence for Policy and Practice Information and Co-ordinating Centre (the EPPI-Centre), at the Institute of Education at the University of London, seeks to provide information on evidence-based practice in health promotion, and the National Institute of Health and Clinical Excellence (NICE) provides evidence of effectiveness in public health. Health information changes rapidly, however: some sources of information are listed in Box 10.2.

Box 10.2 Selected online sources of evidence and systematic reviews

Department of Health
Website: http://www.dh.gov.uk

NHS Centre for Reviews and Dissemination
Website: http://www.york.ac.uk/instcrd

National Institute of Health and Clinical Excellence: Public Health Excellence
Website: http://www.publichealth.nice.org.uk

Evidence from systematic reviews of research relevant to implementing the 'wider public health' agenda
Website: http://www.york.ac.uk/inst/crd/wph.htm

The Evidence for Policy and Practice Information and Co-ordinating Centre (EPPI-Centre)
Website: http://eppi.ioe.ac.uk/EPPIWeb/home.aspx

Wales Centre for Health
Website: http://www.wales.nhs.uk/sites3/home.cfm?orgid=369

Health Scotland
Website: http://www.hebs.scot.nhs.uk

Health Promotion Agency for Northern Ireland
Website: http://www.healthpromotionagency.org.uk/

Health Technology Assessment Database (HTA)
Website: http://nhscrd.york.ac.uk/htahp.htm

NHS Economic Evaluation Database (NHS EED)
Website: http://nhscrd.york.ac.uk/nhsdhp.htm

International Union for Health Promotion and Education (IUHPE)
Website: http://www.iuhpe.org

Reviews of health promotion and education online (RHP&EO)
Website: http://rhpeo.org

The Cochrane Collaboration
Website: http://www.cochrane.org

This site includes access to Abstracts of Cochrane Reviews and the Cochrane Library, which provides access to a number of databases, such as the Cochrane Databases of Systematic Reviews and the Database of Abstracts of Reviews of Effectiveness.

Cochrane Health Promotion and Public Health Field
Website: http://www.vichealth.vic.gov.au/cochrane

Campbell Collaboration
Website: http://www.campbellcollaboration.org

WHO Reproductive Health Library
Website: http://www.update-software.com/RHL

(Adapted from Tones and Green, 2004, p. 169)

Evidence is used to inform practice in a number of ways, including:

- information about an intervention's effectiveness in meeting its goals
- information about how transferable this intervention is thought to be (to other settings and populations)
- information about the intervention's positive and negative effects
- information about the intervention's economic impact
- information about barriers to implementing the interventions.

(Supplement to *American Journal of Preventative Medicine*, 2000, p. 36; cited in McQueen, 2001, p. 264)

However, although the need for evidence is widely discussed and debated in relation to evaluating multidisciplinary public health interventions, Tones and Green (2004) have argued that little attention has been paid to the way in which evidence is used by practitioners in planning interventions. Nutbeam (1996) suggested that there were three different levels of practice with regard to the way in which practitioners used evidence in planning health promotion interventions, and termed them: 'planned', 'responsive' and 'reactive'. These are outlined in Figure 10.1 (p. 304) and are based on an assumption that planned approaches utilise most research evidence.

Nutbeam argued that 'the planned approach to health promotion practice' was based on 'a rational and systematic assessment of the best available evidence concerning population health needs, effective interventions, and the organizational and administrative context for successful intervention' (Nutbeam, 1996, p. 320). On the other hand, responsive approaches placed highest value on the role of the community in defining health needs and solutions, where there may be conflict between community needs analysis to identify expressed needs and priorities identified through more traditional epidemiological analysis. In this approach the use of research evidence is only one of several elements involved in decision making.

Thinking point   think of the recent public health initiative to encourage the consumption of fruit in primary school children – which category does it fit into: planned, responsive or reactive?

Often public health interventions are reactive – that is, rather than being based on a systematic review of the evidence, they are a response to an immediate problem or crisis and a more political agenda. Examples of this in the 1980s were high-profile campaigns about HIV/AIDS which were funded by central government. A more recent example is obesity, particularly childhood obesity and physical activity, for which public health interventions may be based on epidemiological information about the problem, but there is limited evidence of effectiveness of interventions (see Chapter 12).

10.2 Using theory and models in planning

In Chapter 4 you explored theoretical perspectives underpinning the promotion of public health, and in the earlier chapters in Part 2 you examined the ways in which different theories inform research methodologies and how these in turn inform the research methods that are adopted. The use of research and theory can vary greatly in multidisciplinary public health interventions (Jones and Donovan, 2004). McQueen (2007) contends that 'Public health and health promotion have been theoretically weak and practice strong'. Tones and Green have argued that, in addition to evidence-based practice being underpinned by empirical evidence, there should also be a greater emphasis on the contribution of theory: 'empirical evidence and theory are not alternatives, but should be inextricably linked. In short, research evidence about the effectiveness of interventions should contribute to the development of intervention theory, which will itself shape subsequent interventions and the ways in which they are evaluated' (Tones and Green, 2004, p. 172).

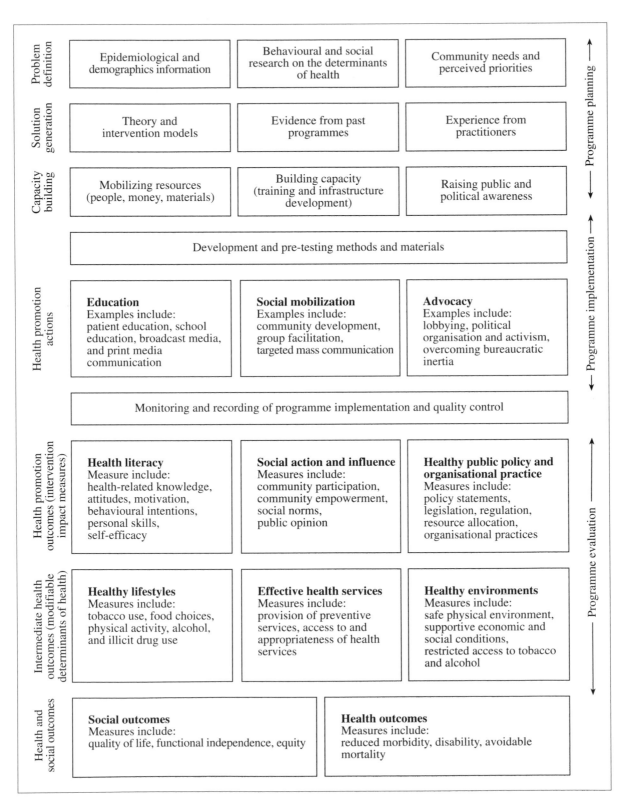

Figure 10.1 Three types of health promotion practice, illustrating variable application of research evidence (Source: Nutbeam, 1996, p. 320, Figure 2)

Nutbeam and Harris suggest that theory can help in the planning and delivery of health-promoting interventions in several ways. It can:

- help us understand better the nature of the problem being addressed;

- describe and explain the needs and motivations of the target population;

- explain or make propositions concerning how to change health status, health-related behaviours and their determinants and;

- inform the methods and measures used to monitor the problem and the programme.

(Nutbeam and Harris, 2004, p. vii)

Effective planning involves developing a systematic approach which incorporates the use of appropriate research methodologies, and the need for public health interventions to be underpinned by clear theoretical perspectives.

10.2.1 Planning models

Multidisciplinary public health practitioners may be placed in a number of different sectors. Whatever the sector – health, local authority, voluntary or private – public health interventions should be based on careful planning. A number of planning models have been developed – including the precede–proceed model (Green and Kreuter, 1999) and the public health decision-making model – PABCAR (Maycock et al., 2001). All models aim to provide a systematic approach to planning, which not only uses epidemiological information in determining priorities for action, but also prioritises the perceived needs of local communities.

Figure 10.2 (overleaf) sets out a planning model for health promotion, which highlights various stages and indicates the potential interconnections between theory and practice.

Thinking point   what message does Nutbeam and Harris's model, given in Figure 10.2, contain about how planning should be undertaken?

This model suggests that the planning process is complex. It sets out five distinct phases in the process:

1 problem definition
2 solution generation
3 capacity building
4 implementation
5 process, impact and outcome evaluation.

Figure 10.2   The use of theory in programme planning and evaluation

Planning phase	Task	Possible use of theory
Problem identification and prioritisation	Clarify major health issues for a defined population, and prioritise in terms of the potential for effective intervention	Clarify what should be the target elements of an intervention, such as individual beliefs, social norms or organisational practices
Planning a solution	Develop a programme plan which specifies programme objectives, strategies and the sequence of activity	Guidance on how, when and where change can be achieved in the target elements of a programme
Mobilising resources for implementation	Generate public and political support, build the capacity of partner organisations and secure resources	Guidance on how to build partnerships, raise public awareness and foster organisational development
Implementation	Execute the programme as planned, utilising multiple strategies (as appropriate to the programme objectives)	Provide a benchmark against which the actual implementation can be compared with the theoretical ideal
Evaluation	Assess the impact and outcome of the programme according to predefined programme objectives	Define outcomes and measurements which could be used at each level of evaluation

(Source: Nutbeam and Harris, 2004, p. 6, Table 1.1)

Although Nutbeam developed this model within the specific context of health promotion, it can be applied more generally to multidisciplinary public health within which health promotion, as one particular type of public health action, is situated.

Problem definition

Defining the problem is a vital first stage of planning in that it informs the development of long-term goals, short-term targets and priorities for any intervention. In order to carry out this phase, first the size and distribution of the particular health problem in the population under consideration needs to be determined (Nutbeam 2001); and second, the determinants of that health problem – for example, social, environmental, or economic factors – must be considered. Nutbeam goes on to describe two further considerations to be taken into account when defining the problem: that of the possibility of changing these determinants, and the community and political priorities which might affect any opportunity to take action (Nutbeam, 2001).

Identification of need is based on behavioural and social research as well as local epidemiological and demographic information. Although epidemiological data may be useful in determining patterns of mortality,

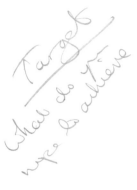

morbidity and specific diseases for public health action, social research is important in determining the specific target of the intervention and the range of possible interventions.

Solution generation

This involves looking at the research evidence and information available to determine the best solutions from a range of possibilities. Decision making should be guided by theoretical perspectives, information on interventions from past intervention programmes, and research evidence.

Capacity building

At this stage there should be an assessment of resource needs for the intervention – including financial and human resources. But limited financial and human resources mean that a range of options is not always possible.

Implementation

Putting the plan into action is the exciting and nerve-racking part. It is always worth making a final check to ensure that no significant changes have occurred during the planning process. At another level, changes in government or NHS policy may need to be taken into account and plans adjusted accordingly. If a lot of effort has been put into a plan, then it can be difficult to jettison or redesign all or parts of it, but the need to adapt and be flexible is essential even after the plan has been put into action. Doggedly going on with a plan when circumstances have changed is a waste of time and resources; monitoring what is going on in order to check that any action is going according to plan is therefore essential. If evaluation is built into each step of the plan, then changes can be integrated and plans revised.

Evaluation

During implementation the evaluation strategy will determine the type of data that needs to be collected. In order for the evaluation to be useful the data needs to be collected rigorously and systematically, with a clear plan at the outset for the collection of both the qualitative data (e.g. notes of meetings, key decisions, changes in the plan) and data from questionnaires or surveys undertaken during the implementation of the intervention – that is, both process information and outcome information. In order to demonstrate the effectiveness of the intervention, often data is collected before the intervention is undertaken. For example, if the intervention is a health education programme in a school on smoking, which aims to improve knowledge about the effects of smoking and to reduce the incidence of smoking among young people, then data will need to be collected on the smoking patterns of young people and their knowledge of smoking before the programme is implemented. Information will also be required on smoking policies in the school before and after the implementation of the intervention. (Chapter 11 is devoted to the issue of evaluation.)

10.3 Developing needs assessment in promoting public health

In order to address Nutbeam's first phase of the planning process, an essential starting point for any intervention is the identification of needs, yet identifying and prioritising needs is complex and resource intensive. Systematic analyses of national and local health status are undertaken by the Chief Medical Officer, the national health promotion bodies, directors of public health, public health observatories and primary care trusts, and they provide much of the data on which decisions on priority setting are based. In the past these analyses have relied on epidemiological enquiry and have been framed within scientific discourse (Bunton et al., 1995). In contrast to this, public health practitioners are increasingly attempting to incorporate the ideas and reflect the needs of lay people.

10.3.1 Assessing need

In Coventry, the planners of a new intervention concerning young people and issues of pregnancy drew upon existing research evidence on the needs of pregnant teenagers and young parents as well as national and local strategies (see Box 10.3).

Box 10.3 Coventry case-study: the Coventry specialist services for pregnant teenagers and young parents project

Although teenage pregnancy is not a recent phenomenon, politically it is an issue that is receiving more attention than ever before. It has been argued that Britain has the highest teenage pregnancy rate in Western Europe – double that of Germany, triple that of France and six times that of the Netherlands (SEU, 1999). The Labour Government commissioned the Social Exclusion Unit (SEU) to study the reasons for such high teenage pregnancy. The ideology underpinning this comes from the Prime Minister, Tony Blair, who suggested that 'The high rate of teenage pregnancy is not inevitable' (SEU, 1999, p. 4). According to the SEU report, each year 90,000 teenagers become pregnant, and of these 7,700 are under sixteen and 2,200 are under fourteen. The National Teenage Pregnancy Strategy is set out in the Social Exclusion Unit report on teenage pregnancy and is a joint Department of Health and Department for Education and Skills Public Service Agreement. The two national targets are:

1   **In terms of prevention to:** halve the under eighteen conception rate in England by 2010 (with an interim reduction target of 15 per cent by 2003 included in the NHS Plan, which is also a manifesto commitment).

2   **In terms of support to:** increase to 60 per cent the participation of teenage mothers in education, training or work by 2010, to reduce the risk of long-term social exclusion.

However, there is an increasing body of work challenging the evidence presented in the SEU report. For example, Arai (2003a, 2003b) highlights the difficulties in comparing British statistics on teenage pregnancy with other European countries.

Political discourses then individualise the problems of teenage pregnancy and parenthood rather than examine the structural factors that affect young people's lives (Phoenix, 1991). Although the Labour Government has in some ways attempted to highlight structural inequalities that affect young people experiencing teenage pregnancy and parenthood, government initiatives can reinforce negative images. By placing the issue of teenage pregnancy and parenthood under the remit of the Social Exclusion Unit, the UK Government is recognising that there can be a detrimental impact on the lives of those involved, but this can also reinforce the pervading notion that teenage pregnancy leads to an inevitable exclusion from mainstream society.

Bradshaw (1972) drew attention to four types of need: normative, comparative, felt and expressed. Normative needs are those defined by professional experts and reflect professional judgements and standards. Using the medical model, for example, doctors may define some people's health or behaviour as falling within a 'normal' range, while others may be entitled to (or required to undergo) treatment on the basis of their identified health needs. Normative definitions of need reflect professional views about the nature of health problems, and there may be considerable discrepancies between these views and those of lay people. Public health practitioners' views will reflect their own judgements about priorities and will be underpinned by values about what constitutes 'good health' and what the goals of public health should be. In addition, health promoters may also assess needs in relation to the services that are provided (Naidoo and Wills, 2000).

Assessing comparative needs usually involves estimation by professionals of which groups are in greater need of available services or resources.

One aspect of national health strategies that many welcomed was that they set out clearer priorities for public health by creating targets for disease reduction and for improving people's quality of life, although some critics have suggested that this unduly restricted the scope of public health activities (Adams, 1994). Whether working to targets or not, it is generally professionals who are assessing people's comparative needs and lay people have, until recently, had little involvement.

Comparative need raises important questions about rationing. Only so many human and financial resources are available and public health practitioners have to prioritise. There has been an extensive debate within public health about how this should be done. There are considerable advantages, for example, in prioritising high-risk groups so that public health interventions can be focused on those in most immediate danger. This runs the risk of stereotyping and stigmatising some groups – for example, teenage mothers – but potentially can deliver more support and advice than general whole population campaigns. Whole population strategies, by contrast, may deliver greater overall benefits without stigmatising particular groups, but at an individual level these benefits may be very small. This has been termed the 'prevention paradox' (Rose, 1981).

Thinking point can you think of ways in which teenage mothers may be singled out for priority treatment, and the stereotypes associated with this?

Box 10.4 Coventry case-study: stereotypes associated with young motherhood

Young mothers are not only stereotyped as a burden on the state (see, for example, Phoenix, 1991; Laws 1996), but despite evidence to the contrary (Phoenix, 1991; Ussher, 2000), teenage mothers are stereotyped as bad mothers and their children as severely disadvantaged. Arguably though, it is not the age of the woman that is the primary issue, but the fact that younger pregnant girls/women are more likely to give birth outside marriage. The stigmatisation of lone parents impacts on the position of mothers more significantly than on fathers, due to the fact that the head of most lone-parent families is female (Robertson Elliot, 1994), and disproportionately affects teenage mothers as 'three-quarters of British women who become mothers in their teenage years do so while single' (Phoenix, 1991, p. 95). Additionally, there is concern that because most pregnancies of unmarried teenagers are unplanned, this will have adverse social and health outcomes for both mother and child (e.g. Finlay 1996).

TMA

Felt needs, the third type of need discussed by Bradshaw (1972), are those that people themselves identify. These may be uncovered by questions addressed to individuals or perhaps by surveys of local residents, but their characteristic feature is that they are perceived by users themselves and generated by their own life experiences. In many cases such needs may be described as hidden or 'latent' because, without knowledge of the services or support that are available, or how needs are being defined in the wider world, people may not believe themselves to be 'in need'. Latent need may be felt by the local population or by groups or families within a local area, but may not show up in a survey of need or be expressed to the public health practitioner.

Expressed need is what people say they need; it is the turning of a felt need into a request, call or even demand for action. For example, people may grumble for years about the restricted opening hours of the local health centre without doing anything about it. However, if they are consulted about opening hours, the grumbles may turn into expressed demands for change. Local mothers may feel the need for a safe crossing place on a busy road and find out that on other roads traffic has been better controlled. This may turn their felt but latent need into an expressed need and they will begin to make demands for traffic controls. Expressed needs may reinforce normative needs because the process of channelling the felt need into an expressed need may itself be mediated by professionals and may reflect the realistic options open for action. Some surveys of people's needs may be fairly closed and focused on professional agendas (Bowling, 2002). On the other hand, people's expressed needs may conflict with public health practitioners' priorities. Attempts to encourage people to cut down their smoking may conflict with users' own expressed needs, such as the need to create pockets of 'time out' in a hectic day of unsupported child care by undertaking the pleasurable activity of smoking a cigarette (Graham, 1988). In addition, expressed needs from users may be in conflict with each other.

Two issues follow from this. First, if public health practitioners use consumer surveys to enable people to 'make their voices heard' in public health planning, then such surveys need to be sensitive and inclusive rather than quick, closed snapshots of local opinion. Second, it is not necessarily the case that expressed need translates easily into normative need or leads to new policy priorities, but it may trigger more research to estimate the 'real' level of concern. A central problem in identifying needs is determining what needs themselves are and, in particular, what types of needs should be regarded as legitimate. Relative needs may be established by comparing the health needs of one locality with another. In any organisation where resources are limited, priorities must be established and an equitable way of achieving this is to measure the relative needs of each area or unit requiring resources. Every organisation makes these policy judgements about priorities, and in recent years they have become more visible and public within healthcare.

In addition to the methodological and ethical issues raised by the methods used to assess health needs, the values given to the needs raised may vary depending on the methodology used. Some policy makers may give more value to needs assessed by large-scale positivist methodologies, while smaller-scale qualitative studies, which aim to involve consumers, may not be given equal value. This raises ethical issues when determining priorities for action: whose needs count?

The Coventry case-study provides an example of the involvement of consumers in developing sexual health services for teenagers (see Box 10.5).

Box 10.5 Coventry case-study: involving consumers

Policy and local context

Coventry Primary Care Trust responded to the targets set in the National Pregnancy Strategy by appointing two teenage pregnancy co-ordinators: one with a focus on prevention and one with a focus on support. A local Teenage Pregnancy Partnership Board (TPPB) was also established to oversee work in this area. In meeting its remit to support young parents, the Coventry TPPB decided to commission some empirical research to find out what it was that pregnant teenagers and young parents felt that they needed. This was a positive step forward because, as Phoenix (1991, p. 86) argues, the debate about teenage pregnancy and young parenthood focuses on the negative, largely because young people have remained silent in much of the discussion. The negative focus is produced by people who are not themselves 'young mothers', but rather are outsiders. There is generally disjunction between 'outsider' and 'insider' perspectives.

The first call for tender by Coventry TPPB was for a project concerned to explore the semi-supported housing needs for lone parents aged under eighteen. The Centre for Social Justice at Coventry University bid for and won this tender and carried out the work in the summer of 2001 (Letherby et al., 2001). They were encouraged by the initiative of Coventry TPPB to attempt to access the 'insider' perspective and were hopeful that their findings would influence policy. In their research bid, they noted that one of the best ways to find out about people's feelings and experiences was to let them tell these themselves (Stanley and Wise, 1993). They planned to collect the data through single and focus group interviews. One-to-one interviewing and small focus group work allow researchers to explore issues in greater depth than would be possible with larger groups (Gilbert, 1993). Although the focus of this project was housing experience and need, as is often the case in social research the

> respondents talked about other aspects of their lives. One issue that emerged, which was of particular concern, was young women's maternity experiences.

In order to obtain the views of groups of people who may have been socially excluded or marginalised in the past, some attention must be paid to the research methodologies and research methods employed. Postal questionnaires may exclude people who have low literacy skills and those whose first language is not English. The response rate for postal questionnaires is known to be much lower than that for face-to-face interviews and they may only be completed by the most motivated people. The issue of language must be considered when undertaking surveys in multilingual and multicultural areas. There is a growing research literature on developing appropriate research methodologies for undertaking research with black and minority ethnic communities (Gunaratnam, 2007; Lloyd, 2007).

Assessing local needs and listening to local voices is not a simple matter. Local people do not speak necessarily with one voice. Although they may share common problems or interests, they may have different agendas and express different needs. Some may speak louder than others, some may find it hard to express themselves, others may not be interested at all. As well as questionnaires, phone-ins and high-street surveys, practitioners have adopted a number of other strategies in an attempt to overcome the difficulties and tap as comprehensive a local voice as possible. These include using key informants and focus groups and setting up health forums.

10.3.2 Listening to local voices

Working with key informants

This resembles the grapevine approach where key individuals are interviewed because they have particular access to local knowledge. They may be formal or informal leaders or the landlord of the local pub who has an 'ear to the ground'. Religious or cultural leaders, or the head teacher at a local school, might be in a similar position.

Thinking point   can you think of possible limitations of this approach?

This approach may provide a distorted or biased view because it may not be possible to disentangle the informant's own interests from the interests of the local population. It may provide only a superficial picture of the local community and not represent the views of minority groups or groups with special concerns.

Focus groups

Focus groups are thought to be a useful way of accessing a range of different interest groups within a community. For example, they may represent the interests of older people, women, or people from a minority ethnic group. Focus groups have been used increasingly as a mechanism for assessing health needs and the experiences of service users. Although a good method for accessing a range of different groups of people, the findings of focus groups must be contextualised and not generalised to the wider population. It is often helpful to use focus groups alongside other methodologies such as surveys.

Health forums

A health forum for a particular locality would comprise a mixture of professionals, members of voluntary organisations, community groups and local residents. It differs from a focus group in that the forum is a cross-section of the community rather than a special interest group. Once set up, a health forum would meet regularly, deal with health issues as they arise, and have a finger on the pulse of the local community and its health needs.

In assessing the needs of communities, both focus groups and health forums have their relative strengths and weaknesses. Focus groups have special access to the needs of specific groups in the community whose voices may not otherwise be heard, but of necessity they have their own agenda which may conflict with that of other groups. Reconciling those different agendas may be very difficult. A health forum can bring together different interest groups, but runs the risk of becoming elitist and dominated by the professionals.

Community profiling

This need not be on a large scale, such as a city-wide profile. Indeed, many general practitioners are being encouraged to adopt a community profiling approach to the services they offer. This community-oriented primary care approach is very much about planning, rather than responding to patients who present themselves at the surgery. The term 'community profile' is broader than an assessment of needs as it also takes into account the resources available within that community to meet those needs. Hawtin et al. have explained 'community profile' as:

> A comprehensive description of the needs of a population that is defined, or defines itself, as a community, and the resources that exist within that community, carried out with the active involvement of the community itself, for the purpose of developing an action plan or other means of improving the quality of life in the community.

(Hawtin et al., 1994, p. 5)

A community profile, then, is more than a health audit; it produces a database of all the resources in the community. For example, in a project in Sandwell in the West Midlands, aimed at assessing the health needs of black and minority ethnic communities in Smethwick, a community profile was developed which included all the voluntary and religious organisations, as well as those statutory organisations that might impact on the determinants of health (Douglas, 1996).

Rapid appraisal

A methodology that has become popular as a way of collecting information upon which priorities can be based is called rapid appraisal. Rapid appraisal does not rely solely on gathering new information but can collect secondary data (from demographers, epidemiologists and large-scale social surveys) as well as information from any source deemed appropriate.

One of the problems that has been identified with rapid appraisal methods is that they rely mainly on key informants who may or may not represent the local population well. It is important that the wider community is involved. Setting priorities *with* rather than *for* people seems eminently sensible if people are to feel committed to a plan of action. But there may also be conflicting interests in the setting of priorities: there are those priorities that are set by others, as well as the practical or real interests on the ground.

Researching the views of consumers

Current public health strategies have enshrined the principle of involving consumers in health planning (DoH, 2004). Awareness of consumers' views and concerns is important when planning public health interventions. Entwistle and Hanley (2001) have identified some other ways of engaging with consumers' views, including holding open meetings; running citizens' juries; inviting consumers to be members of project teams, working groups or committees; inviting consumers to comment on drafts of project plans, research proposals, advertising ideas and information leaflets; and asking consumers to lead or undertake projects themselves.

Participatory appraisal

Participatory appraisal is another method of involving local communities in assessing and appraising their own needs, identifying problems and determining the priorities for solving those problems. In the example given in Box 10.6, participatory rapid appraisal was used in the Ardoyne area of North Belfast to define the health and social needs of women and to formulate joint action plans between the residents and service providers.

> ## Box 10.6 Revealing the hidden 'troubles' in Northern Ireland: the role of participatory rapid appraisal
>
> The PRA [participatory rapid appraisal] team carried out interviews with key informants including local health and social service professionals, voluntary organizations, and community groups ...
>
> Twenty members of the community participated in two focus group discussions. Each group had 10 members of the community, and was led by a skilled facilitator and a researcher to record the findings. A semi-structured interview schedule was prepared, which took the form of a broad framework of issues ... The goal was to elicit the community views and opinions of the locality through a guided questioning route, and for the sub-team to emerge from the focus group with a deeper understanding of the 'community's' priority health and social need issues. The group also discussed how to improve the uptake of existing services and new ways to meet gaps in services.
>
> [...]
>
> ... In Ardoyne, where health and social services management is largely localized, PRA provided a powerful vehicle for active participation of civil society in planning and evaluating services.
>
> (Lazenbatt et al., 2001, pp. 571, 576)

The nature of information on needs is dependent on the research methodology or methodologies chosen. Cross-sectional epidemiological surveys will provide general information about a population – how many people smoke, for example, and their knowledge of the effects of smoking. However, if a greater understanding of when and why people smoke is required, then qualitative methodologies will be more valuable.

You explored quantitative and qualitative methodologies in earlier chapters, and you were introduced to the idea of combining methodologies in multidisciplinary public health research to enable a better understanding of the diverse and complex factors that influence health and health behaviour. Baum (1995, 2007) argues that, because of the increasing complexity of problems facing public health, a range of methodological strategies is required. Public health practitioners therefore need skills in understanding and utilising research findings from diverse perspectives, and to be aware of the range of methodologies available in order to choose the most appropriate combination for a public health research project (Tones and Green, 2004). Green suggests that combining qualitative and quantitative

methodological strategies within research programmes can contribute in the
following ways:

- using qualitative data to inform quantitative studies

- using qualitative work to add depth to statistics, or to explore
  why variables are related – using qualitative methods to
  examine epidemiological findings

- using quantitative work (such as a survey) to test the
  generalisability of small scale qualitative studies (such as a
  focus group)

- using qualitative and quantitative work in tandem to help
  validate findings.

(Green, 2005, p. 157)

The Coventry case-study used two qualitative methods – in-depth single
interviews and focus group interviews, as outlined in Box 10.7 – to elicit
the views of local women.

Box 10.7 Coventry case-study: methods used

- Single, face-to-face interviews: with both teenage mothers and
  service providers.

- Focus group meetings: with teenage mothers and service
  providers.

- Observations of the service provided for teenage mothers.

So far, this chapter has concentrated on the first of Nutbeam's planning
stages: that of problem definition and investigating and assessing needs.
The next section focuses on the second and third phases: those of solution
generation and capacity building.

10.4 Setting priorities and objectives

After defining the problem, Nutbeam identifies the next phase of planning
as that of solution generation, and we will now consider this in terms of
setting priorities and aims and objectives.

10.4.1 Setting priorities

In many situations, a number of influences impact on the setting of public
health priorities. These might include:

- the managers decided on this policy some time ago

- it is an established and long-standing initiative

- public pressure
- political pressure
- someone's hobbyhorse
- a response to a crisis
- it was necessary to demonstrate that the organisation was responding to the issue
- work done in this area had proven effective
- there is a national initiative (e.g. World AIDS day)
- a staff member had expertise in this area
- the unit had to economise and be more efficient
- a change in national policy
- new evidence of need
- national and local targets
- availability of funding.

(Adapted from Ewles and Simnett, 2003, p. 115)

This indicates that setting priorities is dependent on the interests of both the people setting up the initiative and outside influences and pressures. For the Coventry case-study it was very much national and local targets on teenage pregnancy and the availability of funding for assessing needs that set teenage sexual health services as a priority.

The next step is to work on the aims and objectives.

10.4.2 Setting aims and objectives

Aims or goals are broad statements that set out what the programme or initiative expects to achieve. Objectives are statements that map out the tasks needed to reach those goals, including a timeframe for the achievement of each task. It is important to set clear aims and objectives: objectives should be specific, measurable, achievable, realistic and time limited (SMART). It is essential that the aims or goals, which provide the framework for the programme planning, reflect not only the normative needs of the health professionals on the planning group, but also the expressed and felt needs of the target population. Box 10.8 identifies some major goals for multidisciplinary public health interventions.

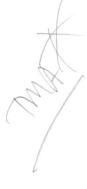

> ## Box 10.8 Goals for interventions which promote multidisciplinary public health
>
> Health education goals
>
> - Related to increased levels of knowledge.
>
> - Concerning attitudes and beliefs.
>
> - Skills or psycho-motor objectives concerning skills acquisition and competence.
>
> Health promotion goals
>
> - Behaviour change including changes in lifestyles and increased take-up of services.
>
> - Aiming for changes in policy.
>
> - Concerning increases in participation and working together.
>
> - Concerning changing the environment to make it more healthy.
>
> (Adapted from Naidoo and Wills, 2000; Ewles and Simnett, 2003)

Other goals for multidisciplinary public health in the twenty-first century would also include organisational and policy changes, and changes in national and global policy. These issues are considered in depth in the companion volume to this book (Lloyd et al., 2007b).

10.4.3 Capacity building

Capacity building is the third stage of planning according to Nutbeam's model and is intricately linked to the previous stages. When defining the objectives of any intervention, it is essential that they are appropriate and precise as well as realistic and manageable. This means being aware of the resources available and identifying likely constraints. Resources exist in a variety of forms, and may include hard cash, availability of volunteers, political responsiveness or particularly useful skills possessed by colleagues, members of the advisory board or the target group.

Setting up an advisory group

It is possible that, for small-scale interventions, the planning and organisation will be taken on by the public health practitioner on their own. Other programme plans may need the participation of a variety of people; the people who are involved in this process are often called stakeholders. All major stakeholders should ideally be involved in planning public health interventions. Tones and Green define primary, secondary and key stakeholders as follows:

- **Primary stakeholders** are the potential beneficiaries – those who are directly affected, either positively or negatively, by the initiative.

- **Secondary stakeholders** are those involved in implementing the initiative.

- **Key stakeholders** are those whose support is essential to the continuation of the initiative – for example, fundholders.

(Tones and Green, 2004, p. 109)

Thinking point   can you think of other likely candidates for an advisory panel for the setting up of a young people's sexual health service?

Box 10.9 Coventry case-study: members of the TPPB

The Coventry Teenage Pregnancy Partnership Board was the planning group that co-ordinated the service development and commissioned the research. Members of the TPPB included representatives from:

- social services
- health visiting
- midwifery services
- Connexions
- the Domestic Violence Partnership.

Once the group is assembled it will be necessary to discuss how the process of planning will work and familiarise the members with public health interventions. As the group becomes oriented, there will of necessity be some role negotiation so that each person understands what contribution they can usefully make. It is essential that each member of the group feels valued and useful otherwise tensions could set in which undermine the goals being pursued. Responsibility for different tasks will need to be delegated bearing in mind the fostering of a group responsibility for the whole undertaking.

10.4.4 Developing proposals for interventions

Whether or not they are applying for funding, practitioners often need to develop proposals for public health interventions. These proposals may need to go to the appropriate local authority committee or board of the primary care trust. Although there is increasing recognition for the need to fund interventions more appropriately, public health practitioners often have to bid competitively for the funding of initiatives. This means that developing clear and coherent funding proposals is essential.

10.4.5 Developing funding proposals

Public health interventions are often funded on a short-term or competitive basis. Examples of projects include Health Action Zone projects and Sure Start projects. In developing a funding proposal it is important to have very clearly stated aims and objectives and very clear timescales as the success of the initiative will be measured against these. There must be a clear rationale for carrying out an intervention, based on prior epidemiological evidence. Funders are increasingly concerned with the relationship of research to theory and practice and ways in which users and the public are involved in developing the programme or proposed research project. Having a clear dissemination strategy is equally important. There are a number of publications on writing and funding proposals, and funding bodies themselves usually give very clear guidance as to what is expected of the person writing the proposal in terms of content. One of the important aspects of developing funding proposals is to ensure that they are properly and realistically costed. A realistic assessment of the resources required and the outcomes expected is extremely important, and plans for evaluating the initiative must be built into the funding proposal.

In some instances there is also a need to develop research proposals. Proposals must have clear research questions and clearly stated aims and objectives. In the past, quantitative research methodologies and quantitative outcomes have been given priority; however, there is an increasing understanding of the value of qualitative research in providing insight into the complexity of public health. Ethical approval will also be required for research projects (this was discussed in Chapter 9).

10.5 Putting it into action: implementing the plan

The next phase in the planning process is the actual implementation of the intervention. In the Coventry example, the following recommendations were made for setting up a specialist service for pregnant teenagers and young parents, which was then implemented (see Box 10.10).

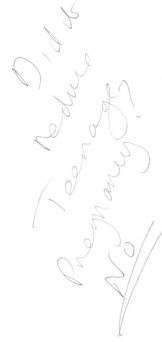

> ## Box 10.10 Coventry case-study: recommendations
>
> The recommendations from the research were that targeted services, both ante- and postnatal, should be organised **at appropriate times**, in **accessible, non-threatening** locations and focused on the particular concerns of young women, and that some young women needed one-to-one as well as group support.
>
> Following the research recommendations, Coventry TPPB:
>
> * established a young parents' forum
>
> * commissioned the Centre for Social Justice at Coventry University to design and deliver a training pack for health and social care professionals, which was produced and presented by the research team that worked on the 2002 project with the help of young mothers
>
> * secured funding for a specialist service aimed at addressing the ante- and postnatal needs of pregnant teenagers and young parents (aged 16–24) in Coventry for an initial period of two years.

Planning can be seen as part of a continuum ending with evaluation, and this chapter forms the bridge between researching health and evaluation. The next chapter explores the ways in which the sexual health service in Coventry was evaluated.

Throughout the planning process it is essential to keep a record of all the decisions that are made and it is useful to prepare a coherent written planning document which will be multipurpose, serving both as a funding document and as a consultation document for discussions with the target and other audiences. This should include an introduction setting out the background to the plan and the assessment of need on which it is based; the aims and objectives, with a statement of the timescale and the tasks to be achieved; and a note of the resources available and of any constraints.

Conclusion

The planning of any intervention needs to be thorough yet to remain flexible. Above all, planning should be based on sound information, and that information should include the knowledge and views of those involved, whether individuals or communities. This chapter has focused on the need for appropriate information and 'evidence' for planning multidisciplinary public health interventions. However, 'evidence' is not the only consideration for public health practitioners. Donnan highlights a number of ethical questions that should be considered when planning public health interventions:

- What should we be doing?

- For whom should we be doing it and at what cost/risk to others?

- Who should decide and how?

(Donnan, 2001, p. 118)

In Chapter 1, you considered the four ethical principles of autonomy, beneficence, non-maleficence and justice. One of the challenges for public health practitioners is to identify and address ethical issues from a population as well as an individual approach, and to achieve the right balance between the rights of the population and the rights of the individual. Involving lay people and users is an essential part of multidisciplinary public health practice. Earlier in this chapter you explored ways in which the views and wishes of a wide range of people could be sought through focus groups, questionnaire surveys, citizens' juries and panels. The ethical issues in relation to planning interventions can be complex and challenging. However, as mentioned in Section 10.3.2, planning should be done *with* rather than *for* people.

Planning and evaluation have been somewhat artificially separated in this and the following chapter. This is because evaluation is a complex and important process, and the next chapter is dedicated to its exploration.

References

Adams, L. (1994) 'Health promotion in crisis', *Health Education Journal*, vol. 53, pp. 354–60.

Arai, L. (2003a) 'British policy on teenage pregnancy and childbearing: the limitations of comparisons with other European countries', *Critical Social Policy*, vol. 23, no. 12, pp. 89–102.

Arai, L. (2003b) 'Low expectation, sexual attitudes and knowledge: explaining teenage pregnancy and fertility in English communities. Insight from qualitative research', The Editorial Board of the *Sociological Review*, vol. 51, no. 2, pp. 199–217.

Baum, F. (1995) 'Researching public health: behind the qualitative–quantitative methodological debate', *Social Science and Medicine*, vol. 40, no. 4, pp. 459–68.

Baum, F. (2007) 'Dilemmas in public health research: methodologies and ethical practice' in Handsley et al. (eds) (2007a).

Bowling, A. (2002) *Research Methods in Health: Investigating Health and Health Services*, Maidenhead, Open University Press.

Bradshaw, J. (1972) 'The concept of need', *New Society*, vol. 19, pp. 640–3.

Bunton, R., Nettleton, S. and Burrows, R. (1995) *The Sociology of Health Promotion: Critical Analyses of Consumption, Lifestyle and Risk*, London, Routledge.

Davies, H.T.O., Nutley, S.M. and Smith, P.C. (2000) *What Works? Evidence Based Policy and Practice in Public Services*, Bristol, Policy Press.

Department of Health (DoH) (2004) *Choosing Health: Making Healthier Choices Easier*, London, The Stationery Office.

Dignan, M.B. and Carr, P.A. (1992) *Programme Planning for Health Education and Promotion*, Philadelphia, PA, Lea and Febiger.

Donnan, S. (2001) 'Ethics in public health' in Pencheon et al. (eds) (2001).

Douglas, J. (1996) 'Developing health promotion strategies with black and minority ethnic communities which address social inequalities and their impact on health' in Bywaters, P. and McLeod, E. (eds) *Working for Equality in Health*, London, Routledge.

Entwistle, V. and Hanley, B. (2001) 'Involving "consumers"' in Pencheon et al. (eds) (2001).

Ewles, L. and Simnett, I. (2003) *Promoting Health: A Practical Guide*, London, Baillière Tindall.

Finlay, A. (1996) 'Teenage pregnancy, romantic love and social science: an uneasy relationship' in James, V. and Gabe, J. (eds) *Health and the Sociology of Emotions*, Oxford, Blackwell.

Gilbert, N. (ed.) (1993) *Researching Social Life*, London, Sage.

Graham, H. (1988) 'Women and smoking in the United Kingdom: implications for health promotion', *Health Promotion*, vol. 3, no. 4, pp. 371–82.

Green, J. (2005) 'Multi-method and multi-disciplinary approaches' in Green, J. and Browne, J. (eds) *Principles of Social Research*, Maidenhead, Open University Press.

Green, L. and Kreuter, M. (1999) *Health Promotion Planning: An Educational and Environmental Approach* (3rd edn), Mountain View, CA, Mayfield.

Gunaratnam, Y. (2007) 'Complexity and complicity in researching ethnicity and health' in Douglas et al. (eds) (2007a).

Douglas, J., Earle, S., Handsley, S., Lloyd, C.E., and Spurr, S. (eds) (2007a) *A Reader in Promoting Public Health: Challenge and Controversy*, London, Sage/Milton Keynes, The Open University.

Hawtin, M., Percy-Smith, J. and Hughes, G. (1994) *Community Profiling: Auditing Social Needs*, Buckingham, Open University Press.

Jones, L., Katz, J. and Sidell, M. (2000) 'Planning health promoting interventions' in Katz, J., Peberdy, A. and Douglas, J. (eds) *Promoting Health: Knowledge and Practice* (2nd edn), Basingstoke, Palgrave Macmillan/Milton Keynes, The Open University.

Jones, S. and Donovan, R. (2004) 'Does theory inform practice in health promotion in Australia?', *Health Education Research*, vol. 9, no. 1, pp. 1–14.

Laws, S. (1996) 'The "single mothers" debate: a children's right perspective' in Holland, J. and Atkins, L. (eds) *Sex, Sensibility and the Gendered Body*, Basingstoke, Macmillan.

Lazenbatt, A., Lynch, U. and O'Neill, E. (2001) 'Revealing the hidden "troubles" in Northern Ireland: the role of participatory rapid appraisal', *Health Education Research*, vol. 16, no. 5, pp. 567–78.

Letherby, G., Brown, G. and Brady, G. (2006) 'Planning and undertaking research: an evaluation of specialist services for pregnant teenagers and young parents', unpublished report, Coventry, Centre for Social Justice, Coventry University.

Letherby, G., Wilson, C., Bailey, N. and Brown, G. (2001) *Supported Semi-Independent Housing for Under 18 Lone Parents: Needs Assessment*, Coventry, Centre for Social Justice, Coventry University.

Lloyd, C.E., Handsley, S., Douglas, J., Earle, S. and Spurr, S. (eds) (2007) *Policy and Practice in Promoting Public Health*, London, Sage/Milton Keynes, The Open University.

Lloyd, C.E. (2007) 'Researching the views of diabetes service users from South Asian backgrounds: a reflection on some of the issues' in Douglas et al. (eds) (2007a).

Maycock, B., Howat, P. and Slevin, T. (2001) 'A decision-making model for health promotion advocacy: the case for advocacy of drunk driving control measures', *Promotion and Education*, vol. VIII, no. 2, pp. 59–64.

McQueen, D. (2001) 'Strengthening the evidence base for health promotion', *Health Promotion International*, vol. 16, no. 3, pp. 261–8.

McQueen, D. (2007) 'The evaluation of health promotion practice: 21st century debates on evidence and effectiveness' in Handsley et al. (eds) (2007a).

Naidoo, J. and Wills, J. (2000) *Health Promotion: Foundations for Practice* (2nd edn), London, Baillière Tindall.

Naidoo, J. and Wills, J. (2005) *Public Health and Health Promotion: Developing Practice* (2nd edn), London, Baillière Tindall.

Nutbeam, D. (1996) 'Achieving "best practice" in health promotion: improving the fit between research and practice', *Health Education Research*, vol. 11, no. 3, pp. 317–26.

Nutbeam, D. (2001) 'Effective health promotion programmes' in Pencheon et al. (eds) (2001).

Nutbeam, D. and Harris, E. (2004) *Theory in a Nutshell: A Practical Guide to Health Promotion Theories* (2nd edn), Sydney, McGraw-Hill.

Pencheon, D., Guest, C., Melzer, D. and Muir Gray, J.A. (eds) (2001) *Oxford Handbook of Public Health Practice*, Oxford, Oxford University Press.

Phoenix, A. (1991) 'Mothers under twenty: outsider and insider views' in Phoenix, A., Woollett, A. and Lloyd, E. (eds) *Motherhood: Meanings, Practices and Ideologies*, London, Sage.

Robertson Elliot, F. (1991) *The Family: Change or Continuity?*, London, Macmillan.

Rose, G. (1981) 'Strategy of prevention: lessons from cardiovascular disease', *British Medical Journal*, vol. 282, pp. 1847–51.

Social Exclusion Unit (SEU) (1999) *Teenage Pregnancy*, London, The Stationery Office.

Stanley, L. and Wise, S. (1993) *Breaking Out Again: Feminist Ontology and Epistemology*, London, Routledge.

Supplement to *American Journal of Preventative Medicine* (*SAJPM*) (2000) 'Introducing the Guide to Community Preventative Services: Methods, First Recommendations and Expert Commentary', *American Journal of Preventative Medicine*, vol. 18, pp. 35–43.

Tones, K. and Green, J. (2004) *Health Promotion: Planning and Strategies*, London, Sage.

Ussher, J.M. (2000) *Women's Health: Contemporary International Perspectives*, Leicester, The British Psychological Society.

Wanless, D. (2004) *Securing Good Health for the Whole Population: Final Report*, London, H.M. Treasury.

World Health Organization (WHO) (1998) *World Health Assembly Resolution WHA51.12 – Health Promotion* [online], http://www.who.int/healthpromotion/wha51-12/en/ (Accessed 29 November 2006).

Chapter 11

Evaluating public health interventions

Revised by Jenny Douglas, Moyra Sidell, Cathy Lloyd and Sarah Earle[1]

Introduction

The previous chapter looked at approaches to planning public health interventions and the importance of building evaluation into the planning process. Increasingly, public health practitioners are required to demonstrate whether or not an intervention has been effective, and the reasons why. Evaluation is an essential part of this.

As you saw in earlier chapters, promoting public health includes a range of diverse activities, such as providing health information and advice, awareness-raising campaigns, influencing public policy, lobbying for change, professional training, community development, management and organisational development and community public health interventions. Although health promotion is an important part of modern multidisciplinary public health, in relation to evaluation both health promotion and the 'new' public health have different (if overlapping) histories: the new public health has often adopted a medical model of health, and health promotion a social model. This is changing, but public health and health promotion have in the past drawn on different sources of evidence, with the result that health promotion has sometimes been seen as not having a sound evidence base (McQueen, 2001). This debate about evidence, which you met in the previous chapter, also permeates discussions about notions of appropriate methodologies for evaluating multidisciplinary public health. Although it is now widely accepted that both quantitative and qualitative methodologies have an important contribution to make in evaluation, it has been argued that health promotion is still evaluated using inappropriate tools (Thorogood and Coombes, 2000). Writing in 1997, Speller et al. contended that, because of the use of inappropriate methodologies, 'the current search for evidence of effective health promotion is unlikely to succeed and may result in drawing

[1] from original chapters by Alyson Peberdy (2000), with contributions from Gayle Letherby, Geraldine Brown and Geraldine Brady

false conclusions about health promotion practices to the long term detriment of public health' (Speller et al., 1997, p. 361).

This chapter considers the application of the research methodologies which were reviewed in previous chapters to the evaluation of interventions that promote public health. It is important to note that, although frameworks for evaluation draw on a range of research methodologies, evaluation is not the same as research. In outlining the differences between research and evaluation, Springett (2001) highlights one of the key differences: that evaluation explicitly involves values.

Following Chapter 10, the same case-study of a project in Coventry in the West Midlands, on using research to plan and evaluate specialist services for pregnant teenagers and young parents (Letherby et al., 2006), is used to illustrate points discussed in this chapter.

The following section begins by exploring the nature and purpose of evaluation. It reflects on who should take responsibility for evaluation, when evaluation should be carried out, and what should be the focus of evaluation. Section 11.2 moves on to consider evaluation design, outlining some of the main methods and approaches to evaluation within modern multidisciplinary public health. In Section 11.3, attention shifts to a discussion of the criteria that can be used to evaluate public health interventions, exploring effectiveness, acceptability, appropriateness, equity and efficiency. The next section returns to the issue of values, exploring the way in which evaluation is essentially a value-driven process. Finally, the chapter concludes by reflecting on changing policy and practice and the implications of this for evaluation in public health.

11.1 What is evaluation?

> [E]valuation is the systematic examination and assessment of features of a programme or other intervention in order to produce knowledge that different stakeholders can use for a variety of purposes.
>
> (Rootman et al., 2001, p. 26)

It is important to begin by recognising that evaluation is something in which practitioners are already actively involved, both professionally and in their daily lives. If evaluation is basically about judging the worth of an activity, then everyone engages in evaluation whenever they reflect critically on their actions in order to decide whether to continue or modify what they are doing. Whenever they ask themselves questions such as 'How did that session go?', 'Did I achieve what I set out to do?', or 'Did the patient or client really understand what I was explaining to her or was she just being polite when she said she did?', they are engaged in evaluating, albeit informally, their activities.

All evaluation has two fundamental elements: identifying and ranking the criteria (values and aims), and gathering the kind of information that will make it possible to assess the extent to which these are being met. Choosing the criteria that will guide the evaluation can be especially complex when there are no clearly stated aims or when the stakeholders have competing or conflicting perspectives. Decisions about the kind of information that should be gathered, and how best to gather it, will need to take into account a large number of practical, ethical and methodological considerations, and will therefore require careful thought and discussion.

A distinctive characteristic of formal (as distinct from informal) evaluation is its potentially public nature. The process and findings can, in principle, be scrutinised and repeated so that it is possible for others to check and confirm or refute them. It is also possible for others to put into action what has been learned and thus to benefit from it. Evaluation should be integral to the development of a particular project and part of an ongoing cyclical process of review and reform, as illustrated in Figure 11.1.

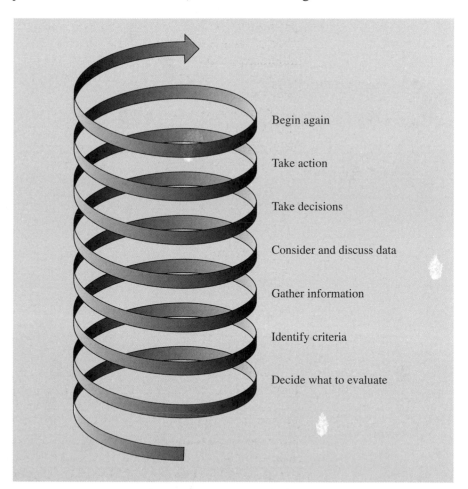

Begin again

Take action

Take decisions

Consider and discuss data

Gather information

Identify criteria

Decide what to evaluate

Figure 11.1   Evaluation cycle (Source: Katz et al., 2000, p. 279, Figure 16.1)

11.1.1 Why evaluate?

Thinking point   why should public health practitioners evaluate interventions?

If you ask a number of people why they evaluate their work they will probably give different answers. Figure 11.2 sets out some of the responses people have given to this question.

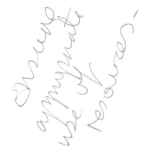

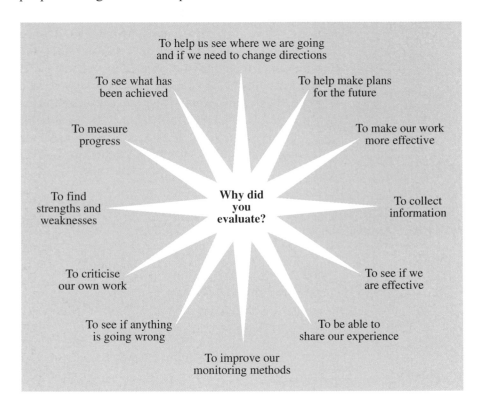

Figure 11.2 Why we evaluate (Source: Katz et al., 2000, p. 280, Figure 16.2)

There are many possible reasons for wanting to evaluate activities aimed at promoting public health. These include questions about effectiveness, the desire to improve practice, and a willingness to be self-critical and do as good a job as possible by consciously learning from experience. In an ideal world, evaluation and planning are inextricably linked as parts of an ongoing cycle. In addition to the desire of individuals to learn lessons that will improve practice, there may also be financial and political pressures that encourage or demand evaluation. Increasingly, projects are required to have an evaluation component in order to be eligible for funding, and the World Health Organization (WHO) (1998) recommends that at least 10 per cent of financial resources in any initiative should be set aside for evaluation. Other commentators argue that it is important for policy makers and practitioners to show that their actions are consistent, accountable and fair, especially in the face of potential legal challenges (Bravo Vergel and Ferguson, 2006). It has also been suggested that the trend towards 'evidence-based medicine' has promoted similar enthusiasm within public health (Kemm, 2006).

Evaluation has become an essential and central tool in a system aimed at providing a rational, evidence-based way of meeting needs. But in a number of important respects, the evaluation of public health interventions tends to be more complex and difficult than the evaluation of health services and therapeutic interventions. Although often judged by the same criteria, public health interventions have rather different tasks and goals which are hard to measure. The effects of the medical treatment of physically sick individuals are more obvious and immediate than the effects of public health interventions on medically well groups and populations. Evaluation is also important in helping to understand why some public health interventions are successful, thus aiding the development of theories about such interventions. Reasons for evaluation are summarised in Box 11.1.

Box 11.1 Some reasons for evaluating public health activities

Public health activities are evaluated in order to:

- secure funding

- check that a programme is having the desired effect

- improve methods, procedures and materials

- assess whether the resources invested are being used efficiently

- demonstrate that an activity is worth continuing

- inform future plans

- assess whether an intervention is ethically justifiable

- increase knowledge and understanding of the value and limitations of health promotion

- develop theory

- ration resources or legitimate budget cuts.

(Adapted from Downie et al., 1990, pp. 73–4)

11.1.2 Who should evaluate?

Evaluation may be carried out either by independent, external researchers or by practitioners. Much evaluation of public health activity is done by the very people who carry out the interventions. There are advantages and

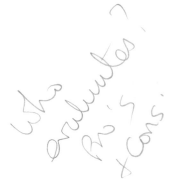

disadvantages with either pattern. An external evaluator may perhaps be fairer and more objective, but may take longer to understand the issues and establish contacts. It can also be argued that, when people evaluate their own practice, they learn more easily what they can improve, and how: but this may be the case only when they are committed to improvement rather than to self-justification. Capitalising on the strengths of both kinds of evaluator, there are those who argue that it is desirable for evaluation to be carried out on both an external and an internal basis on the grounds that this approach can stimulate useful debate and reflection (Beattie, 1990).

A further and important consideration, which was raised in Chapter 7, is the participation of users and clients. To what extent are the people for whom the intervention or service is designed going to play an active part in evaluating it? Will they act as evaluators themselves; as consultants to the evaluation, helping to shape and guide it; or as one source of information among others; or will they be completely passive recipients? Where they are being used as informants, how might they respond differently to external and internal evaluators? There are several possibilities here that require exploration. Sometimes people feel able to talk more freely to external evaluators, perhaps because external evaluators are seen as more neutral. Sometimes external people are mistrusted, and sometimes their unfamiliarity with the project and project workers means that communication proves too difficult. These and other possibilities have to be considered in relation to particular groups and contexts.

11.1.3 When and what to evaluate?

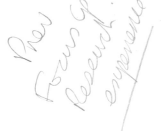

The question of when to evaluate is closely bound up with the kind of role an evaluation is to play. Is it to be the final judgement about an intervention, or a contribution to the intervention process? Box 11.2 lists three common types of evaluation.

Box 11.2 Three common types of evaluation

1   **Formative:** guides the development of the intervention.

2   **Summative (process):** documents the process of the implementation of the intervention.

3   **Summative (outcome):** documents the impact of the intervention.

Both summative forms of evaluation together provide a judgement about the intervention.

(Adapted from Hyndman and d'Avernas, 2004, Slide 11)

Formative evaluation   A formative evaluation will usually involve stage-by-stage comparison between stated objectives or criteria and what is actually happening, which has the advantage of creating opportunities for things to be changed for the better before the form of intervention is entirely fixed. Formative evaluation assesses the process of planning and developing an intervention. It helps to ensure that interventions are developed in accordance with stakeholder/community needs. In addition, formative evaluation identifies how and why key decisions were made.

Process evaluation   Process evaluation usually involves feedback during the course of a project, when things are still taking shape. Process evaluation assesses the procedures and tasks involved in implementing an intervention (i.e. what is happening?). It is sometimes called implementation assessment. Components of process evaluation might include: the number and type of people reached by an intervention; what participants thought about the intervention; the quantity and type of activity/service provided; and a description of how services are provided and the quality of services provided (participant satisfaction). Process evaluation can be carried out at, or near, the end of a project, documenting the process of implementing the project.

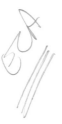

Outcome evaluation   Considering the worth of an intervention when it has reached its final form is known as an outcome evaluation. Outcome evaluation assesses the extent to which an intervention has achieved its intended purpose (i.e. did the desired change take place?). In public health, outcome evaluations are usually linked to the achievement of the objectives of the intervention. Hyndman and d'Avernas suggest that possible components of outcome evaluations are:

- Changes in awareness
- Changes in knowledge
- Changes in attitudes
- Changes in behaviours
- Changes in policy
- Changes in social/physical environment
- Changes in morbidity/mortality rates
- Cost effectiveness/cost benefit analysis

(Hyndman and d'Avernas, 2004, Slide 16)

Many evaluations incorporate both process and outcomes by having two aspects or phases, one focusing on the process (the way things are done) and the other on the outcomes (the consequences). Some evaluations are entirely concerned with process. In the field of health education, for instance, an evaluation might focus solely on the quality and nature of the communication between professionals and their clients by asking questions such as: 'Is the communication culturally appropriate?', 'Is the information perceived as credible and relevant?', or 'Is there a good match between the aims of the professional and the needs of the client?'.

When an evaluation is primarily concerned with outcomes, decisions about timing will need to take into account questions about the short- or long-term nature of the outcomes. Then, the immediate effects of an intervention are described as the impact and longer-term effects as the outcomes. Decisions about the focus of the evaluation and, in particular, whether to concentrate on process, impact or outcome will depend on the resources and funding available, the underlying questions and, most importantly perhaps, the criteria guiding the evaluation. Qualitative research methods are often used in process evaluation, whereas outcome evaluation often uses quantitative methods. Triangulation (which was explained in Chapter 7, Section 7.6.2) can bring together data from a number of different sources such that process and outcome evaluation can complement each other.

Monitoring　Monitoring involves the systematic and continuous surveillance of particular aspects of a project or service. Often it is required in relation to externally set targets and, as such, is not part of an evaluation process, though it may alert people to problems calling for further investigation. Sometimes, however, monitoring is an integral part of a formative evaluation. Evaluation is always wider than monitoring: it not only gathers information but also involves judgements about values. One way of summing up the difference is to say that evaluation responds to the question: 'Are we doing the right things?', while monitoring is concerned with answering the narrower question: 'What are we doing and are things progressing according to plan?'. Hence, monitoring is an essential part of determining how the intervention is proceeding.

If monitoring refers to a smaller-scale activity than evaluation, quality assurance is broader, referring to both the undertaking of evaluation and the implementation of findings. Regardless of the scale and level of an evaluation, there are certain fundamental questions that need to be considered before beginning to plan an evaluation.

Thinking point　can you think of any questions that should be considered before you plan an outcome evaluation?

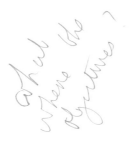

The following are examples of questions that would seem to be essential in any evaluation. A few examples of answers are also suggested.

- What are the purposes of the evaluation? (Check effectiveness; plan the next stage; justify continued funding; understand what is happening.)
- What criteria will be used? (Achieving aims and objectives; cost-effectiveness; acceptability to clients; open access.)
- What information is required? (Views of clients; annual accounts; referral rates.)

- What methods can be used to gather the information? (Postal surveys; group discussions; interviews; consulting records.)
- How should the information be reported and used to achieve the original purpose? (Verbally at a meeting with your line manager; by written report; at a staff workshop; at a community meeting.)

It is important to consider these questions from the outset so that any evaluation is both coherent and feasible. Other, more specific questions are given in Box 11.3.

Box 11.3 Checklist for planning an evaluation

- Who are the principal groups and individuals involved?
- What is the purpose of the evaluation?
- What approach, model or framework will be used to provide direction?
- What are the main evaluation questions or issues?
- What political and ethical considerations need to be taken into account?
- By what standards or criteria will the evaluation be judged?
- What resources are available for the evaluation?
- Who should carry it out?
- What sort of data (information) is needed?
- What will be the methods of enquiry?
- How is the data to be analysed?
- How will the data be checked for its validity and reliability?
- How will the findings be presented?
- To whom are the findings to be made available?

(Adapted from Phillips et al., 1994, p. 67)

11.2 Evaluation design

Multidisciplinary public health involves a range of different, complex activities and thus the evaluation method must be appropriate to the aims and objectives of the intervention.

Thinking point   are some methods more appropriate than others for evaluating multidisciplinary public health interventions?

In earlier chapters in this part of the book you explored quantitative and qualitative research methodologies. In deciding on the methodology to use for an evaluation, the methodology must be appropriate to the research questions posed in the evaluation (Morgan, 2006). Although randomised controlled trials have been held up as the gold standard in the evaluation of public health interventions, it has become increasingly clear that this method is not always appropriate (Springett, 2001). Some evaluations will require different quantitative methods, or a mix of both qualitative and quantitative research methodologies (see Figure 11.3).

Figure 11.3 Commonly used research methods for different evaluation types	
Type	Commonly used methods
Formative	Focus groups
Process	Documentation review Interviews with programme delivery agents Interviews/surveys of clients Focus groups
Outcome	Population surveys Client/user surveys

(Source: adapted from Hyndman and d'Avernas, 2004, Slide 18)

Very different views exist as to the best way of carrying out evaluation. Some of the differences can be highlighted by contrasting two different approaches to knowledge and understanding. On the one hand, there is the perspective that tries to apply the rules and procedures of the physical and medical sciences to the area of evaluation; on the other, there is a more holistic, qualitative approach which challenges the appropriateness of applying physical science methods to complex human phenomena.

You will recall from Chapter 1 that multidisciplinary public health includes many different approaches and methods. This means that people involved in funding, managing and carrying out particular kinds of public health activity will have certain expectations and assumptions about what evaluation means and what kind of evaluation is needed in relation to their areas of work. So, for example, where there is an emphasis on medical approaches to public health, evaluation will tend to be regarded as a way of demonstrating reductions in mortality and morbidity that can be attributed to public health interventions. In contrast, client-centred approaches might expect evaluation to describe and illuminate health-promoting interactions so that practitioners can reflect on the way they work and understand more about the processes involved.

Designing a formal evaluation means choosing a research plan that is appropriate to the purposes of the evaluation, and, as just noted, this choice will be influenced by the kind of public health intervention being pursued and the values and assumptions underlying it. There are three broad (and, in practice, often overlapping) categories from which to choose: (quasi-) experimental designs concerned to establish cause and effect, survey designs which aim to identify significant patterns, and qualitative designs which focus on description and interpretation. It is important to be aware of the choices that are available and the possibilities and problems inherent in each. As mentioned earlier, in Chapter 10 you explored the development of a needs assessment to develop a specialist service for pregnant teenagers and young parents in Coventry. In Box 11.4 below, the evaluators give their account of evaluating the service using a range of qualitative methods.

Box 11.4 Coventry case-study: evaluating a specialist service

One year into the pilot provision of the specialist service, it was decided that it was necessary to find a way to continue to resource this service. With this in mind, a proposal was put forward to undertake an evaluation of the service. This provided the opportunity to identify the extent to which such provision assists in breaking down the barriers that have traditionally characterised pregnant teenagers' and young parents' experience of ante- and postnatal services, and, it was hoped, to contribute further to improving their health and wellbeing.

The aims of the evaluation were to identify (1) whether current specialist services meet the needs of pregnant teenagers and young parents, and (2) how specialist services can be improved. In order to achieve these aims, the evaluation adopted a multi-method qualitative approach which involved the following:

- observation of the service

- examination of the internal evaluations

- single interviews and focus group interviews.

The intention was to collect data from the perspective of respondents and to give respondents the opportunity to reflect on the service and their role within it. The 'triangulation' (use of multi-methods) approach adopted enabled the researchers not only to collect different types of data, but to 'double check' issues and themes using different approaches (Miller and Brewer, 2003). The single and focus group interviews took place with pregnant teenagers and young mothers aged sixteen to twenty-four who were currently/or had previously accessed specialist services in Coventry, and professionals

> (including both managers and key workers) who provide specialist services to pregnant teenagers or young mothers and expectant fathers or young fathers in Coventry.

This example demonstrates the range of qualitative evaluation methods that can be used. The evaluators of the Coventry case-study used observation, documentary reports, individual interviews and focus groups. Thus, they were able to explore the various kinds of data obtained using different methods, in the light that each method shed on the experience that service users had of the sexual health service. In planning any particular evaluation it might be appropriate and useful to adopt a mixture of qualitative and quantitative methodologies; for example, to use a qualitative methodology to inform the design of a large sample survey and fill out the detail of a general pattern revealed by that survey.

11.2.1 Pluralist methodology

The choice of design has very practical consequences because it influences the kind and range of information or data that the evaluation will consider relevant. It will be linked partly with the extent to which an evaluation is intended to be concerned either with measurable outcomes or with evaluating the process. It may also be affected by the extent to which the terms of reference are internal or external in origin. Each design has to be decided according to its appropriateness to each new undertaking. An evaluator needs to be aware of the choices available so that the advantages associated with each feature of the design may be balanced against any sacrifices that each choice entails.

Thinking point   what difficulties could there be in using a combination of methods or approaches to evaluation?

Many evaluations in the field of public health use a mixture of designs and methods and may be described as pluralist (in varying degrees), although, as was noted in Chapter 9, combining qualitative and quantitative methodologies is not without its critics. Some researchers (e.g. Lincoln and Guba, 1985) have argued that the logic, values and rules underlying experimental and quantitative design, on the one hand, and qualitative, illuminative design, on the other, are so different that the two cannot, with integrity, be added together. However, others (e.g. Baum, 2007), while remaining sensitive to the differences, have accepted the value of mixing methods. Baum (2007) suggests that this enables particular public health research questions to be answered and that the use of multiple methods enables triangulation between the methods and allows a more detailed understanding of complex issues. The European Guidelines on Evaluation

(WHO, 1998) stress the importance of using a range of methodologies and not focusing on randomised controlled trials. For example, a range of qualitative and quantitative methodologies was used to evaluate an arts and health project in Northern Ireland: the Dreams Art and Health Project (Arts Council of Northern Ireland, undated), based at the Mater Hospital in Belfast. Some of the evaluation tools included an enjoyment survey and the use of video documentation and observational diaries, as well as physiological measurements such as blood pressure, pulse and respiration rates.

11.3 Evaluation criteria

It has already been noted that evaluation necessarily involves identifying criteria against which to measure or assess the worth of the activities being evaluated. Frequently, the aims or goals of the activity, project or programme provide the criteria, although it is also possible to assess worth in relation to external standards and values such as public acceptability, cost-effectiveness or efficiency.

Consider the influential attempt to identify a general set of criteria for evaluating quality, given in Box 11.5. Originally designed for healthcare, rather than for public health, it provides a checklist which is introduced here to illustrate the kinds of evaluative question that might be asked.

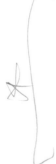

Box 11.5 Evaluation criteria

Effectiveness: the extent to which aims and objectives are met.

Acceptability: to the people concerned and society at large.

Appropriateness: relevance to need.

Equity: equal provision for equal needs.

Efficiency: the ratio of costs to benefits.

(Adapted from Phillips et al., 1994, p. 19)

Effectiveness lies at the heart of evaluation and tends to be what most people have in mind when they hear or use the word 'evaluation'.

11.3.1 Effectiveness

Effectiveness is concerned with whether an activity has achieved what it set out to do. This is sometimes described as the evaluation of outcomes in relation to aims and objectives. Aims are the planned, or hoped for, effects of an activity and outcomes are the actual effects, both intended and unintended. It will also need to take note of other outcomes that were not part of that aim. Some may be welcome (e.g. increased understanding of how HIV is transmitted), but others may not be (e.g. a group of parents withdrawing their children from a school).

Thinking point   are there differences between aims and objectives?

In everyday conversation the terms 'aims' and 'objectives' are often used interchangeably. In principle, there is an important difference, though in practice it is sometimes difficult to draw a clear distinction. Aims tend to be general, and they may be broken down into specific objectives which contribute to the aim. Often they include intentions and hopes about the way a project will operate (the process), as well as about its outcomes, and sometimes the focus is almost entirely on style and ethos when this is the desired immediate outcome or impact. Figure 11.4 illustrates the relationship between aims and objectives, and Box 11.6 shows the aims and objectives of the Coventry project.

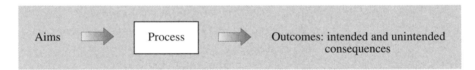

Figure 11.4   The relationship between aims and outcomes (Source: Katz et al., 2000, p. 285, Figure 16.3)

Box 11.6 Coventry case-study: aims and objectives

Aim 1: to identify whether current specialist services meet the needs of pregnant teenagers and young parents.

Objectives:

- to identify factors influencing pregnant teenagers' and/or young parents' decisions to access services

- to identify potential barriers that pregnant teenagers and/or young parents may experience in accessing the services provided

- to explore pregnant teenagers' and/or young parents' perception of the services provided

- to identify what factors professionals view as influencing use of specialist services

> - to identify what professionals view as potential barriers for take up of specialist services
>
> - to explore professionals' perception of the services provided.
>
> Aim 2: to identify how specialist services can be improved.
>
> Objectives:
>
> - to identify areas of service provision that pregnant teenagers and or young parents view as positive and negative.
>
> - to identify ways in which service users and professionals feel the service needs to be developed.

Identifying aims and objectives is not always straightforward. Certain kinds of aims and objectives are, by their nature, easier to describe than others, and not all programmes and projects have an explicit and agreed set of aims, although if there is to be an evaluation of effectiveness it is important that the various parties involved should try to be explicit and specific about what they are aiming to achieve. In Chapter 10 you were introduced to the acronym 'SMART' as a way of describing objectives (Tones and Tilford, 2001).

For evaluation to take place, aims have to be testable (operationalised), which involves not only identifying smaller-scale objectives that contribute to an aim, but also finding a way of assessing or measuring the extent to which these objectives have been achieved. Objectives should be clearly understood, should state what is to be accomplished and should be measurable. To be useful in evaluation the objectives should include:

- the outcome to be achieved, or what will change

- the conditions under which the outcome will be observed, or when the change will occur

- the criterion for deciding whether the outcome has been achieved, or by how much it has changed

- the priority population, or who will change.

Indicators of effectiveness provide ways of measuring outcomes; sometimes they provide evidence of steps believed to be essential stages in reaching the desired aim or goal and sometimes they indicate whether procedures and processes are going as planned. They may be either quantitative or qualitative, and decisions about the kinds of indicator to use will be influenced by the values and assumptions underlying the various approaches to health promotion and evaluation already outlined.

Deciding what will be an appropriate and feasible measure of effectiveness or change is a crucial step in planning and carrying out an evaluation. Where it is difficult to gather information directly about the outcome of an activity, and where it is not possible to demonstrate a direct link between public health activities and the desired outcome, intermediate and indirect indicators are often used.

In the area of large-scale plans and healthy public policy, indicators should be explicitly related to and closely linked with targets and goals, or to the change pathways leading to these goals. Identifying indicators for community development projects as distinct from public policy programmes presents equally interesting but not insurmountable challenges. Measurable objectives and intermediate indicators can be selected even where an activity's or project's main aim is something as general and seemingly abstract as empowerment, although in such situations it may be important for the manner of selection to reflect the aim. A reviewer of community intervention evaluation suggests this can be done by:

> an interactive dialogue between evaluator and program workers which shows how a common but indistinct objective ... 'to empower residents' can be broken down and translated into more practical and recognisable terms ... (which) represent specific things happening to specific people. There may, for example, be attitudinal changes across the community as a whole, skills changes within the immediate group involved, changes in the makeup of advisory boards or groups.
>
> (Hawe et al., 1994, p. 205)

Identifying and using indicators is possible not only in areas that do not appear to lend themselves to quantification; it may enhance the whole activity by stimulating discussion and debate about the direction being followed.

11.3.2 Acceptability

An important but sometimes overlooked evaluation criterion is acceptability. There are a number of reasons why, and levels at which, questions about acceptability may be relevant and important in an evaluation. For instance, an intervention that has been acceptable to a particular population may encounter difficulties elsewhere if, in a different geographical, economic, cultural or ethnic context, the language and imagery prove highly problematic.

Methods can be generally effective without being generally acceptable in relation to aesthetic, religious, or moral values.

11.3.3 Appropriateness

The criterion of appropriateness differs from that of acceptability. Here the question is whether an activity is appropriate to the particular health needs of the people being targeted rather than culturally and ethically acceptable to their world view. As discussed in earlier chapters, appropriate targeting is central for the social marketing approach to health education. Also needs assessment, described in Chapter 10, provides the foundation for making informed decisions about appropriateness. It is important to remember that external and internal perceptions of need may differ greatly, so evaluations may have to distinguish between people's own perceptions of their needs and those held by others, such as doctors or health workers, who are drawing on a different understanding or model of health. In the Coventry case-study, the perceptions of young people in relation to teenage pregnancy and the specialist services were quite different from those of the health workers (see Box 11.7).

Box 11.7 Coventry case-study: perceptions of teenage pregnancy and specialist services

Using qualitative methods – in-depth single and focus group interviews – the researchers spoke to thirty-eight young mothers, seven grandmothers and forty-nine professionals. Their key findings were:

- There are myths and stereotypes on both sides (e.g. both professionals and young people hold stereotypes about each other), *but* professionals have more power and therefore the stereotypes they hold are more significant.

- With reference to contraceptive use, young people (especially girls/young women) are 'damned if they do and damned if they don't' as contraceptive use defines a girl/young woman as sexually active and 'looking for sex', and lack of contraceptive use marks a girl/woman as irresponsible.

- Contrary to popular myth some of the babies of teenagers are planned and certainly, for all the young women the researchers spoke to, all babies were wanted.

- Encounters with professionals are often structured by misunderstandings and frustration which means that access to services is non-existent or meaningless.

11.3.4 Equity

Many public health interventions are concerned with addressing inequalities in health. At the minimum, concern for equity involves asking how accessible to all a particular public health intervention is. Evaluation criteria will include not just the numbers of people who have been involved in a project, but also an identification of the socio-economic composition of the population reached. For example, part of the evaluation will be concerned with assessing the extent to which socially excluded communities have participated in the public health intervention.

11.3.5 Efficiency

Questions about the relation between costs and effectiveness in the field of multidisciplinary public health are important. In a world of limited resources, costs clearly have to be taken into account. If, for instance, a health education programme is entirely effective in changing the health behaviour of a small group of people, but achieves this success by drawing on an enormous amount of human and financial resources, this fact is relevant in evaluation. Once cost is made explicit, a number of comparisons become possible, in principle at least. For example, a comparison may be made between a project and equally effective but cheaper projects, between this project and projects that are slightly less effective but considerably cheaper, between this and projects that reach larger numbers with similar success and similar cost, and so on.

In this context there are two main forms of analysis of which you need to be aware. Cost-effectiveness analysis (CEA) compares the costs of similar interventions that achieve a given goal (e.g. smoking cessation clinics compared with family doctors providing routine advice on giving up smoking). If different interventions meet with similar success then it becomes important to know which is cheaper. But the comparison becomes more complex if there are differences in degrees of success and differences in cost, as well as differences in types of outcome, and in such a case a calculation needs to be made in terms of 'cost per unit of effect' or 'effects per unit of cost'. Here cost–benefit analysis (CBA) provides a way to compare the cost of the intervention with the financial benefits resulting from achieving the goal (e.g. the cost of various kinds of anti-smoking advice with the financial benefits of giving up smoking). The two are summarised in Box 11.8.

Box 11.8 Cost-effectiveness and cost–benefit analysis

1   Cost-effectiveness analysis compares the efficiency of similar interventions to achieve a given goal by stating the different financial costs involved.

2   Cost–benefit analysis not only states the costs but also seeks to place a monetary value on the benefits accruing from a programme. A calculation of the cost per given benefit is then possible (typically expressed as a cost–benefit ratio).

(Adapted from Tones and Tilford, 2001, p. 117)

It could be argued that at one level an informal use of these ideas is already part of a practitioner's everyday decision making. Whenever a decision is made about how much time to spend on a particular activity or person, the practitioner is implicitly applying a cost–benefit analysis (perhaps based more on guesswork than on evaluation). For example, a community worker may find they have to choose between a range of requests made on their limited time; for instance, between spending six hours a week counselling a small number of adults who want support in losing weight, and using the same amount of time setting up a playgroup for children living in a very overcrowded area with no play facilities. Deciding which of these is going to be a better use of their time, and therefore of their employer's budget, involves trying to calculate the long-term health benefits of the two projects.

One important limitation of purely economic cost-effectiveness and cost–benefit analyses is the assumption that economic costs and benefits matter to the exclusion of other dimensions. This means that the calculations that purchasers, managers and practitioners make when deciding how best to use scarce economic resources may well need to include non-economic considerations, such as pleasure and anxiety, as well as the more obvious ones relating to money. For instance, one invisible cost of a screening programme could be the raising of anxiety levels to a degree that impairs not only people's sense of wellbeing, but also their health as medically defined. An evaluation that failed to take into account such apparently non-economic effects would provide an unsatisfactory basis for planning. The formal application of economic analysis to health promotion is a quite recent phenomenon and raises the question of values in evaluation.

11.4 Values and evaluation

Public health is, essentially, a value-driven process. As such, there are different views on why evaluation takes place, and different ways of conceptualising the relationship between values and the approach taken to evaluation. Three of these views are summarised below.

11.4.1 Managerial evaluation

One line of argument is that the ideal of efficiency in evaluation works in the interests of managers and government and this is the main reason for its official popularity. Some commentators argue that managerial evaluation, with its pressure to measure and record performance against set criteria and to establish cause and effect relationships, has the consequence of discouraging people from asking the kinds of questions about worth and purpose which might threaten the status quo (Everitt, 1995). Thus, managerial evaluation might be said to preclude moral debate and to support or intensify the existing distribution of power, driving values 'into the critical unconscious, where they continue to exercise force but without being available for analytical scrutiny' (Connor, 1993, p. 34). What alternatives exist? This is of particular relevance to current debates about inequalities in health, where adopting a managerial approach may militate against evaluation methodologies that can demonstrate whether inequalities have been reduced by a particular intervention.

11.4.2 Critical evaluation

In contrast to managerial evaluation, critical evaluation attempts to foster moral debate by recognising the impact of power differentials and using dialogue as a method of consciousness raising and empowerment. In this view, emancipatory dialogue – the process of critical action and reflection – is the way of arriving at truth. Going one step further, critical postmodernist thinkers would argue that, as truth is inextricably linked with power, evaluation, far from being a way of revealing the truth, in fact contributes to its construction by means of deconstructing ways of knowing that consistently render some people less powerful than others (Everitt, 1995). But postmodernism has been criticised for lapsing into total relativism. If there is no truth, just many 'truth claims' constructed through discourses, then is there any way of knowing whether an activity intended to promote public health is worthwhile? In response to this dilemma, Everitt simultaneously argues for the centrality of values and warns against the dangers of absolutism: 'values must be treated with care ... we must strive for making judgements in the direction of the "good", just as we must strive for "truth" but we must be tentative about the status of "a value" and "the truth"' (Everitt, 1995, p. 15).

A central value in evaluation is that of helping to give a voice to those who are least heard. This has a number of implications for the conduct of evaluation. The evaluator, far from being a neutral middle-person, actively seeks out the experience and perspectives of the least powerful parties or 'stakeholders'. The task is not simply to ensure that less influential people are given a chance to answer questions, but also to find ways of enabling them to shape decisions about the nature and purpose of the evaluation.

11.4.3 Participatory evaluation

Participatory evaluation places great emphasis on the importance of participation and working in ways which value process as much as outcome. Questions about who conducts evaluation and whose interests evaluation serves have been most directly acknowledged and addressed in community health interventions. Participatory methods, as discussed in Chapter 7, are regarded as valuable because they offer relatively powerless groups and individuals an opportunity to articulate and reflect on their experience, influence what happens and develop new skills, knowledge and confidence. They do, in short, actively promote public health.

In participatory evaluation all the participants (community members, project workers, funders and managers) are involved in evaluating the community health intervention (Tuhiwai Smith, 2001). Participatory methodologies involve all the team members in training, where they prepare and plan for the evaluation by defining the objectives of the evaluation, the data collection, and designing and developing evaluation tools. This could involve analysis of existing records and documentation, focus group discussions, observation, and meetings with staff and key informants. Training would involve all the team in the methodologies agreed. The analysis and development of recommendations would also involve all members of the team.

One of the essential aspects of participatory evaluation is to effect some change, and hence dissemination of the findings of the evaluation is key. As well as producing formal reports, dissemination to other community members using innovative approaches such as drama, poetry or songs is encouraged. For many funders, participatory evaluation is perceived as costly as it is very time consuming and funders may not appreciate its value or methodological validity, preferring quantitative statistical information. The benefit of participatory evaluation is that it can engender community involvement in changing services or approaches to health, which are then embedded in a community so that the effects are much longer term.

An example of a public health intervention which has adopted a participatory evaluation approach is the Powys Sure Start Programme in Wales. Powys and Ceredigion Health Promotion Unit was commissioned in April 2000 to undertake the evaluation of the programme until March 2002. It was agreed that the evaluation would focus on the process and impact of Sure Start, given that the focus of targets set at a national level is on outcomes. Box 11.9 outlines some of the aims and methods used in this Sure Start programme evaluation.

Box 11.9 Evaluating Powys Sure Start, Wales

The aim of the evaluation is to:

- ... evaluate the effectiveness of the programme at addressing national targets.
- ... assess the process of developing the Sure Start programme at a local level in line with local objectives, with a focus on the development of the partnerships between organisations and the mechanics of this.

- Regularly canvass parental and worker views regarding their perspectives of Sure Start at a local level.

- Develop mechanisms for evaluation to continue to be conducted for the lifetime of the programme that can be continued in-house.

So far, the evaluation has involved:

- An initial consultation with Sure Start key stakeholders as part of team building sessions to agree on the aims, objectives and evaluation questions of local programmes.

- Individual interviews with Sure Start key stakeholders to gain an understanding of the different perspectives of stakeholders and their parent organisation.

- An identification and review of parent support literature.

- Circulation of reports on the initial findings for discussion amongst stakeholders to enable actions to be taken as agreed by stakeholders.

- Interviews with parents referred for Sure Start services in one area regarding their needs and expectations.

- Reviewing minutes of meetings and other secondary data that shows the process of day-to-day working.

- Canvassing of parental and worker views regarding their perspectives of Sure Start at a local level.

(Bird, 2001, p. 3)

11.5 Changing policy and practice

Complex community initiatives, such as Sure Start programmes, require evaluation methods that can assess a range of activities at several different levels. In evaluating such initiatives the external policy context is also of particular importance (Barnes et al., 2005) because evaluation is often directed at changing policy and practice, as well as at assessing the effectiveness of specific interventions.

In order for evaluation to make a difference at any level, it is important not only to build in evaluation of public health interventions at the planning stage, but also to ensure that resources are allocated for dissemination. Dissemination can take many forms and must be targeted to the specific audience. While primary care trust and local authority boards may require short reports, other stakeholders may wish to have more detailed information and this information should also be accessible to local people who have been involved in the intervention. Fullilove et al. (2006) suggest that much more attention needs to be paid to methods of dissemination if

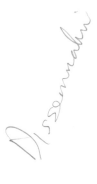

public health is to be improved. They argue that when ideas fit into mainstream thinking, then dissemination is often straightforward enough. However, when ideas fit 'outside the box', then more novel strategies need to be employed; for example, they suggest that films and site visits can be novel strategies for the dissemination of new and challenging ideas. Stuttaford et al. (2006) have also developed different methods of dissemination. For example, when reporting on an evaluation of a stroke prevention initiative in South Africa, they used the method of applied theatre.

In the example of the Coventry project, how evaluation of the teenage pregnancy service led to specific recommendations in terms of changing and developing policy and practice was clear to see. These recommendations are detailed in Box 11.10.

Box 11.10 Coventry case-study: recommendations

The project evaluation led to the following recommendations:

1   Provide a service that meets ante- and postnatal needs.

2   Encourage participants to 'move-on' to other services – perhaps the young parents' forum or other 'mainstream' mothers and toddlers type groups.

3   Provide a service that is attractive to and meets the needs of *all* young mothers and young fathers.

4   Secure new, larger accommodation.

5   Adhere to health and safety regulations which will necessitate appropriate training for all participating professionals.

6   Review session length and content.

The sustainability or development of a service or an initiative is often determined by political imperatives and the external context. Although evaluation is crucial to implementing public health interventions, a demonstration of effectiveness will not necessarily guarantee continued funding or support for the initiative. In the case of the Coventry teenage pregnancy project, the evaluation identified several problems and challenges and, as identified in Box 11.10, made a number of recommendations. However, since presentation of the full evaluation report in 2005 (Brown et al., 2005), only two of the recommendations have, in fact, been implemented (Recommendations 3 and 4). Similarly, although early findings from the national evaluation of Sure Start demonstrated that it was succeeding in making a difference, it could be argued that the funding for Sure Start had ceased before the outcomes of the initiative could be fully embedded into mainstream provision. Finally, it is important to be cautious when implementing changes to policy or practice since the process of research, planning, implementation and evaluation is essentially a politically and ideologically driven one. As Kemm argues:

> all too often the phrase 'evidence-based' introduces not a tightly constructed argument from evidence but an attempt, by those who have no knowledge of evidence or understanding of rigour, to pretend that highly contestable propositions are beyond dispute. Claims that something is evidence-based should always be treated as invitation to scrutinize evidence and the inferences that are drawn from it and never as settling the merits of the proposal.
>
> (Kemm, 2006, p. 323)

Conclusion

Evaluation of public health interventions is currently receiving much attention and has come to be regarded as an essential and central tool in the provision of a rational, evidence-based way of meeting health needs. Such a view rests on the belief that the findings of evaluations somehow add up in a way that can improve our understanding of how public health works and, in particular, our knowledge about the effectiveness of particular kinds of intervention.

Views about what counts as good evaluation are likely to be influenced by, among other things, definitions of health and the values ascribed to public health promotion. It will also be influenced by the settings in which evaluation takes place and the people – lay and professional – involved. This brings us round full circle to the issues that were raised in the first part of this book. For instance, people who draw on a predominantly medical model of health will usually be concerned with disease reduction and risk factor analysis, and regard establishing relationships of cause and effect through randomised controlled trials as the ideal approach to evaluation. Quantification and objectivity will be emphasised and the role of social structures minimised or completely overlooked. However, the question of how values such as participation, empowerment, holism and critical awareness can be built into the process of evaluation could usefully be placed higher on the agenda, especially by those who regard the medical model of health as insufficient.

This chapter has argued that the 'high status' and apparently most rational approaches to evaluation are, in many contexts, not productive. It may well be that instead of devoting more time and money to such projects, the way forward is to adopt a more creative approach which acknowledges the centrality of values and makes no claim to be neutral. So, although few would argue about the principle that all public health practice should have its basis in sound evidence, there exists a continuing and lively debate about exactly what this means and what are the best ways of achieving it.

References

Arts Council of Northern Ireland (undated) Evaluation of the Dreams Art and Health Project: forthcoming, http://www.artscouncil-ni.org/subpages/strategyandpolicies.htm (Accessed 23 October 2006).

Barnes, M., Bauld, L., Benzeval, M., Judge, K., Mackenzie, M. and Sullivan, H. (2005) *Health Action Zones: Partnerships for Health Equity*, London, Routledge.

Baum, F. (2007) 'Dilemmas in public health research: methodologies and ethical practice' in Douglas, J., Earle, S., Handsley, S., Lloyd, C.E., and Spurr, S. (eds) *A Reader in Promoting Public Health: Challenge and Controversy*, London, Sage/Milton Keynes, The Open University.

Beattie, A. (1990) 'Community development for health: the British experience' in Smithies, J. and Adams, L. (eds) *Community Participation in Health Promotion*, London, Health Education Authority.

Bird, S. (2001) *A Participatory Evaluation of Powys Sure Start, Annual Report to March '01*, Powys, Powys & Ceredigion Health Promotion Unit.

Bravo Vergel, Y. and Ferguson, B. (2006) 'Difficult commissioning choices: lessons from English primary care trusts', *Journal of Health Services Research and Policy*, vol. 11, no. 3, pp. 150–4.

Brown, G., Brady, G. and Letherby, G. (2005) *An Evaluation of Specialist Services for Pregnant Teenagers and Young Parents*, Coventry, Centre for Social Justice, Coventry University.

Connor, S. (1993) 'The necessity of value' in Squires, J. (ed.) *Principled Positions: Postmodernism and the Rediscovery of Value*, London, Lawrence & Wishart.

Downie, R.S., Fyfe, C. and Tannahill, A. (1990) *Health Promotion Models and Values*, Oxford Medical Publications, Oxford, Oxford University Press.

Everitt, A. (1995) 'Developing critical evaluation', unpublished paper, Social Welfare Research Unit, University of Northumbria at Newcastle.

Fullilove, M.T., Green, L.L., Hernández-Cordero, J.J. and Fullilove, R.E. (2006) 'Obvious and not-so-obvious strategies to disseminate research', *Health Promotion Practice*, vol.7, no. 3, pp. 306–11.

Hawe, P., Degeling, D. and Hall, J. (1994) *Evaluating Health Promotion: A Health Worker's Guide*, Sydney, MacLennan and Petty.

Hyndman, B. and d'Avernas, J. (2004) 'Introduction to evaluating health promotion programs', Workshop, 23–24 November, Toronto, The Health Communication Unit, Centre for Health Promotion, University of Toronto.

Katz, J., Peberdy, A. and Douglas, J. (eds) (2000) *Promoting Health: Knowledge and Practice*, London, Palgrave/Milton Keynes, The Open University.

Kemm, J. (2006) 'The limitations of "evidence based" public health', *Journal of Evaluation in Clinical Practice*, vol. 12, no. 3, pp. 319–24.

Letherby, G., Brown, G. and Brady, G. (2006) 'Planning and undertaking research: an evaluation of specialist services for pregnant teenagers and young parents', unpublished report, Coventry, Centre for Social Justice, Coventry University.

Lincoln, Y. and Guba, E. (1985) *Naturalistic Inquiry*, Thousand Oaks, CA, Sage.

McQueen, D. (2001) 'Strengthening the evidence base for health promotion', *Health Promotion International*, vol. 16, no. 3, pp. 261–8.

Miller, R.L. and Brewer, J.D. (2003) *The A–Z of Social Research: A Dictionary of Key Social Science Research Concepts*, London, Sage.

Morgan, A. (2006) 'Evaluation of health promotion' in Davies, M. and Macdowall, W. (eds) *Health Promotion Theory*, Maidenhead, Open University Press.

Peberdy, A. (2000) 'Evaluation in health promotion: why do it?', and 'Evaluation design' in Katz et al. (eds) (2000).

Phillips, C., Palfrey, C. and Thomas, P. (1994) *Evaluating Health and Social Care*, Basingstoke, Macmillan.

Rootman, I., Goodstadt, M., Potvin, L. and Springett, J. (2001) 'A framework for health promotion evaluation' in Rootman, I., Goodstadt, M., Hyndman, B., McQueen, D.V., Potvin, L., Springett, J. and Ziglio, E. (eds) *Evaluation in Health Promotion: Principles and Perspectives*, Copenhagen, World Health Organization Regional Office for Europe.

Speller, V., Learmonth, A. and Harrison, D. (1997) 'The search for evidence of effective health promotion', *British Medical Journal*, vol. 315, pp. 361–3.

Springett, J. (2001) 'Appropriate approaches to the evaluation of health promotion', *Critical Public Health*, vol. 11, no. 2, pp. 139–52.

Stuttaford, M., Bryanston, C., Hundt, G.L., Connor, M., Thorogood, G. and Tollman, S. (2006) 'Use of applied theatre in health research dissemination and data validation: a pilot study from South Africa', *Health: An Interdisciplinary Journal for the Social Study of Health, Illness and Medicine*, vol. 10, no. 1, pp. 31–45.

Thorogood, M. and Coombes, Y. (2000) *Evaluating Health Promotion: Practice and Methods*, Oxford, Oxford University Press.

Tones, K. and Tilford, S. (2001) *Health Promotion: Effectiveness, Efficiency and Equity*, Cheltenham, Nelson Thornes.

Tuhiwai Smith, L. (2001) *Decolonizing Methodologies*, London, Zed Books.

World Health Organization (WHO) (1998) *Health Promotion Evaluation: Recommendations to Policy-Makers*, Report of the World Health Organization European Working Group on Health Promotion Evaluation, Copenhagen, World Health Organization Regional Office for Europe.

Chapter 12

Understanding obesity

Sarah Earle

Introduction

Obesity is widely regarded as a threat to public health, but it is not an uncontroversial topic. Indeed, amid considerable debate concerning the treatment and prevention of obesity, the classification of obesity as a disease has been questioned. The purpose of this chapter is, therefore, two-fold. First, it aims to deconstruct the classification of obesity as a disease, exploring how different ways of knowing have contributed to an understanding of obesity as a threat to public health. Second, it examines the evidence base for different approaches to obesity prevention.

The chapter begins by exploring why obesity is perceived to be a threat to public health and asks the question: is obesity and overweight really a public health issue? Section 12.2 then examines different ways of thinking about obesity and overweight, considering issues of definition, measurement, representation and experience. Section 12.3 explores approaches to treatment and prevention, examining how, until very recently, attention was focused on biological research and the clinical management of obesity in individuals, rather than on the prevention of obesity and overweight in populations. Finally, and focusing especially on food and physical activity, Section 12.4 considers the challenges of planning, implementing and evaluating strategies to prevent obesity and promote public health in the twenty-first century.

12.1 Obesity and overweight: a public health issue?

Obesity was first classified as a disease in 1985, but its classification remains disputed; some commentators have suggested that obesity is simply a risk factor for diseases such as diabetes or coronary heart disease and not a disease in and of itself (Gard and Wright, 2005). Similarly, others suggest that it has more in common with medical conditions such as hypertension; that is, not all people who are obese or overweight are ill: in fact, some are very healthy indeed – just as some thin people are ill and others are healthy. Conway and Rene (2004) argue that the classification of obesity as a disease is complex and is influenced by values, politics, economics, science and semantics. Concurring with this, Gard and Wright go further to suggest that it is simply nonsense to describe obesity as a disease: 'Calling obesity a disease because obesity is associated with various non-communicable diseases is like identifying short men as ill because of the established association between short stature and ischaemic heart disease' (Gard and Wright, 2005, p. 95).

Prior to the 1960s, obesity was uncommon, but in the last thirty to forty years the prevalence of obesity has grown to what can be described as epidemic proportions. There is now concern that it is a major contributor to the global burden of disease, accounting for between at least 2 and 7 per cent of total healthcare costs. In England alone, the conservative, estimated total cost of obesity is thought to be well over 3 billion pounds (see Figure 12.1).

Figure 12.1   The estimated cost of obesity in England, 1998 and 2002 (£millions)

	1998 (National Audit Office)	2002
Treating obesity		
GP consultations	6.8	12–15
Ordinary admissions	1.3	1.9
Day cases	0.1	0.1
Outpatient attendances	0.5	0.5–0.7
Prescriptions	0.8	13.3
Total cost of treating obesity	*9.5*	*45.8–49.0*
Treating the consequences of obesity		
GP consultations	44.9	90–105
Ordinary admissions	120.7	210–250
Day cases	5.2	10–15
Outpatient attendances	51.9	60–90
Prescriptions	247.2	575–625
Total cost of treating the consequences of obesity	*469.9*	*945–1,075*
Indirect costs		
Lost earnings due to attributable mortality	827.8	1,050–1,150
Lost earnings due to attributable sickness	1,321.7	1,300–1,450
Total indirect costs	*2,149.5*	*2,350–2,600*
Total cost of obesity	**2,628.9**	**3,340–3,724**

(Source: adapted from House of Commons Health Committee, 2004, p. 129)

Globally, there are now more than one billion overweight adults, 300 million of whom are obese (WHO, 2003). Indeed, the majority of adults in the USA and the countries of the European Union are overweight or obese. Figure 12.2, which depicts obesity levels in Europe, shows that England, Wales and Scotland have relatively high levels of obesity prevalence compared with other European countries. The number of overweight and obese people has increased and is growing further.

In England, for example, the proportion of women categorised as obese rose by 8 per cent between 1993 and 2003, and the proportion of men rose by nearly 10 per cent (DoH, 2004c). Obesity is increasingly seen as a 'disease of excess', but it is not solely restricted to the richer, developed countries; it is also found in developing countries, including those where people suffer from malnutrition and starvation. For example, in sub-Saharan Africa, obesity and malnutrition coexist not just in the same country, but within the same community (Voûte and Fuster, 2005). In low-income countries obesity is common among middle-class women and people of higher socio-economic status, whereas in more affluent countries obesity is common not only among middle-aged people, but also among children and young adults (WHO, 2003). Within this debate, of course, it is important to recognise that there are cultural differences in the way in which fatness is perceived. Indeed, some would argue that interest in obesity and overweight reflects, in particular, the concerns of white western cultures, rather than those of black, Asian or Hispanic cultures. As De Casanova (2004) argues, an understanding of the body must be located within the context of race and class, as well as gender.

The global increase in childhood obesity and overweight is of particular concern to policy makers, researchers and health workers. Worldwide, 155 million school-age children are severely overweight, as are a further 22 million children aged under five. In the European Union, there are 14 million overweight school-age children, three million of whom are obese. Childhood obesity and overweight have increased significantly in the UK with a marked upward trend since the mid-1980s (see Figure 12.3 for trends in England). In 2002 in the UK, 22 per cent of boys and 28 per cent of girls aged two to fifteen were either overweight or obese (BMA, 2005).

Obesity and overweight pose risks for increased rates of premature mortality and morbidity related to chronic diseases such as type 2 diabetes, cardiovascular disease, stroke and certain types of cancer (WHO, 2003). Metabolic syndrome, which (although contested) denotes a cluster of

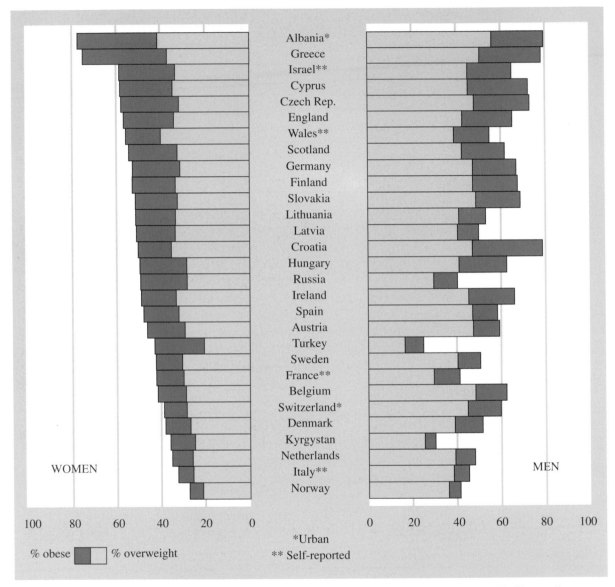

Figure 12.2   Obesity in Europe (Source: House of Commons Health Committee, 2004, p. 15, Figure 1)

conditions, including high levels of blood pressure, blood sugar and cholesterol, and abdominal obesity, also greatly increases the risk of cardiovascular disease and type 2 diabetes (BMA, 2005). Indeed, obesity and diabetes are so linked that the term 'diabesity' has come into use, reflecting the greatly increased risk of diabetes for obese people. Health risk varies according to level of obesity or overweight, with a greatly increased risk for conditions such as diabetes and a slightly increased risk for some cancers (see Figure 12.4).

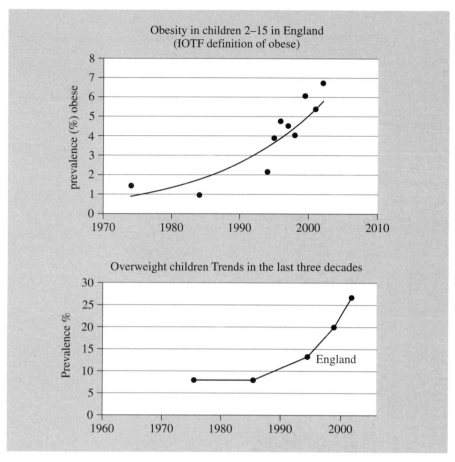

Figure 12.3   Trends in childhood obesity and overweight in England
(Source: IOTF, 2004)

Figure 12.4   Obesity and the relative risk of health problems

Greatly increased risk	Moderately increased risk	Slightly increased risk
Breathlessness	Coronary heart disease	Anaesthetic risk
Diabetes (type 2)	Gout	Cancer (e.g. colon cancer)
Gall bladder disease	Hypertension	Foetal defects
Sleep apnoea	Osteoarthritis	Polycystic ovary syndrome

(Source: adapted from WHO, 2000, p. 43, Table 4.1)

In children, similar patterns of co-morbidity are seen. For example, increasing numbers of young children are presenting with the early symptoms of metabolic syndrome. Type 2 diabetes, which was usually found in adults, is now increasingly being seen in children as a consequence of increasing rates of obesity. Early onset of diabetes increases the risk of complications, such as visual impairment, kidney failure and peripheral vascular disease, in later life. There is also some evidence to suggest that weight gain in childhood is a risk factor for developing coronary heart disease in later life (BMA, 2005).

Thinking point   to what extent is obesity an individual or a societal problem?

There is increasing awareness that obesity is not just an individual problem and a personal responsibility, but a societal issue caused by increased industrialisation, urbanisation and mechanisation. Most people work longer hours, rely on cars to get around, have less time to prepare foods from fresh, have sedentary jobs and perform little physical activity. People live in obesogenic – or obesity-promoting – societies in which they eat more and are less physically active than is healthy to maintain an appropriate body weight.

12.2 Defining, measuring and exploring obesity

Not only is the classification of obesity disputed but so, too, are the nature and existence of the obesity epidemic. We explore this controversy here by thinking about ways in which obesity is defined and measured, and by looking at experiences and representations of obesity and overweight.

12.2.1 The biomedical classification of obesity

Epidemiology contributes essential information for understanding the incidence and prevalence of obesity and overweight in society which, in turn, influences the actions taken to promote public health. Epidemiology and the biomedical classification of obesity have dominated, and continue to dominate, thinking about obesity and overweight. However, epidemiological research, like any other, relies on reliable systems of classification and measurement.

The World Health Organization (WHO, 2000, p. 6) defines obesity as: 'a condition of abnormal or excessive fat accumulation in adipose tissue, to the extent that health may be impaired'. However, although obesity is widely recognised by some members of the medical and scientific community as one of the largest unmet public health crises of the twenty-first century, there is, in fact, little consensus on how to measure fatness. Obesity is most commonly measured by using body mass index (BMI), which is defined as weight in kilograms divided by square height in metres (kg/m^2):

$$BMI = \frac{\text{Weight (kilograms)}}{\text{Height (metres)}^2}$$

According to WHO (2000), people with a BMI under 18 kg/m^2 are considered underweight. Those with a BMI over 25 kg/m^2 are defined as overweight, and people with a BMI of 30 kg/m^2 or over are defined as obese, with associated levels of co-morbidities (see Figure 12.5). Average adult BMI levels of 25–27 kg/m^2 are found in Europe and the USA, whereas lower levels of 22–23 kg/m^2 are more prevalent in Africa and Asia (WHO, 2003).

Figure 12.5   Classification of weight in adults according to body mass index

Classification	BMI	Risk of co-morbidities
Underweight	<18.5	Low (but risk of other clinical problems increased)
Normal range	18.5 – 24.9	Average
Overweight	≥25.0	
Pre-obese	25.0 – 29.9	Increased
Obese class I	30.0 – 34.9	Moderate
Obese class II	35.0 – 39.9	Severe
Obese class III	≥40	Very severe

< = less than.

≥ = greater than or equal to.

(Source: adapted from WHO, 2000, p. 9, Table 2.1)

Other anthropometric (body) measurements of overweight are also used in obesity research. For example, skinfold thickness at various sites of the body can be used, as can measurement of lean body mass (the weight of the body, less the fat). Body circumferences, especially waist circumference, are also used. Waist circumference, in particular, is seen as a convenient measure which correlates closely to BMI, and the ratio of waist-to-hip circumference is a good approximate index of both intra-abdominal fat and total body fat (or central obesity). Increases in waist circumference correlate to increased risk for various chronic conditions (WHO, 2003). Body mass index is commonly used in epidemiological measurements of obesity. However, at the individual level, BMI is thought to be questionable and waist measurement may, in fact, be a more accurate indicator of health risk. This is the basis of the National Obesity Forum's campaign *Waist Watch Action* (see Figure 12.6).

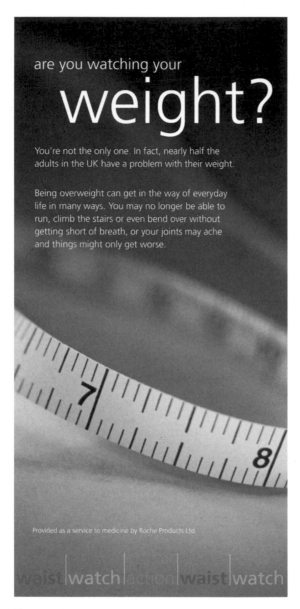

Figure 12.6   Waist Watch Action: a campaign launched by the National Obesity Forum, encouraging people to check their waist measurement

However, anthropometry is not without its critics. For example, Gard and Wright (2005, p. 94) suggest that much caution is needed if 'science fiction' is not to be represented as 'science fact'; there is also much criticism of the use of anthropometry in the health surveillance of populations. In its White Paper *Choosing Health* (DoH, 2004a), the government has pledged to reintroduce the school medical – the annual weighing and measuring of children in primary schools – in England, although the Royal College of Nursing (RCN), among others, is opposed to this measure, arguing that it will further embarrass and stigmatise young people (Templeton, 2005, p. 5).

Thinking point   why is measuring obesity important?

Although universal acceptance of measurement systems does not exist, the effective measurement of obesity is useful for selective interventions in public health and for the symptomatic treatment of individuals who are obese. Agreed systems of measurement and classification are also necessary to ensure accurate measurement over time and across populations, to provide baseline data (initial information), and to give a basis for evaluation (WHO, 2000).

Given the seemingly increasing prevalence of childhood obesity and the fact that obesity in children generally follows into adulthood, it is important that obesity prevention should begin in childhood. However, there is currently no universally accepted system for the classification of childhood obesity, although several BMI-based systems are available, including that of the WHO and the International Obesity Taskforce (IOTF). Figure 12.7 outlines some of the problems associated with BMI measurement in children.

Figure 12.7   Problems associated with BMI as an indicator of, or screening measure for, adiposity (fat deposit) in childhood and adolescence

Problem	Explanation
Age and sex	BMI varies with age and sex during childhood
BMI component increases	Increases in BMI during childhood growth are mainly attributable to increases in lean body mass, especially in boys
Maturation	Maturation patterns differ between countries and between sexes
Ethnicity	The relationship between BMI, fatness and risk is not identical across ethnic groups
Validity of BMI as proxy for fatness	Validity studies using BMI to identify children with excess adiposity have generally documented low to moderate sensitivities for BMI
BMI and fatness over time	The relationship between BMI and fatness may not be stable over time
Evidence of risk	Insufficient evidence from prospective studies linking excess fatness in childhood with morbidity and mortality

(Source: Neovius et al., 2004, p. 106, Table 1)

Creating a universal classification system for obesity is problematic for both children and adults, particularly given the ethnically diverse world population. Techniques that have been developed for the measurement of body fat have been validated largely on Caucasian populations and, hence, given the differences between ethnic groups, may not be valid for non-Caucasian individuals (Deurenberg and Deurenberg-Yap, 2001). These ethnic differences are evident both in terms of body fat distribution and in relation to the correlation between percentage body fat and disease risk (Neovius et al., 2004). In a study of BMI and percentage body fat in different population groups of Asians, Deurenberg et al. (2002) found that Asians had a higher percentage body fat at lower BMI compared with Caucasians. This means that, for comparisons of obesity prevalence between ethnic groups, universal BMI cut-off points are inappropriate and different ones should be used. The same study also found considerable differences between Asian groups – for example, between Chinese and Indonesians – and between ethnic groups living in different locations – for example, Chinese groups living in New York, Beijing and Hong Kong.

12.2.2 Social science understandings of obesity

As discussed in Chapter 7, knowledge of the world is not 'neutral', or 'real', but is shaped by different ways of measuring and looking at the social world. For example, while epidemiological research focuses on the measurement of overweight and obesity in and across populations, and biomedical research focuses on the measurement and treatment of obesity in individuals, social scientific knowledge is more concerned with exploring the meaning of obesity in relation to the individual and society. The social sciences can, thus, offer a critical perspective on the biomedical classification of fat people as 'overweight' or 'obese' and on the clinical treatment of people who are labelled as such.

Social science research has highlighted the way in which obesity can lead to psychological distress, such as depression, in both adults and children (Sjoberg et al., 2005; Heo et al., 2006) and to poorer quality of life (Brownell, 2005). Research also suggests that obese and overweight people can find themselves discriminated against in employment and education, as well as in other aspects of their daily lives (Carr and Friedman, 2005). However, not all researchers agree. For example, Wardle and Cooke (2005) argue that studies typically report poorer psychological wellbeing and depression among treatment seekers and that obese children in the general population are unlikely to be depressed. Similarly, a study of over 9,000 obese and overweight adults (Doll et al., 2000) found that, in general, obese people did not experience a deterioration of psychological wellbeing as a result of obesity or overweight, and that such findings in other studies could be explained with reference to other co-morbidities.

Feminist writers, beginning from the standpoint that the 'personal is political', have also explored the issue of obesity and overweight. Drawing on the idea of patriarchal power – the oppression of women by a society dominated by male power – Bordo (1995) has suggested that culture maintains a firm grip on women's bodies, defining fatness as bad and thinness as good. From a psychological perspective, writers such as Chernin (1981) and Orbach (1988) have expressed concern about the prevalence of eating disorders such as anorexia and bulimia nervosa among women, arguing that women become damaged by a patriarchal society that places unrealistic expectations on women and girls. As Gard and Wright (2005) argue, although not everyone agrees with these feminist perspectives, they have been influential in shaping views about obesity and overweight.

Writing from a disability rights perspective, Cooper (1997), who describes herself as an 'able-bodied fat woman' defines obesity, or fatness, as a disability. Writing critically of feminist perspectives, she argues that feminism has variously (and fallaciously) defined all fat people as either sufferers of eating disorders or as primordial goddesses. Drawing on a social model of disability to identify similarities between disabled people and fat people, and between disability politics and fat politics, Cooper writes:

> The bodies of fat and disabled people share low social status ... Like people with mobility impairments, many fat people are disabled by a lack of access in the physical environment, for example, clothes don't fit, seats are too small, turnstiles are impossible to navigate. Fat and disabled people encounter discrimination in all areas of our lives ... where we are constantly reminded that there is something wrong with us.
>
> Most blatantly congruent are our experiences of medicalisation. ...
>
> [...]
>
> When we conceptualise fatness as a disease, we also assume that somehow it must be cured in order for our bodies to function normally.

(Cooper, 1997, pp. 36, 37)

Thinking point   in what ways are obesity and disability similar?

Although obesity and disability share some similarities, disabled people are often positioned as the victims of their impairment. In contrast, overweight and obese people are often seen as being personally responsible for their body size, shape and weight. Goffman's (1963) work on stigma provides a useful way of understanding this distinction. Stigma refers to an attribute that is deeply discrediting (Goffman, 1963), disqualifying a person from full participation in society, and setting them aside as deviant, rather than 'normal'. Goffman makes the distinction between individual physical attributes that are discreditable and those that are discrediting. Discreditable attributes are those that can usually be easily hidden from others; for example, diabetes or HIV. Discrediting attributes cannot be hidden from others and are immediately stigmatising for the individual concerned. Examples of this might include physical impairment, obesity and overweight. Goffman suggests that the attribution of responsibility for stigma is important in that individuals are more likely to be stigmatised if they are seen as responsible for their stigma. Overweight and obese people are often seen as responsible for their weight – they may be perceived as greedy, lazy and lacking in willpower. For obese people, fatness can become what Goffman terms their 'master status' – the quality or characteristic above all others that defines the individual. In this respect, disability and obesity are positioned very differently.

Sontag's work (1979, 1989) on illness and metaphor can also be a useful way of understanding the meaning of obesity within contemporary western societies, and it has been influential in social science understandings of chronic illness and the body. In her discussion of cancer and HIV she showed how certain illnesses, particularly those which are poorly understood, come to be defined as more than just an illness. For example, the word 'cancer' (or the 'Big "C"') became synonymous with death, and those who lived with cancer were often seen as 'fighters'. Sontag argued that willpower – or metaphors of empowerment which are implicit in the rhetoric of cancer treatment and research – adds greatly to the suffering of people living with cancer because it implies a personal and moral responsibility for recovery. Similarly, obesity has become a metaphor for sloth, greed and abundance.

In this way, obesity is regarded not just as a disease but as the scourge of modern urban life. Writing in the Guardian, Parry (2005) argues:

> To be overweight is said to be the product of a breakdown in family values and of slothful kids. Low-income groups are more likely to be obese, and so it is assumed that children living in poverty must watch more TV than rich children. But telling parents to restrict TV viewing is easier than dealing with health inequalities caused by poverty, a more likely cause of obesity than daytime TV, no matter how damaging that might seem.
>
> (Parry, 2005)

Writing specifically about the relationship between fatness and health, Robison (2005) suggests that concerns over the obesity epidemic have, themselves, reached epidemic proportions. He argues that this new rhetoric is harmful (see Box 12.1) and, drawing on the Health at Every Size movement, challenges the biomedical response to obesity. The Health at Every Size movement, an US movement which began to take form in the 1970s, encourages the recognition of natural diversity in body shape and size and the notion that it is possible to be healthy at every weight. This position is supported by organisations such as the National Association to Advance Fat Acceptance (NAAFA) in the USA. Robison argues that neither the relationship between obesity and morbidity, nor the relationship between weight loss and improved health, have been proven. Furthermore, he argues that the promotion of weight loss may actually violate the principle of non-maleficence (doing no harm).

Box 12.1 Obesity epidemic hysteria

Obesity is seen as a modern day scourge because of:

- the biased reporting of research which claims causality between obesity and illhealth

- the continuous pressure on individuals to lose weight

- a public that is misinformed, concerned, and afraid about food and health.

(Adapted from Robison, 2005)

Thinking point   how might the promotion of weight loss violate the principle of non-maleficence as suggested above?

Promoting weight loss may seem to be a fundamentally worthwhile activity and, indeed, some people are likely to agree with this. However, the medicalisation of obesity and overweight has helped to further regulate the way in which individuals think about their bodies and their lifestyles, placing the 'blame' for obesity firmly on the shoulders of individuals rather than on the society in which they live (see the discussion of medicalisation in Chapter 2).

12.2.3 Representing and experiencing obesity and overweight

As discussed in earlier chapters, lay understandings of health and illness often draw on various bodies of knowledge, including biomedicine and social science, as well as 'common sense' and popular views, such as those derived from the mass media. The media draw on scientific knowledge in their representations of obesity but, although there are many ways in which this knowledge can be interpreted, such reporting is usually warning of a catastrophic global obesity epidemic in which everyone, everywhere, is at risk (Gard and Wright, 2005). The media also represent obesity using metaphors of war. For example, the words 'victory' and 'fighting' are often used in representations of obesity (see Box 12.2).

Box 12.2 The 'war' on obesity

The following are examples of newspaper headlines:

Hormone raises hope of victory in war on obesity
(Alok Jha, *Guardian*, 11 November 2005)

US sugar barons 'block global war on obesity'
(Jo Revill and Paul Harris, *Observer*, 18 January 2004)

Employers urged to help fight obesity
(Debbie Andalo, *Guardian Society*, 6 May 2004)

The media are also responsible for perpetuating the myth that obesity and overweight are not just medical conditions but moral problems, and that the obesity epidemic is caused by individual and familial gluttony and sloth. This is certainly the message put forward by television programmes such as *Fat Families* (ITV1, in 2005) and *Honey We're Killing the Kids* (BBC Three, in 2005):

> Do you have young children? Take a look at them. Now, can you imagine being introduced to them ... when they're grown up?
>
> What if the future you'd imagined for them hasn't quite gone to plan? How would you react if you discovered that, as adults, your children have under-achieved, have serious health problems and have a much lower than average life expectancy? And, as their parents, it's all **your** fault!
>
> (BBC Three, *Honey We're Killing the Kids*, 2005)

Of course, such moralising is not new – there is a long cultural history of the association between fatness and morality and the responsibility of individuals and families – especially mothers – for food and health (Gard and Wright, 2005). Indeed, moral failings are perpetuated not just within the media but elsewhere. For example, the House of Commons report, Obesity, has a section entitled, 'Gluttony or sloth', which cites Prentice and Jebb who argue that:

> It is certain that obesity develops only when there is a sustained imbalance between the amount of energy consumed by a person and the amount used up in everyday life. But which side of this energy balance equation has been most altered in recent decades to produce such rapid weight gain? Should obesity be blamed on gluttony, sloth, or both?

(Prentice and Jebb, 1995, quoted in House of Commons Health Committee, 2004, p. 23)

Mass media representations of obesity are important. They can influence the way in which lay people (and others) understand and experience obesity, although they never reflect the totality of these experiences. The views of obese and overweight people are also important but, in spite of this, very little research has been conducted to explore their experiences. A qualitative Scottish study of thirty-six obese, overweight and 'normal' weight young people (Wills et al., 2006), for example, found that the participants seldom referred to the terms obesity or overweight when talking about body shape or size. Instead, the young people in this study referred to being 'fat', both as a description of body size or shape and as a term of abuse. Approximately half of the participants in this study who were obese or overweight also reported being bullied because of their weight. Such findings can be useful when thinking about promoting the health of children and young people and how best to communicate with them. In an in-depth qualitative study of nine obese women living in New Zealand, Carryer (2001) discusses women's experiences of chronic reduction – or yo-yo – dieting, obsessions with food, and feelings of shame and stigma. She also discusses the impact of obesity on women's access to health and healthcare. For example, one respondent describes the way in which obesity curtails her enjoyment of physical activity in the outdoors:

> I absolutely love it up the mountain, I love the air, the snow the sensation of skiing and all I could think of [is] what would I wear cause I've got nothing that will fit me on the ski field and if I fall over and break my leg, how humiliating to be carried off the mountain by two zippy ski instructors.
>
> (Quoted in Carryer, 2001, p. 96)

Another respondent describes the humiliation of medical treatment:

> Once going into A & E [emergency room] with suspected appendicitis, I was feeling really miserable. They left me there and then poked and prodded around of course and this doctor came in and he said of course you are overweight, and I thought well that was a brilliant deduction, I said 'so it can't possibly be appendicitis then, you know it's just fat?'
>
> (Quoted in Carryer, 2001, p. 95)

The biomedical classification of obesity, and epidemiological approaches to obesity and overweight, have dominated the obesity agenda to the exclusion of other approaches. Bodies of knowledge, while complex and often overlapping, have a profound effect on understandings of obesity and overweight. These ways of knowing have influenced how 'obesity' is classified, quantified, experienced and represented and, together, they have contributed to the concerns – justified or otherwise – with an obesity epidemic. The next section in this chapter considers the issue of treatment and prevention – focusing on the different approaches that can be adopted at a range of levels – and looks at the evidence for each of these.

12.3 Approaches to treating and preventing obesity

Until quite recently, treatment of obesity and overweight had been at an individual level and focused on biological research and clinical management. However, given the seemingly increasing number of overweight and obese people, and associated levels of co-morbidity, the treatment of both conditions is not an affordable option for most health systems in the long term. In the light of this, there is a growing awareness on the part of governments, policy makers, practitioners and researchers, of the need to focus on long-term prevention and on initiatives that emphasise environmental change rather than behavioural change. The potential for preventing obesity is expressed diagrammatically in Figure 12.8, which shows that, at present, efforts are devoted largely to an investigation of factors in the upper boxes, whereas the most likely arena for a long-lasting approach to obesity lies in the lower boxes.

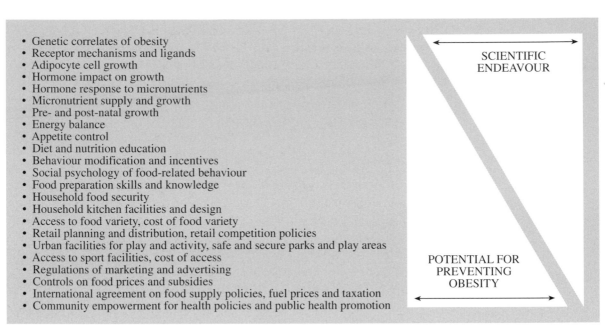

- Genetic correlates of obesity
- Receptor mechanisms and ligands
- Adipocyte cell growth
- Hormone impact on growth
- Hormone response to micronutrients
- Micronutrient supply and growth
- Pre- and post-natal growth
- Energy balance
- Appetite control
- Diet and nutrition education
- Behaviour modification and incentives
- Social psychology of food-related behaviour
- Food preparation skills and knowledge
- Household food security
- Household kitchen facilities and design
- Access to food variety, cost of food variety
- Retail planning and distribution, retail competition policies
- Urban facilities for play and activity, safe and secure parks and play areas
- Access to sport facilities, cost of access
- Regulations of marketing and advertising
- Controls on food prices and subsidies
- International agreement on food supply policies, fuel prices and taxation
- Community empowerment for health policies and public health promotion

SCIENTIFIC ENDEAVOUR

POTENTIAL FOR PREVENTING OBESITY

Figure 12.8   The potential for preventing obesity (Source: Lobstein et al., 2004, p. 70, Figure 37)

However, although prevention is important – and is addressed later in this subsection – the need to support those who are overweight and obese is still of major individual and public concern. The increasing burden of obesity and overweight has lead to growing numbers of commercial weight loss programmes – such as Weight Watchers and Slimming World and, more recently, a range of online programmes and diet tools – which, according to Hamilton and Greenway (2004) have seldom been adequately evaluated. This lack of evaluation, they argue, has been influenced by a range of factors including a fear that (negative) research results would place programmes at a disadvantage. In this regard, anxiety about an obesity epidemic may force change: 'The silver lining inside the black cloud of the international obesity epidemic is that, at long last, weight management has become a major public health issue. One positive consequence of this new priority is the increased interest in and funding for comparative trials of weight loss diets' (Winkler, 2005, p. 199). But, Winkler argues, one of the main problems with weight loss trials is the inability to measure what people actually eat, given that people often misreport what and how much they eat, with overweight people – he claims – misreporting up to 40 per cent of consumption.

Thinking point   what other factors might influence the evaluation of weight loss programmes?

Although measuring individual behaviour and weight loss is not without difficulties, these are insignificant compared with those associated with measuring the success of population-level interventions such as policy or environmental change. Promoting an evidence-based public health approach to obesity prevention is, therefore, problematic. The Prevention Group of the International Obesity Task Force (IOTF, 2004) has developed a key set of policy and programme issues that form the basis of a prevention framework for planning, implementing and evaluating obesity interventions. Each issue has a different set of evidence requirements and outputs to support policy and programme decision making. Unlike clinical decision making, which is often based on evidence drawn from randomised controlled trials, the IOTF argues that the evidence base for obesity prevention must draw on many different types of evidence (see Figure 12.9). Given the dearth of evidence available, some argue that action to prevent obesity should be based on the 'best evidence available', as distinct from the 'best evidence possible' (Swinburn et al., 2005).

Figure 12.9   Developing a framework for evidence-based obesity action

Issue (implied question)	Policy/programme relevance	Relevant evidence and information	Examples of outputs
I. Building a case for action on obesity (Why should we do something about obesity?)	Showing urgency of taking action on obesity Comparing costs, health burden, and gains from prevention with other risk factors and diseases Addressing prioritization of obesity over others issues Identifying populations of special interest Setting benchmarks and population goals	Monitoring and surveillance data (e.g. prevalence, trends) Observational studies (e.g. relative risks, occurrence rates in different populations) Economic analyses (e.g. costs of obesity, DALYs lost) Informed opinion (e.g. for modelling assumptions)	Prevalence estimates including projected trends Estimates of the social and economic burden of obesity (direct, indirect, intangible costs) Comparative health burdens in terms of years or DALYs lost Estimated potential reductions in burden with interventions
II. Identifying the contributing factors and points of intervention (What are the causative and protective factors that could potentially be targeted by interventions?)	Identifying targets for intervening Relating obesity issues to other existing agendas Identifying congruent and conflicting policies and activities Identifying the key government, NGO and private sector stakeholders that are central to obesity prevention	Observational studies (e.g. cohort studies of diet and activity patterns on weight gain) Experimental studies (e.g. diet trials) Indirect evidence (e.g. advertising investment on marketing foods to children) Monitoring and surveillance data (e.g. on food supply, behaviour trends) Informed opinion (e.g. on what factors are modifiable)	Evidence reviews of specific modifiable determinants of obesity including levels of certainty and the likely size of impact Identified drivers of environmental charge and pathways to weight gain or loss

III. Defining the range of opportunities for action (How and where could we intervene?)	Providing coherence, coordination, and comprehensiveness to planned actions Creating the links and overlaps with existing plans, policies, and programmes Identifying the settings and sectors and key strategies needed for action Demonstrating the feasibility of a population approach to obesity prevention Outlining the multidimensional nature of the action needed	Parallel evidence from other public health initiatives (e.g. tobacco control) Pre-existing frameworks for action (e.g. Ottawa Charter, settings approaches) Informed opinion (e.g. about other successful frameworks, modifiable and feasible strategies) Information on current relevant initiatives Programme logic and theory	Coherent obesity prevention strategic framework either as a stand-alone or as part of a broader plan of action for nutrition and physical activity, and/or non-communicable diseases Short and long-term population goals Identified settings, sectors, and support actions
IV. Evaluating potential interventions (What are the specific, potential interventions and their likely effectiveness and cost-effectiveness?)	Describing potential interventions in concrete terms Estimating their likely effectiveness in the target population (where possible) Identifying resource implications Progressing specific obesity initiatives through the necessary processes (engaging stakeholders, identifying capacity, setting agendas, etc.)	Experimental studies Observational studies Effectiveness analyses (including modelling where data are sparse) Economic analyses Programme logic and theory Programme evaluation (e.g. from existing community of demonstration interventions)	Specific descriptions of potential interventions and support actions Estimates of effectiveness, cost-effectiveness, or cost-utility for the interventions Sensitivity and uncertainty parameters around the above estimates
V. Selecting a portfolio of specific policies, programmes and actions (What is a balanced portfolio of initiatives that is achievable yet sufficient to reduce obesity?)	Gaining stakeholder input into judgements on the policy and implementation implications Gaining stakeholder input into and support for priority interventions with the portfolio Taking action	Estimates of effectiveness and cost-effectiveness of interventions and their associated sensitivity and uncertainty (above) Informed opinion on specific interventions and actions about their: Feasibility Sustainability Other potential positive of negative effects Effects on equity Acceptability to stakeholders	Balanced portfolios of specific policies, programmes and other actions to prevent obesity

NGO, non-governmental organisation; DALY, disability-adjusted life year

(Source: Swinburn et al., 2005, p. 26, Table 2)

The epidemiological triad, used successfully in managing other health epidemics, has been put forward as one of the ways in which an obesity epidemic could be managed (also see Chapter 8). The epidemiological triad, which has been applied to non-infectious epidemics since the 1980s, uses a model that identifies the hosts of any epidemic, its agents, vectors (or vehicles) and environments (see Figure 12.10). When applied to obesity and overweight the 'hosts' include individuals who are obese and overweight as well as those who are of 'normal' weight (see also Swinburn and Egger, 2002).

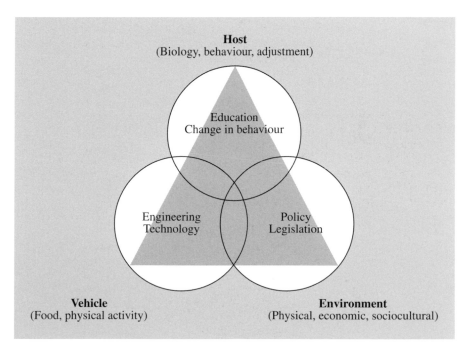

Figure 12.10   Obesity and the epidemiological triad (Source: Egger and Swinburn, 1997, Figure 2)

It is suggested that individuals who are obese can be influenced by a variety of techniques, ranging from health education, skills training and behaviour modification, to medical and surgical intervention for those who are very obese (Egger and Swinburn, 1997). In the case of obesity, the agent can refer to the over-consumption of food. The vectors (or vehicles) relate to both sides of the energy balance equation: energy intake and energy expenditure. Action would, therefore, need to be taken both to reduce energy intake and to increase energy expenditure. In the final part of the triad, environments become the focus for action. However, recognising that environments are complex systems, the ANGELO (analysis grid for environments linked to obesity) framework has been devised as a means of analysing the obesogenic elements of both micro- and macro-environments. This is illustrated in Figure 12.11, in which the first column lists the physical, economic, policy and socio-cultural aspects of the environment. Each of these has a related question which can be used to interrogate the extent to which settings and/or sectors are obesogenic in relation to food and/or physical activity.

Figure 12.11   The ANGELO model: an approach to environmental diagnosis

Aspects of the environment	Micro-environment (settings)		Macro-environment (sectors)	
	Food	Physical activity	Food	Physical activity
Physical	What is available?			
Economic	What are the financial factors?			
Policy	What are the rules?			
Socio-cultural	What are the attitudes, beliefs, perceptions, values?			

(Source: adapted from Egger et al., 2003, p. 118, Figure 3)

Obesity prevention is widely recognised as complex and requiring a multifactoral approach. Such an approach is illustrated by the list in Box 12.3 on tackling obesity in children, which emphasises the importance of lifestyle 'choice' as well as other public health measures.

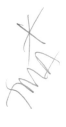

Box 12.3 Tackling obesity in children: healthier environments

- Regulation of food marketing; 'fat tax' on high-fat, high-sugar food and beverages.

- Schools to become health-supporting environments.

- Restaurants, food and beverage companies must continue to improve product offerings for children, reduce portion sizes and make healthy choices more fashionable.

- The media should reinforce healthy lifestyle choices through advertising, television, film and the internet.

- Safe parks and playgrounds.

(Adapted from Voûte and Fuster, 2005)

However, although the relevance of a public health agenda for obesity is acknowledged, many are sceptical. Antipatis et al. (1999) conducted a study assessing the views of twenty-five professionals working in the field

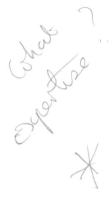

What Expertise?

of obesity on public health approaches to obesity prevention. Most respondents either had an academic background with expertise in obesity, public health nutrition or epidemiology (the majority), or were health professionals, health planners or representatives of the commercial sector (the minority). The results from the survey showed that those working in the obesity prevention field had more confidence in the usefulness and feasibility of implementing strategies aimed at changing individual behaviour than in structural approaches aimed at changing obesogenic environments (see Figure 12.12).

Figure 12.12   Views on public health approaches to obesity prevention

Potential strategy	Usefulness	Feasibility
Predominantly food-related		
1. Increase food industry development, production, distribution and promotion of products low in dietary fat and energy	No clear trend	+
2. Use pricing strategies to promote purchase of healthy foods	+	-
3. Improve quality of food labelling	No clear trend	+
4. Increase mass media promotion of healthy foods	+	+
5. Promote water as the main daily drink	+ +	+ +
6. Promote development and implementation of appropriate nutrition standards and guidelines for catering establishments	+	No clear trend
7. Regulate food advertising and marketing practices aimed at children	+ +	–/+
8. Provide land in towns and cities for 'family' growing of vegetables, legumes and other healthy produce	No clear trend	–/–
Predominantly activity-related		
9. Improve public transport to reduce dependence on the motor car	No clear trend	No clear trend
10. Promote cycling as a means of transport	+ +	+ +
11. Promote walking as a means of transport	+ +	+ +
12. Change building codes to promote use of stairs instead of elevators and escalators	+	–/+
13. Increase provision of affordable local exercise/recreational facilities and programmes	+	No clear trend

14. Provide flexible working arrangements to allow time for exercise and to (decrease reliance on convenience processed foods)	No clear trend	No clear trend
15. Provide exercise and changing facilities at work	No clear trend	No clear trend
16. Use interactive videos and programs to get children active watching television	No clear trend	No clear trend
17. Promote learning and practice of healthy physical activity (and nutrition) habits through schools	+ +	+ +
Health sector-related		
18. Mass media public awareness campaign on need to maintain a healthy weight throughout life	+	+ +
19. Build economic incentives into health insurance plans	+	No clear trend
20. Provide adequate training in obesity prevention and management for physicians and other healthcare workers	+ +	+

N.B. + + clear positive trend; + general positive trend; - - clear negative trend; - general negative trend; –/+ bi-modal trend.

(Source: Antipatis et al., 1999, p. 1005, Table 1)

In this subsection we have examined some approaches to obesity prevention. However, whichever approach is favoured, it is important to recognise that, although considerable knowledge of the 'static epidemiology' (i.e. the incidence and prevalence of people who are obese or overweight in terms of demographic and health-related characteristics) of obesity exists, little is known about its 'dynamic epidemiology' (i.e. patterns of weight gain and loss over time in individuals and populations). As Jonas (2004) notes, there are many unanswered questions. Who gains weight, how much and why? Who is at risk? Who is not at risk? Are there different patterns of weight gain? However, two key issues need to be at the forefront of obesity prevention: namely, food and physical activity. These are considered below, in particular by focusing on some of the interventions designed to address the problem of energy imbalance, and by considering the evidence base for each.

12.3.1 Food and the prevention of obesity

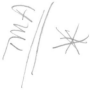

Food, or, more specifically, the over-consumption of foods that are high in sugars and fats, has been identified as one of the leading causes of obesity and overweight. The WHO (2003) report on *Diet, Nutrition and the Prevention of Chronic Diseases* concludes that there is convincing evidence to suggest that high intake of these energy-dense, micronutrient-poor foods increases the risk for obesity and weight gain. It also concludes that the heavy marketing of such foods is a probable risk factor for obesity. Larger portion sizes and widespread availability of such foods were identified only as possible risk factors for obesity.

Changing people's eating behaviour through health education is, therefore, often seen as one of the key ways to halt the increasing prevalence of obesity in society. However, it is widely recognised that the majority of people do not follow the nutritional guidelines that have been issued by health professionals over several years (FPH, 2003). This perspective, of course, assumes that individuals are rational actors who, with professional guidance, will make the 'right' health decisions. As discussed in earlier chapters, changing health behaviours is far more complex than this. This perspective also assumes that healthy food information is linear and unambiguous. However, given the range of sources of health information, this is not the case; consumers are often quite confused about what, when and how much they should be eating.

In England, the 5 A DAY programme (DoH, 2003a), which encourages people to eat at least five portions of fruit and/or vegetables each day, has five strands of activity, all of which are underpinned by an evaluation and monitoring programme:

1   National School Fruit Scheme

2   Local 5 A DAY initiatives

3   National/local partners – Government Health Consumer Groups

4   Communications programme including 5 A DAY logo

5   Work with industry – producers, caterers, retailers.

(DoH, 2003a)

Thinking point   why is working with industry important in promoting healthier eating?

In a consumer society, branding – which sends social messages to consumers – becomes increasingly important. For example, Schwartz and Puhl (2003) suggest that chocolate and sweets are strongly associated with holidays and parties. Some brands of chocolate and soft drinks also claim, or have claimed, to 'help you work, rest and play', 'satisfy your hunger' or 'give you energy'. It is not surprising, then, that the marketing and branding of unhealthy foods has come under particular scrutiny. Food portions, packaging, labelling and marketing are an important part of a public health strategy to prevent obesity and overweight, with greater calls either for self-regulation by the food industry itself or for legislative action by governments. The White Paper, *Choosing Health* (DoH, 2004a), for example, expresses a commitment to develop a strategy to restrict the advertising and promotion of foods high in fat, salt and sugar to children via both broadcast and non-broadcast media, sponsorship, brand sharing, point-of-sale advertising and labels, wrappers and packaging. However, as with most public health strategies to prevent obesity and overweight, there is little evidence to support such initiatives (Livingstone, 2004).

Evaluation of the 5 A Day pilot initiatives (DoH, 2002) concluded that community initiatives could stem a fall in fruit and vegetable consumption (against national trends) if those interventions were sustained. However, the evaluation also reported that the initiatives had not increased overall fruit and vegetable intake. Evaluation of the National School Fruits Scheme, which involved both teachers and parents, has shown some positive changes in the eating habits and attitudes of young children and their families, particularly among young parents (DoH, 2003b). However, reported in the Guardian, many commentators are critical and argue that the scheme has not tackled the wider issues concerning children's diets (Lawrence and Carvel, 2006).

In England, the Food in Schools Programme, which consists of eight projects piloted across England between 2003 and 2004, is designed to promote healthy eating at key points during the school day (see Figure 12.13). Some similar initiatives can be found across Scotland, Wales and Northern Ireland. The National Healthy Schools Programme, jointly funded by the Department for Education and Skills (DfES) and the Department of Health (DoH) is part of the government's drive to reduce health inequalities, promote social inclusion and raise educational standards. *Choosing Health* (DoH, 2004a) stated that the eight projects piloted by the Food in Schools Programme would be rolled out across all schools as part of the National Healthy Schools Programme.

Figure 12.13   The Food in Schools Programme's eight pilot projects

Project/Region	Aim
Breakfast Clubs West Midlands	To improve the nutritional quality of food and drink provided and consumed via Breakfast Clubs, as well as improving knowledge about healthy eating.
Healthier Tuck Shops South West	To improve the nutritional content and quality of food and drink provided in school tuck shops, and improve knowledge about healthy eating.
Healthier Vending Machines East of England	To provide the nutritional content and quality of food and drink provided in vending machines in schools.
Healthier Lunchboxes South East	To develop an effective, sustainable approach to improving the nutritional content of packed lunches which can be widely disseminated.
Cooking Clubs North West	Using the medium of cookery clubs to increase pupil and family awareness and understanding of the importance of a balanced diet, food hygiene and safety.

Growing Clubs London	To provide children in schools with the opportunity to learn and participate in food growing activities, linking the food chain, nutrition and health.
Dining Room Environment York and Humber	To improve the physical dining room environment factors contributing to an increased uptake of school meal services. To identify ways that this may improve knowledge about and promote healthy eating.
Water Provision East Midlands and North East	To develop a whole school approach to increase water consumption and address accessibility issues.

(Source: FPH, 2003, p. 11, Figure One)

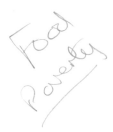

Other activities have focused on the issue of food poverty; this is defined by the Food Poverty Network as a lack of money, inadequate shopping facilities, conflicting information about food and health and poor transport which, either combined or in isolation, mean that people are denied healthy food choices. For example, those on a low income are more likely to be influenced by pricing and food promotions such as BOGOFs (Buy-One-Get-One-Free) which may adversely affect health choices. Given shopping and retail distribution patterns, those without a car may have reduced access to fruit and vegetables and will often pay higher prices for similar products found in out-of-town supermarkets. The poor availability of good food in restaurants and in settings such as schools and workplaces can also affect health negatively. Drawing on a critical perspective which focuses on issues of food production, consumption and sustainability, food poverty is seen as a barrier to good health.

Strategies to prevent food poverty might include the mapping of 'food deserts' with the aim of setting up alternative supplies through food projects such as home delivery services, transport-to-supermarket schemes, community cafés, food co-operatives, community farms and allotments. Box 12.4 describes a community farm and café project in Wales.

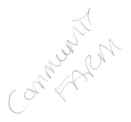

Box 12.4 Ffaldau Farm, Wales

At Ffaldau Farm, a community food-growing project was set up in a community centre welcoming all local people. The project provides a community café and community allotments for growing vegetables and herbs. Users include disadvantaged children, young people, women, older people, mental health service users, and those with learning disabilities.

(Adapted from Courtauld, 2003, p. 54)

Thinking point   to what extent can food projects eradicate food poverty?

Although local food projects may go some way to alleviate food poverty, they are unlikely to eradicate it. Public policy initiatives in the areas of transport and urban planning, among others – as well as general poverty reduction measures – are also necessary. However, in writing about the role of such strategies to prevent obesity, Crawford argues that: 'Although common sense suggests that such interventions will have a positive impact, they are yet to be implemented in studies designed to prevent obesity, and we therefore lack evidence of their effectiveness' (Crawford, 2002, pp. 728–9).

Agreeing with this, Jain (2004) suggests that this problem is further compounded by the inability to measure food intake and energy expenditure accurately; this, he argues, is especially vital in health policy research which seeks to measure the effects of interventions among large groups of people.

Public health action on food also includes the lobbying and campaigning work of organisations such as the Tescopoly Alliance (Figure 12.14). This organisation seeks to highlight and challenge the negative impact of all major British supermarkets on small businesses, communities and the environment, calling for national and international legislation to curb the market power of large supermarkets. The Tescopoly Alliance and other organisations such as Friends of the Earth, the New Economics Foundation and Grassroots Action on Food and Farming also seek to stimulate and support public health action at a local level. Campaigners argue that big supermarkets harm small business, communities and the environment both locally and globally.

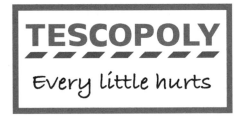

Figure 12.14   The Tescopoly Alliance

Next we consider the role of strategies to promote physical activity and the evidence that exists to support these.

12.3.2 Physical activity and the prevention of obesity

Attempts to reduce energy intake have some support, but combating sedentary lifestyles and increasing physical activity are seen as equally (if not more) important in preventing obesity and overweight. Indeed, many commentators (e.g. Robison, 2005) would argue that the focus should be on fitness, not fatness.

Physical activity may be associated with positive health benefits, especially for adults, decreasing risks for coronary heart disease, stroke, diabetes and hypertension, as well as obesity. In older people, physical activity is also thought to prevent falls. However, as Gard and Wright (2005) have pointed out, it is important to avoid the nostalgic view that things 'ain't what they used to be'. That said, there is widespread agreement – by governments and policy makers in particular – on the need to increase physical activity by changing behaviour as well as by public health policies that promote physical activity.

French (2007) has argued for the increasing use of social marketing as a public health strategy and, indeed, there has already been considerable interest in the use of the mass media to increase physical activity, particularly among children. For example, VERB – a social marketing campaign co-ordinated by the US Department of Health and the Human Service's Centers for Disease Control and Prevention – has been launched to advertise physical activity as 'cool and fun' among 'tweens' (9–13-year-olds). A prospective, longitudinal study of the VERB campaign using self-reporting measures shows some positive results (Huhman et al., 2005). Mass media campaigns have also been used in the UK, especially in Scotland. The first Scottish television campaign, launched in 1998, focused on walking and promoted a number of 'interesting facts' about physical activity. Evaluation of this campaign showed that awareness was very high. However, this increased knowledge had no measurable impact on walking (WHO, 2004). Many researchers are pessimistic about the value of health media campaigns to increase physical activity, arguing that they ignore the complex processes of media communication and the way in which knowledge and awareness translates into action (Finlay and Faulkner, 2005).

Just as there is often confusion about healthy food messages, so too messages about levels of physical activity can also be confusing. Questions they give rise to, for example, include: What physical activity is required to prevent obesity and overweight? For how long should people undertake physical activity, how often and at what intensity? Current UK guidelines on physical activity are based on the prevention of cardiovascular disease, rather than on the prevention of obesity. A review of the literature suggests that physical activity levels will need to increase if society is to avoid unhealthy weight gain (Erlichman et al., 2002). The levels of physical activity currently recommended (at the time of writing in 2006) are 30 minutes of moderate exercise on at least five days each week; however, it is recognised that this may not be enough to prevent unhealthy weight gain (WHO, 2004).

Most countries have reported a decline in participation in physical activity by their populations, apart from Canada, Finland and New Zealand which have reported increases (see WHO, 2004). Some of the factors common to those countries which have successfully encouraged a greater uptake of physical activity are outlined in Box 12.5.

Box 12.5 The characteristics of countries with increased physical activity levels

- Physical activity – especially the 'great outdoors' – is an important part of national culture.

- The use of both bottom-up and top-down approaches.

- Increased funding for local initiatives.

- Well-funded and imaginative mass media campaigns adopting consistent messages.

- The promotion of 'moderate' activity.

- The setting of realistic, rather than ambitious, targets.

- Collaboration across different sectors.

- Demonstration of the links between good health and increasing physical activity.

(Adapted from WHO, 2004, pp. 6–7)

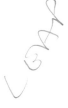

At local level, efforts are being made to promote physical activity. For example, in England, Local Exercise Action Pilots (LEAPs) – which are locally run pilot programmes to test and evaluate new ways of encouraging people to take up more physical activity – were launched in 2004. Ten primary care trusts in neighbourhood renewal areas across England have been selected to run these pilot programmes. LEAP is jointly funded by the Department of Health, the Countryside Agency and Sport England and the programmes include a wide range of activities reaching various target groups, from activity camps for children to community walking programmes for older people recovering from strokes (for an example, see Box 12.6).

> ## Box 12.6 The Dudley LEAP project
>
> The Dudley LEAP project aims to increase the use of parks for physical activity as an alternative to indoor gym or leisure facilities. In collaboration with an activity referral scheme, the project adopts a whole-population approach to increasing levels of physical activity in Dudley. Typical activities include: health walks, children's activity clubs, sports and recreation clubs, fun days and improved provision of facilities and equipment hire.
>
> (Adapted from DoH, 2006a)

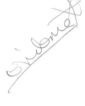

An interim evaluation of the LEAP programmes indicates that community interventions in physical activity can engage participants who would otherwise be sedentary (DoH, 2006b). This evaluation recommends that primary care trusts, local authorities and other agencies should ensure that future community health initiatives include adequate resourcing for physical activity interventions.

Many people would agree that increasing physical activity is not just a behavioural issue that can be dealt with at a local level, but one that relies on partnership working and collaboration at all levels. Physical activity is also a social issue because participation levels vary according to differences in gender, age, ethnicity and socio-economic status. The Department for Culture, Media and Sport's *Game Plan* (DCMS, 2002), a strategy for delivering the government's sport and physical activity objectives, sets out to increase participation in sport and physical activity to 70 per cent of the population by 2020. Currently, only 31 per cent of the English population are physically active (DoH, 2004b); similar levels are found in Scotland and slightly lower levels (28 per cent) in Northern Ireland and Wales (WHO, 2004). The strategy recognises that young white men comprise the group most likely to participate in physical activity and sport, whereas women, manual workers and people from minority ethnic groups are far less likely to do so:

- women are 19% less likely to take part in sport and physical activity than men;

- the impact of social group is significant, with levels of participation almost three times higher among professional groups than among manual groups; and

- ethnic minority participation is 6% lower overall than the national average.

(DCMS, 2002, p. 13)

In England, the Department for Culture, Media and Sport and the Department of Health are developing a national delivery plan for physical activity and sport which sets out to increase participation in physical activity and sport among economically disadvantaged groups, school leavers, women and older people.

Thinking point   can you think of other strategies to promote physical activity?

Strategies to promote physical activity should also consider wider public policy such as the use of urban spaces, the development of transport policy and healthy employment policies, among others. Urban spaces, for example, should be safe areas in which people can participate in physical activity. Access to the countryside and the 'right to roam' are also important aspects of planning for health, especially given the emphasis on the 'great outdoors' in countries with high levels of physical activity. If people are to walk or cycle part of the way to work, then appropriate provision must be made for safer routes, cycle pathways or 'park and walk' schemes. The building of new housing and the locating of new industrial or commercial sites also influence the likelihood of people being able to walk or cycle to and from work or school. Employers, too, can empower employees to integrate physical activity into the work day. Kumanyika et al. (2002) argue that obesity prevention objectives should be integrated into all relevant policies and programmes at local, national and international levels.

Understanding why people do or do not participate in physical activity is complex. Many public health interventions have not been fully evaluated and those that have sometimes show increases in health awareness, rather than changes in health behaviours. Also, while it is possible to identify some of the characteristics of physically active populations, such as the outcomes of much research and evaluation, these characteristics may not be easily transferable to other settings.

Conclusion

This chapter has focused on two key issues. First, it has shown that, although concern over an 'obesity epidemic' continues to grow, this epidemic remains a contested scientific and social fact. In doing so, it has explored how different ways of knowing have, and can, contribute to debates on obesity and overweight. Given the nature of these debates, it is important to take one step back from what Robison (2005) has described as the epidemic of concern with the obesity epidemic. After all, although obese and overweight people may become ill, many would argue that they are not, in effect, ill because they are fat.

Second, even if concern with an obesity epidemic is to be accepted at face value, this chapter has questioned the evidence base for the treatment and prevention of obesity and overweight. Until now, obesity has remained firmly within the medical lexicon, with most interventions focusing on treatment or individual behaviour modification. It is only recently that measures have been put into place to tackle obesity and overweight at population levels. However, very little evidence exists to support the majority of initiatives designed either to decrease energy consumption or to increase energy expenditure, although some commentators have argued for the focus of obesity prevention programmes to be on fitness, not fatness.

The challenge is therefore two-fold. Action to promote public health must continue to question the scientific and value base which supports a concern with an obesity epidemic. At the same time, it must also seek to create the evidence to support change.

References

Andalo, D. and agencies (2004) 'Employers urged to help fight obesity', *Guardian Society*, 6 May [online], http://business.guardian.co.uk/print/0,,4917905-108725,00.html (Accessed 21 July 2006).

Antipatis, V.J., Kumanyika, S.K., Jeffery, R.W., Morabia, A. and Ritenbaugh, C. (1999) 'Confidence of health professionals in public health approaches to obesity prevention', *International Journal of Obesity*, vol. 23, pp. 1004–7.

BBC Three (2005) *Honey We're Killing the Kids* [online], http://www.bbc.co.uk/bbcthree/tv/killing_the_kids.shtml (Accessed 9 April 2006).

Bordo, S. (1995) *Unbearable Weight: Feminism, Western Culture and the Body*, London, University of California Press.

British Medical Association (BMA) (2005) *Preventing Childhood Obesity*, London, British Medical Association.

Brownell, K.D. (2005) 'The chronicling of obesity: growing awareness of its social, economic, and political contexts', *Journal of Health Politics, Policy and Law*, vol. 30, no. 5, pp. 955–64.

Carr, D. and Friedman, M.A. (2005) 'Is obesity stigmatizing? Body weight, perceived discrimination, and psychological well-being in the United States', *Journal of Health and Social Behavior*, vol. 46, no. 3, pp. 244–59.

Carryer, J. (2001) 'Embodied largeness: a significant women's health issue', *Nursing Inquiry*, vol. 8, no. 2, pp. 90–7.

Chernin, K. (1981) *Womansize: The Tyranny of Slenderness*, London, The Women's Press.

Conway, R. and Rene, A. (2004) 'Obesity as a disease: no lightweight matter', *Obesity Reviews*, vol. 5, pp 145–51.

Cooper, C. (1997) 'Can a fat woman call herself disabled?', *Disability and Society*, vol. 12, no. 1, pp. 31–41.

Courtauld, C. (2003) *Community Food Projects: A Directory* [online], http://www.sustainweb.org/pdf/pov_directory.pdf (Accessed 12 May 2006).

Crawford, D. (2002) 'Population strategies to prevent obesity', *British Medical Journal*, vol. 325, pp. 728–9.

De Casanova, E.M. (2004) '"No ugly women" – concepts of race and beauty among adolescent women in Ecuador', *Gender and Society*, vol. 18, no. 3, pp. 287–308.

Department for Culture, Media and Sport (DCMS) (2002) *Game Plan – A Strategy for Delivering the Government's Sport and Physical Activity Objectives*, London, Cabinet Office.

Department of Health (DoH) (2002) *Five-A-Day Pilot Initiatives: Executive Summary of the Five-A-Day Pilot Initiatives Evaluation Study*, London, The Stationery Office.

Department of Health (DoH) (2003a) *5 A DAY: Just Eat More (fruit & veg)*, London, Department of Health.

Department of Health (DoH) (2003b) *Research Report: A Study into Parents' and Teachers' Views of the National School Fruit Scheme*, London, The Stationery Office.

Department of Health (DoH) (2004a) *Choosing Health: Making Healthy Choices Easier*, London, The Stationery Office.

Department of Health (DoH) (2004b) *Choosing Health? Choosing Activity: A Consultation on how to Increase Physical Activity*, London, The Stationery Office.

Department of Health (DoH) (2004c) *Health Survey for England 2003*, London, Stationery Office.

Department of Health (DoH) (2006a) *Dudley Beacon and Castle with Dudley South Primary Care Trust* [online], http://www.dh.gov.uk/PolicyAndGuidance/HealthAndSocialCareTopics/ HealthyLiving/LocalExerciseActionPilots/LocalExerciseActionPilotsGeneralArticle/fs/ en?CONTENT_ID=4133546&chk=n7J2zV (Accessed 19 September 2006).

Department of Health (DoH) (2006b) *Local Exercise Action Pilots (LEAP): Summary of the Interim Findings*, London, The Stationery Office.

Deurenberg, P. and Deurenberg-Yap, M. (2001) 'Differences in body composition assumptions across ethnic groups: practical consequences', *Current Opinion in Clinical Nutrition and Metabolic Care*, vol. 4, pp. 377–83.

Deurenberg, P., Deurenberg-Yap, M. and Guricci, S. (2002) 'Asians are different from Caucasians and from each other in their body mass index/body fat percent relationship', *Obesity Reviews*, vol. 3, pp. 141–6.

Doll, H.A., Peterson, S.E.K. and Stewart-Brown, S.L. (2000) 'Obesity and physical and emotional well-being: associations between body mass index, chronic illness and the physical and mental components of the SF-36 questionnaire', *Obesity Research*, vol. 8, no. 2, pp. 160–70.

Egger, G. and Swinburn, B. (1997) 'An "ecological" approach to the obesity pandemic', *British Medical Journal*, vol. 315, pp. 477–80.

Egger, G., Swinburn, B. and Rossner, S. (2003) 'Dusting off the epidemiological triad: could it work with obesity?', *Obesity Reviews*, vol. 4, pp. 115–19.

Erlichman, J., Kerbey, A.L. and James, W.P.T. (2002) 'Physical activity and its impact on health outcomes. Paper 2: Prevention of unhealthy weight gain and obesity by physical activity: an analysis of the evidence', *Obesity Reviews*, vol. 3, pp. 273–87.

Faculty of Public Health (FPH) (2003) *ph.com*, The Newsletter of the Faculty of Public Health, London, Faculty of Public Health [online], http://www.fph.org.uk/ policy_communication/downloads/publications/phcom/2003/decph.com03/ph.com Dec%202003.pdf (Accessed 9 April 2006).

Finlay, S.J. and Faulkner, G. (2005) 'Physical activity promotion through the mass media: inception, production, transmission and consumption', *Preventive Medicine*, vol. 40, no. 2, pp. 121–30.

French, J. (2007) 'The market-dominated future of public health?' in Douglas, J., Earle, S. Handsley, S., Lloyd, C.E., and Spurr, S. (eds) (2007) *A Reader in Promoting Public Health: Challenge and Controversy*, London, Sage/Milton Keynes, The Open University.

Gard, M. and Wright, J. (2005) *The Obesity Epidemic: Science, Morality and Ideology*, London, Routledge.

Goffman, E. (1963) *Stigma: Notes on the Study of a Spoiled Identity*, London, Penguin.

Hamilton, M. and Greenway, F. (2004) 'Evaluating commercial weight loss programmes: an evolution in outcomes research', *Obesity Reviews*, vol. 5, pp. 217–32.

Heo, M., Pietrobelli, A., Fontaine, K.R., Sirey, J.A. and Faith, M.S. (2006) 'Depressive mood and obesity in US adults: comparison and moderation by sex, age and race', *International Journal of Obesity*, vol. 30, no. 3, pp. 513–19.

House of Commons Health Committee (2004) *Obesity: Third Report of Session 2003–04, Volume 1*, London, The Stationery Office.

Huhman, M., Potter, L.D., Wong, F.L., Banspach, S.W., Duke, J.C. and Heitzler, C.D. (2005) 'Effects of a mass media campaign to increase physical activity among children: year–1 results of the VERB campaign', *Paediatrics*, vol. 116, no. 2, pp. 277–84.

International Obesity Task Force (IOTF) (2004) *Obesity in Children and Young People: A Crisis in Public Health* [online], http://www.iotf.org/childhoodobesity.asp (Accessed 9 April 2006).

Jain, A. (2004) 'Fighting obesity', *British Medical Journal*, vol. 328, p. 1327.

Jha, A. (2005) 'Hormone raises hope of victory in war on obesity', *Guardian*, 11 November [online], http://www.guardian.co.uk/print/0,,5330884-103526,00.html (Accessed 21 July 2006).

Jonas, S. (2004) 'The "dynamic epidemiology" of obesity: knowledge to help improve our ability to manage the condition', *American Medical Athletic Association Journal*, Summer, pp. 5–17.

Kumanyika, S., Jeffery, J.W., Morabia, A., Ritenbaugh, C. and Antipatis, V.J. (2002) 'Public health approaches to the prevention of obesity. Working Group of the International Obesity Taskforce. Obesity prevention: the case for action', *International Journal of Obesity*, vol. 26, no. 3, pp. 425–36.

Lawrence, F. and Carvel, J. (2006) 'Free fruit and veg scheme for young pupils hits problems', *Guardian*, 28 January [online], http://society.guardian.co.uk/health/story/0,,1696884,00.html. (Accessed 10 May 2006).

Livingstone, S. (2004) *A Commentary on the Research Evidence Regarding the Effects of Food Promotion on Children*, London, London School of Economics.

Lobstein, T., Baur, L. and Uauy, R. (2004) 'Obesity in children and young people: a crisis in public health', *Obesity Reviews*, vol. 5 (suppl. 1), pp. 4–85.

Neovius, M., Linné, Y., Barkeling, B. and Rössner, S. (2004) 'Discrepancies between classification systems of childhood obesity', *Obesity Reviews*, vol. 5, pp. 105–14.

Orbach, S. (1988) *Fat is a Feminist Issue*, London, Arrow Books.

Parry, V. (2005) 'Fat versus fiction', *Guardian*, 16 June [online], http://www.guardian.co.uk/life/lastword/story/0,,1506961,00.html (Accessed 9 April 2006).

Prentice, A.M. and Jebb S.A. (1995) 'Obesity in Britain: gluttony or sloth?', *British Medical Journal*, vol. 311, pp. 437–9; also available online at: http://bmj.bmjjournals.com/cgi/content/full/311/7002/437 (Accessed 29 September 2006).

Revill, J. and Harris, P. (2004) 'US sugar barons "block global war on obesity"', *Observer*, 18 January [online], http://www.guardian.co.uk/print/0,,4838847-110418,00.html (Accessed 21 July 2006).

Robison, J. (2005) 'Health at every size: antidote for the "obesity epidemic"', *Health at Every Size*, vol. 19, no. 1, pp. 3–10 [online], http://www.gurze.com/client/client_images/PDFs/HAES19-1.pdf (Accessed 9 April 2006).

Schwartz, M.B. and Puhl, R. (2003) 'Childhood obesity: a societal problem to solve', *Obesity Reviews*, vol. 4, pp. 57–71.

Sjoberg, R.L., Nilsson, K.W. and Leppert, J. (2005) 'Obesity, shame, and depression in school-aged children: a population-based study', *Pediatrics*, vol. 116, no. 3, pp. 389–92.

Sontag, S. (1979) *Illness and Metaphor*, London, Allen Lane.

Sontag, S. (1989) *AIDS and its Metaphors*, London, Penguin.

Swinburn, B. and Egger, G. (2002) 'Preventive strategies against weight gain and obesity', *Obesity Reviews*, vol. 3, pp. 289–301.

Swinburn, B., Gill, T. and Kumanyika, S. (2005) 'Obesity prevention: a proposed framework for translating evidence into action', *Obesity Reviews*, vol. 6, pp. 23–33.

Templeton, S.K. (2005) 'Nurses fight weight test for children', *Sunday Times*, 17 July, p. 5.

Voûte, J. and Fuster, A. (2005) 'Fatness to fitness', *Global Agenda*, vol. 3, pp. 214–6.

Wardle, J. and Cooke, L. (2005) 'The impact of obesity on psychological well-being', *Best Practice and Research: Clinical Endocrinology and Metabolism*, vol. 19, no. 3, pp. 421–40.

Wills, W., Backett-Milburn, K., Gregory, S. and Lawton, J. (2006) 'Young teenagers' perceptions of their own and others' bodies: a qualitative study of obese, overweight and "normal" weight young people in Scotland', *Social Science and Medicine*, vol. 62, no. 2, pp. 396–406.

Winkler, J.T. (2005) 'The fundamental flaw in obesity research', *Obesity Reviews*, vol. 6, pp. 199–202.

World Health Organization (WHO) (2000) *Obesity: Preventing and Managing the Global Epidemic*, WHO Technical Report Series 894, Geneva, World Health Organization.

World Health Organization (WHO) (2003) *Diet, Nutrition and the Prevention of Chronic Diseases: Report of a Joint WHO/FAO Expert Consultation*, Geneva, World Health Organization.

World Health Organization (WHO) (2004) *Promoting Physical Activity: International and UK Experiences*, Geneva, World Health Organization.

Acknowledgements

Grateful acknowledgement is made to the following sources:

Figures

Figure 1.2: Copyright © Getty Images; Figure 1.3: Copyright © Getty Images; Figure 1.4: Copyright © Getty Images; Figure 1.5: Adapted from: Seedhouse, D. (2002) *Ethics The Heart of Health Care*, John Wiley & Sons Ltd; Figure 2.1: Hughner, R.S. and Kleine, S.S. (2004) 'Views of health in the lay sector a compilation and review of how individuals think about health', *Health: An Interdisciplinary Journal for the Social Study of Health, Illness and Medicine*, Vol 8 (4) 2004, Sage Publications; Figure 3.2: Dahlgren, G. and Whitehead, M. (1991) *Policies and Strategies to Promote Social Equity in Health*, Institute for Futures Studies, Stockholm; Figure 3.3: Office for National Statistics (2005) Social Trends 35, Income and Wealth. Crown copyright material is reproduced under Class Licence Number C01W0000065 with the permission of the Controller of HMSO and the Queen's Printer for Scotland; Figure 3.4: Taken from National Statistics Online, http://www.statistics.gov.uk.(2005) Crown copyright material is reproduced under Class Licence Number C01W0000065 with the permission of the Controller of HMSO and the Queen's Printer for Scotland; Figure 3.5: Film Images/The Advertising Archives; Figure 3.6: Copyright © Epilepsy Action; Figure 3.7: Lader, D. and Goddard, E. (2005) 'Smoking-related behaviour and attitudes 2004: Smoking behaviour and habits'. Crown copyright material is reproduced under Class Licence Number C01W0000065 with the permission of the Controller of HMSO and the Queen's Printer for Scotland; Figure 3.8: Office for National Statistics (2004) 'Adults exceeding weekly benchmarks of alcohol'. Taken from National Statistics Online, http://www.statistics.gov.uk. Crown copyright material is reproduced under Class Licence Number C01W0000065 with the permission of the Controller of HMSO and the Queen's Printer for Scotland; Figure 4.1: © Nick Cobbing / Rex Features; Figure 5.5: Kwok-Cho Tang, Don Nutbeam, et al. (2005), 'Building capacity for health promotion-a case study from China', *Health Promotion International*, Vol 20, No 3 March 2005, Oxford University Press; Figure 5.7: Courtesy of The Advertising Archives; Figure 5.10: Ewles, L. and Simnett, I. (2003) *Promoting Health: A Practical Guide*, Elsevier Science Ltd; Figure 5.12: Downie, R.S., Fyfe, C. and Tannahill, A. (1994) *Health Promotion: Models and Values*, Oxford University Press; Figure 5.13: Adapted from: Gabe, J., Calnan, M. and Bury, M. (eds) (1991) *The Sociology of the Health Service*, Routledge; Figure 5.15: Adapted from Caplan, R. (1993) 'The importance of social theory for health promotion: from description to reflexivity', *Health Promotion International*, Vol 8 no 2, Oxford University Press; Figure 6.1: Babb, P., Martin, J. and

Haezewindt, P. (2004) 'Focus on Social Inequalities', National Statistics 2004. Crown copyright material is reproduced under Class Licence Number C01W0000065 with the permission of the Controller of HMSO and the Queen's Printer for Scotland; Figure 6.2: Macfarlane, A., Stafford, M. and Moser, K. (2004) 'The Health of Children and Young People', National Statistics 2004. Crown copyright material is reproduced under Class Licence Number C01W0000065 with the permission of the Controller of HMSO and the Queen's Printer for Scotland; Figure 6.3: Gordon, B., Mackay, R. and Rehfuess, E. (2004) *Inheriting the World: The Atlas of Children's Health*, World Health Organization, Geneva; Figure 6.4: Graham, H. and Power, C. (2004) 'Lifecourse framework linking childhood disadvantage to poor adult health', *Child: Care, Health and Development*, Blackwell Publishing Ltd.; Figure 8.3: 'Health at a Glance, OECD indicators 2003'. OICD; Figure 8.4: Myer, T., Corbin, T., Tortoriello, M., and Devis, T. (2006) United Kingdom Health statistics UK, No.2 2006 edition. Office for National Statistics. Copyright © Crown copyright 2006. Crown copyright material is reproduced under Class Licence Number C01W0000065 with the permission of the Controller of HMSO and the Queen's Printer for Scotland; Figure 8.5: Williams, H., Dodge, M., Higgs, G. et al (1997) Mortality and Deprivation in Wales, Cardiff University of Wales. Reproduced with permission; Figure 8.6: Crayford, T., Hooper, R., Evans, S. (1997) 'Death rates of characters in soap operas on British television: is a government health warning reguired?', *British Medical Journal*, Vol 315, December 1997; Figures 8.7 and 8.8: www.hpa.org.uk, *Renewing the focus HIV and other Sexually Transmitted Infections in the United Kindom in 2002*, November 2003, Health Protection Agency; Figure 8.9: Singleton, N., Bumpstead, R., O'Brien, M., Lee, A., Meltzer, H. (2001) 'Prevalence of mental disorders and substance misuse, National Statistics, Psychiatric morbidity among adults living in private households'. Crown copyright material is reproduced under Class Licence Number C01W0000065 with the permission of the Controller of HMSO and the Queen's Printer for Scotland; Figure 8.10: *Health and Mortality A Concise Report* (1998) United Nations; Figure 8.11: Copyright © Health Education Authority; Figure 8.12: adapted from Miller, R. E. (2002) *Epidemiology for Health Promotion and Disease Prevention Professionals*, Copyright © 2002 The Haworth Press; Figure 8.13: The Kings Fund (2004) 'The role of the Government', Research Report June 2004. Copyright © Kings Fund; Figure 10.1: Nutbeam, D (2001) *Direct Action, Oxford Handbook of Public Health Practice*. Copyright © 2001 Oxford University Press. By permission of Oxford University Press; Figure 10.2: Nutbeam D. (2004) *The Use of Theory in Program Planning and Evaluation Theory in a Nutshell*, McGraw Hill Education; Figure 11.1: adapted from Edwards J. (1991) *Valuation in Adult and Further* Education A Practical Handbook for Teachers and Organisers, The Workers Education Association; Fig 11.2: Figure 16.2 adapted from Feuerstein M.T. (1986) *Partners In Evaluation*

Development and Community Programmes with Participants, Macmillan Press Ltd; Figure 12.1: House of Commons Health Committee Obesity Third Report of Session 2003–04. Crown copyright material is reproduced under Class Licence Number C01W0000065 with the permission of the Controller of HMSO and the Queen's Printer for Scotland; Figure 12.2: House of Commons Health Committee Obesity Third Report of Session 2003–04. Crown copyright material is reproduced under Class Licence Number C01W0000065 with the permission of the Controller of HMSO and the Queen's Printer for Scotland; Figures 12.2 and 12.3: Taken from www.iotf.org/childhoodobesity, International Association for the Study of Obesity, International Obesity Taskforce; Figure 12.5: WHO Technical Report Series (2000) 'Obesity: Preventing and Managing the Global Epidemic' World Health Organization, Geneva 2000; Figure 12.7: Neovius, M. et al. (2004) 'Discrepancies between classification systems of childhood obesity', *Obesity Reviews*, Reviews 5, 2004, The International Association for the Study of Obesity; Figure 12.8: ASO (2004) 'Obesity in children and young people', *Obesity Reviews*, Review 5 (Suppl 1) 2004, International Association for the Study of Obesity; Figure 12.9: Swinburn, B. et al. (2005) 'Obesity prevention evidence framework', *Obesity Reviews*, Review 6, 2005, International Association for the Study of Obesity; Figure 12.10: Egger, G. and Swinburn, B. (1997) 'An "ecological" approach to the obesity pandemic', 1997, 315, *British Medical Journal*, BMJ Publishing Group; Figure 12.8: Antipatis, V. et al. (1999) 'Confidence of health and professionals in public health approaches to obesity prevention', *International Journal of Obesity*, 23. Copyright © 1999, Stockton Press.

Text

Box 6.8: Hilpern, K. (2000) 'Lets talk about sex, baby', The Guardian, 28 June 2000, by permission of Kate Hilpern; pp. 224–5: Nedra Kline Weinreich (1996) *Integrating Quantitative and Qualitative Methods in Social Marketing Research*, Weinreich Communications.

Every effort has been made to contact copyright holders. If any have been inadvertently overlooked the publishers will be pleased to make the necessary arrangements at the first opportunity.

Index

absence of disease, health as 43–4

absenteeism 90–1

acceptability 339, 342

accommodation instability 88–9

Acheson Report 72–3

action research 279, 286

Action on Smoking and Health (ASH) 15

adulthood, transition to 164–5

advisory group 319–20

age 72, 76–81
 children's concepts of health and 175
 and consent 165
  hazardous drinking 249–50
  lifecourse and 80–1

age-specific death rates 241

age-specific incidence rate 246

ageing population 92

agencies promoting public health 102–12

Agenda 21 94, 111

AIDS/HIV 82, 175, 240, 250, 303

aims 299
 evaluation and 339–42
 setting 318–19

alcohol consumption patterns 83, 85

allied health professionals (AHPs) 116

analytic epidemiology 253–5

analytical models of health promotion 155–7

ANGELO (analysis grid for environments linked to obesity) framework 373–4

anthropometry 360–3

anti-bullying policies 180–1

approaches to health 46–60

appropriateness 339, 343

Ardoyne, Northern Ireland 315–16

Armagh and Dungannon energy efficiency HAZ project 120

artefact explanation 71

Association of Public Health Observatories (APHO) 109

attitudes 134, 260–1, 277

authenticity 291–3

autonomy, respect for 27–8

Bangkok Charter for Health Promotion in a Globalised World 18–19, 123

behaviour 71
 child health behaviours 171
 children's knowledge of health and 174–5
 theories explaining change in 132–8
 see also lifestyle

behavioural approach 130–1, 151–2

behavioural immunology 49

beneficence 25–6

Berwick Borough Sure Start 178

biomedicine 130–1
 classification of obesity 360–3
 knowledge 201–2, 202–3, 205
 research 205, 209–11

biophilia thesis 93–4

biopsychosocial model 56, 58

birth weight 167–8

births, registrations of 235

Births and Deaths Registration Act 1874 237

Black Report on Inequalities in Health 15, 71

body mass index (BMI) 360–1, 363–4

Boolean searching 220–1

breastfeeding 166

Breathing Space, Edinburgh 139

Bristol Pregnancy and Domestic Violence Programme 114

British Medical Association (BMA) 15

British Social Attitudes (BSA) survey 260

bullying 180–1

cancer 256, 366

cancer registers 248

capacity building 140, 306, 307, 319–21

Care and Repair England 119

carers, children as 173

caring 292

Cartesian dualism 44

case-control studies 255–6

causal variables 254–5

cause-specific death rates 242

causes of death 237

census, national 232–5

Central Board of Health 11

Central Council for Health Education 13

Centre for Public Health Excellence 106, 216

Chadwick Report 68

Chamberlain, Joseph 11–12

change agents 146

Chicago Southeast Diabetes Community Action Coalition 141

childbirth 50, 201

childhood 163–4

Children Act 2004 176

children and young people 27–8, 163–93

cancers in adolescent girls 256

diversity, inequalities and health 167–9

health education in early 20th century 13

health and illness 172–7

healthy child 165–6

injury prevention 177–80

mental health promotion in schools 180–2

obesity 94, 166, 357, 359, 363–4, 374

politics of health of 165–77

promoting health of 177–89

reasons to focus on health of 169–72

road safety 108

sexual health 182–9, 290

in a social context 163–5

Stepping Out programme 280–1

Children's Centres 118, 178

Children's Commissioner 176

Children's Research Centre 173–4

Children's Trusts 176–7

China 140

chlamydia 246, 247, 254

choice 83–5

cholera 240

Choosing Health: Making Healthier Choices Easier 20, 73, 91, 110–11, 112, 121, 297–8, 362, 377–8

citizenship 2–5

clarity 292

client-centred approach 151–2, 336

clustering of health risk 171

Cochrane Centre 301, 302

Cochrane Library 216, 302

codes of ethics 29

coherence 227

sense of 49–50

cohort studies 256

collaborative working 117–18

combining search terms 220–1

Commission for Patient and Public Involvement in Health (CPPIH) 120

communication theories 143–50

communicative resonance 292, 293

community 54–5

community action 16, 179

community change theories 138–43

community competence 142

community development 139, 155–7, 342

community empowerment 17

community farm and café project 379

community networks 72, 85–8

community participation 209

community profiling 314–15

community public health nurse 22

Community Strategy 110

comparative needs 309–10

complementary and alternative medicine 56, 276

comprehensiveness 207

conscientisation 206–7

consent 165, 288

consumer involvement 312–13, 315

contribution 292

control, locus of 83

Convention on the Rights of the Child 182

coping 49–50

coronary heart disease (CHD) 80

cost-benefit analysis (CBA) 344–5

cost-effectiveness analysis (CEA) 344–5

Coventry 4–5

  specialist service for pregnant teenagers and young parents 308–9, 310, 312–13, 317, 320, 321–2, 337–8, 340–1, 343, 349

credibility 292

criteria for evaluation 339–45

critical consciousness 142

critical evaluation 346

critical perspectives 212–13, 279

cross-sectional studies 255

crude death rates 241

cultural perspectives 213–14, 280

culture 200, 357

and regulation of sexuality 184–5

and smoking in children 172

street culture 276, 280, 285, 293

data analysis 288–91

data collection

  qualitative research 286–8

  quantitative research 217–23

Data Protection Act 1998 233

databases 216

death certificates 235–9

deaths, registration of 235–9

decision making, ethical 29–30

Deeside, Scotland 46

demography 231, 231–9

  census 232–5

  registration systems 235–9

Department for Communities and Local Government 105

Department for Culture, Media and Sport (DCMS) 384

Department for Environment, Food and Rural Affairs (DEFRA) 105, 108

Department of Health (DoH) 105, 280, 301, 384

  Chief Medical Officer's section of website 217

  'flu jab campaign 135

Department for Transport (DfT) 108

depression 93, 364

descriptive epidemiology 247–52

developing countries 7, 164, 251, 357

devolution 108–9

diabetes 358, 359–60

diffusion of innovations 145–6

Directors of Public Health 21, 112

disability

obesity and 365
    regulation of sexuality 184–5
discourse 47, 201, 286
disease 41–3
    changing patterns over time 51
    health as absence of 43–4
    measures of disease frequency 245–7
dissemination 348–50
distributive justice 28–9
diversity 10, 167–9, 170
doctors 29, 114–15, 256
domestic violence 114
downstream determinants of health 52–3, 72
Dreams Art and Health Project 339
drug education campaign 145
drug trials 257
Dudley LEAP project 382–3
Duncan, William Henry 11

Earth Summit 1992 94
economic empowerment 207
Economic and Social Research Council
(ESRC) 204, 224, 280
education 86–7, 104, 117
    see also health education
effectiveness 339, 339–42
efficiency 339, 344–5
emotional literacy 182
employers 122–3
employment 5–6, 384
empowerment 16–17, 142, 152–3, 203, 207
end in itself, health as 5–7
energy efficiency 120
English Regions Network 109
environment 11–12, 68, 69–70, 71
    children's health 169, 170

general socio-economic and environmental
    conditions 72, 92–5
    living and working conditions 72, 88–92
    supportive environments 16, 18, 179
environmental health action 94–5
environmental health practitioners (EHPs)
112–14
epidemiological triad 253–5, 373
epidemiology 48, 131–2, 231, 239–59
    analytic 253–5
    descriptive 247–52
    early studies 240–1
    morbidity statistics 245–7
    mortality statistics 241–5
    types of epidemiological studies 255–9
Epilepsy Action 'Take Control Campaign' 83
epistemology 204
equity 28, 339, 343–4
ethical grid 29–30
ethics 24–30, 113–14
    planning interventions 322–3
    principles of ethical research 224
    qualitative research 284–6
ethnicity
    birth weight and 167–8
    genetics and health 76–7
    and obesity measurement 363
    and wealth 75
ethnographic research 280, 286
Europe, obesity levels in 357, 358
evaluation 306, 307–8, 327–53
    changing policy and practice 348–50
    checklist for planning 335
    criteria 339–45
    cycle 329
    design 335–9

information found in search 223
pluralist methodology 338–9
reasons for 330–1
of research 226–7, 262–3, 291–4
types of 332–4
values and 345–8
who should evaluate 331–2
Every Child Matters 176, 186
Every Child Matters: Change for Children 176–7
Every Child Matters: Next Steps 176
evidence 23–4
in planning 300–3, 304
evidence-based obesity action 371–2
evidence-based resources 216, 219
Evidence for Policy and Practice Information and Co-ordinating Centre (EPPI-Centre) 301
exchange 147
experimental approach 256–8, 336
Expert Patients' Programme 60
expressed needs 311
external evaluators 331–2

factors affecting health 70–3, 76–95
age, sex and heredity 72, 76–81
general social and environmental conditions 72, 92–5
individual lifestyle 72, 81–5
living and working conditions 72, 88–92
social and community networks 72, 85–8
family 120, 121
Fazil study on advocacy for Asian families with disabled children 275, 279, 284–5, 292
fear-arousing messages 144–5
felt needs 311
feminist perspectives on obesity 364–5
Ffaldau Farm, Wales 379

5 A Day programme 377, 378
5Cs 292
Flowers study of gay men's relationships 275, 279, 284, 288, 289, 293
focus groups 287, 314, 317
foetal programming 74, 169
food 94, 174
and prevention of obesity 376–80
food poverty 379–80
Food in Schools Programme 378–9
Food Standards Agency (FSA) 106
formative evaluation 332, 333, 336
formula milk 166
Forthview Primary School, Edinburgh 182
Framework Convention on Tobacco Control 103
freedom 4–5
Freire, P. 17, 141–2, 206–7
fuel poverty 81
'fully engaged' scenario 20, 107
funding proposals 321

Game Plan strategy 383
gatekeepers 283, 287
gay men's relationships 275, 279, 284, 289, 293
gender 6
hazardous drinking 249–50
regulation of sexuality 185
sex, gender and health 79–80
General Household Survey (GHS) 259, 260
General Practice Research Database 248
generalisability 227
generic workers 57
genetic testing 25–6
geneticisation 77–9
genetics 69–70, 76–9

genital herpes simplex 247

geography of disease patterns 250–1

gonorrhoea 247

government, role of 261

grey literature 215

health 37–65

    changing understandings of 67–9

    defining by children and young people 172–7

    definitions 2, 41–6

    determinants of 71–2

    factors affecting *see* factors affecting health

    key concepts 39, 40

    means to an end vs end in itself 5–7

    models and approaches 46–60

    politics of child health 165–72

    as a right 3

    self-reported 235, 236, 260

Health Action Model 137–8

Health Action Zones 119, 120, 138, 142

Health Belief Model 133–4, 137

'Health Challenge Wales' 73

health consciousness 5–7

health development 8, 9

Health Development Agency (HDA) 105–6

health–ease–disease continuum 49, 50

health education 9, 82, 151–2, 319

    models of health promotion 152–5

    and obesity 377

    rise of in early twentieth century 12–14

Health Education Authority (HEA) 15, 106

Health Education Council (HEC) 13–14, 15

Health at Every Size Movement 366

health field concept 15, 69–70

Health for All by the Year 2000 2, 16

health forums 314

Health Impact Assessment (HIA) 280–1

health improvement 8, 9

health inequalities 70–6

    contemporary explanations 73–6

health information sources 215–17, 300–2

    identifying appropriate source 219

Health and Lifestyles Survey 38–9

Health of the Nation: A Strategy for Health in England 71, 110

health persuasion 144, 155–7

health policy 9

health professionals 114–16

health promotion 8, 9, 16–19, 319

    drivers of 23–4

    guiding principles 54

    models of 151–7

    values in 22–3

Health Promotion Agency for Northern Ireland 106, 301

health promotion specialists (HPSs) 115–16

Health Promotion Teams 111–12

health protection 9, 28, 153–5

Health Protection Agency (HPA) 106, 247

health scares 118–19

Health Scotland 106, 109, 301

health services 17, 69–70, 179

Health Survey for England (HSFE) 259, 260

health surveys 231, 259–68, 273, 282, 337

    characteristics of 262–3

    critical views of 266–8

    questions 264–6

    sampling 263–4

    scope 260–2

Health 21 2

health visitors 12, 13, 22

'Health, Work and Wellbeing Strategy' 91

healthy ageing (positive ageing) 80–1

Healthy Cities projects 53–4

Healthy Living Centres 142

healthy public policy 9, 16, 18, 179

Healthy Respect 188

heart disease 80, 130–1

Helsinki Declaration on medical ethics 257

heredity 72, 76–81

HIV/AIDS 82, 175, 240, 250, 303

holistic approach to health 56–8

homophobia 181, 184

hospital episode statistics 248

housing 53, 117

Human Genome Project (HGP) 76–9

humanist approach 157

iatrogenesis 52

Illawarra Healthy Cities project 53–4

illness 41–3
  changing understandings of 67–9
  and metaphor 366
  see also disease

immigrant populations 251

implementation 306, 307, 321–2

incidence rates 245–6

income inequality 74–5, 75–6

individual empowerment 17

individuals
  responsibility for health 3–4, 68
  see also behaviour; lifestyle

industry, working with 377–8

inequalities
  global and child health 167–9, 170
  health 70–6

infant feeding 166

infant mortality rate (IMR) 167, 241–2

infectious diseases 5, 12, 51, 251–2

informal public health workers 119–23

information search 217–23
  sources of health information 215–17

informed consent 288

injury prevention, childhood 177–80

innovations, diffusion of 145–6

insecticide-treated bed nets 277–8

internal evaluators 331–2

International Classification of Diseases, Injuries and Causes of Death (ICD) index 41, 237

International Covenant on Economic, Social and Cultural Rights 1–2

International Monetary Fund (IMF) 7, 105

International Obesity Task Force (IOTF) 363, 370–1

international organisations 7, 103–5
  see also under individual names

internet 114, 203

interpersonal communication 148–50

interpretive phenonmenological analysis (IPA) 279, 289

interpretivism 212

intervention studies 256–8

interview schedules 264–6

interviews 282, 286–7, 317

Intute website 217

inverse care law 89

issue selection 142

Japanese population in the USA 251

journals 216

justice 2–3, 28–9

key informants 313

key words 219–20

King's Fund Public Attitudes to Public Health Policy survey 3–4, 261

knowledge

bodies of 200–1
knowledge base of research 201–4
knowledge sharing 207–8

Lalonde Report 15, 67, 69–70, 95
language 150, 313
lay beliefs 58
lay epidemiology 59, 206
lay experts 59–60
lay knowledge 58–9, 201–2
lay people
    accounts of health 58–60
    concepts of health 38–9
    experiences and social model 52–4
    informal public health workers 119–23
lay research 205–9
legislative action 155–7
leisure services staff 117
life expectancy 79
lifecourse 74
    age and 80–1
    childhold disadvantage and adult health
    169, 171
lifestyle 69–70, 130–1
    factors and health 72, 81–5
limiting scope of research 221
listening 149–50
Liverpool Stepping Out programme 280–1
living and working conditions 72, 88–92
lobbying 121–2
local authorities 110–11
Local Exercise Action Pilots (LEAPs) 382–3
local food projects 379–80
Local Involvement Networks (LINks) 120
local organisations 110–12
Local Strategic Partnerships (LSPs) 110
local voices, listening to 313–17

locality development 140
locus of control 83
Long Hours Working Partnership Project 92
long-term conditions 5, 116, 117
longitudinal studies 234, 256
looked after children 183–4

madness 213–14
male youth street culture 276, 280, 285, 293
managerial evaluation 345–6
marketing 147
    food 377–8
    social 147–8, 381–2
mass media see media
means to an end, health as 5–7
media 118–19
    campaigns to promote physical activity
    381–2
    mass media communication 144–5
    representations of obesity 367–8
media advocacy 119
medical approaches 151–2, 336
medical assistance, factors in seeking 42–3
medical model of health 47–9, 67, 69, 130–1
    social model and 55–6
medical officers of health (MOHs) 11
Medical Research Council (MRC) 204, 280
medicalisation 51–2, 201, 367
medicine
    and public health 48–9
    see also doctors
mental health 41–2, 213–14
    children's views 175–6
    environment and 93
    promoting positive mental health in schools
    180–2
    surveys 248

metabolic syndrome 357–8, 359

metaphor 366

methodology 278–80

  pluralist and evaluation 338–9

miasma theory 68

midwives 114–15

models

  of health 46–60

  of health promotion 151–7

  planning models 305–8

modern multidisciplinary public health *see* public health

monitoring 334

morbidity statistics 245–7, 247–8

mortality statistics 235–7, 241–5

mosquito nets 277–8

multidisciplinary public health *see* public health

National Advisory Committee on Nutritional Education (NACNE) 15

national census 232–5

national director for occupational health 91

National Food Survey 259

National Health Service (NHS)

  Centre for Reviews and Dissemination 301

  introduction of 69

  local organisations promoting public health 111–12

National Healthy Schools Programme 180, 378

National Institute for Health and Clinical Excellence (NICE) 106, 216, 301

National Library for Public Health 215

National Obesity Forum 361, 362

national organisations 105–10

National School Fruits Scheme 377, 378

National Service Framework for Children, Young People and Maternity Services 177

National Service Framework for Older People 117

National Statistics Online 216–17

National Statistics Socioeconomic Classification (NS-SEC) 232–3

National Teenage Pregnancy Strategy 183, 308–9

nature, domains of 93–4

needs assessment 305, 306–7, 308–13

  listening to local voices 313–17

  single assessment process 117

Neighbourhood Statistics 217

neo-materialist explanations 74–6, 92

neonatal mortality rates 242

networks 72, 85–8, 119–23

New Labour 72–3

'new' public health movement 9, 15–16

Newsholme Report 13

NHS Direct 203

NHS Plan 120

non-governmental organisations (NGOs) 105

non-maleficence 25–6

non-random sampling 264

normative models 151–5

normative needs 309

norms 134

Northern Ireland 60, 108–9, 117, 177, 339

  children and smoking 172

  Speakeasy project 188

Northern Ireland Assembly 108, 109

notifiable diseases 248–9

nurses 114–15

Nursing and Midwifery Council 21–2

nutrition 174, 376–80

obesity 94, 213, 303, 355–89
    approaches to treating and preventing 369–84
    biomedical classification 360–3
    children and young people 94, 166, 357, 359, 363–4, 374
    cost of 356
    evidence-based action 371–2
    food and prevention 376–80
    physical activity and prevention 381–4
    public health issue 355–60
    representing and experiencing 367–9
    social science understandings 364–7
    views of professionals working in the obesity field 374–6
objectives 299
    evaluation and 339–42
    setting 318–19
objectivity 210–11, 223
Office for National Statistics (ONS) 235, 237, 259, 260
Office for Population Censuses and Surveys (OPCS) longitudinal study 234
'old' public health 9, 11–14
older people 57, 92
    Beattie's model of health promotion 156
    causes of death 239
    fuel poverty 81
    income polarisation 80–1
    medical care and social care 117
Organisation for Economic Co-operation and Development (OECD) 238
Ottawa Charter for Health Promotion 16–18, 19, 28, 46, 70, 103, 179
Our Health, Our Care, Our Say 117
outcome evaluation 332, 333–4, 336
overweight 361
    public health issue 355–60

representing and experiencing 367–9
    see also obesity

paradigm shift 210
parent/teacher associations (PTAs) 86–7
parents, and sex education 187–8
participant observation 280, 287–8
participation 10, 120–1, 142, 177
participatory action research (PAR) 274, 288, 290
participatory appraisal 315–16
participatory evaluation 346–8
participatory research 206–9
Partnership for Care 110–11
Patient Advice and Liaison Service (PALS) 120–1
Patient and Public Involvement (PPI) forums 120
Pavis and Cunningham-Burley study of youth street culture 276, 280, 285, 293
Peckham Health Centre 68
peer-led SRE 186
perceived behavioural control 134
period prevalence rate 247
perinatal mortality rates 242
personal characteristics 249–50
personal counselling 155–7
personal hygiene era 12–14
personal skills, developing 16, 17, 179
personal, social and health education (PSHE) 186–7
personal trainers 121
pertussis (whooping cough) 251–2
pharmacists 116
phenomenological research 279, 286, 289
philosophy 278–80
physical activity 87, 381–4
planned behaviour, theory of 134–5

planned interventions 302–3, 304

planning document 322

planning interventions 297–326

   assessing need 305, 306–7, 308–13

   capacity building 306, 307, 319–20

   developing funding proposals 321

   developing needs assessment 308–17

   developing proposals for interventions 321

   evidence in planning 300–3, 304

   implementation 306, 307, 321–2

   listening to local voices 313–17

   reasons for planning 299–300

   setting aims and objectives 318–19

   setting priorities 317–18

   terminology 299

   using theory and models in 303–8

planning models 305–8

pluralist theories of community change 141

point prevalence rate 247

police officers 117

policy 299

   evaluation and changing 348–50

   public involvement in policy process 121–2

   qualitative research and 277

polio elimination programme 103

political empowerment 207

poor health, effects of 5–6

Population Act 1840 232

population at risk 239

   see also epidemiology

positivism 211–12

postal questionnaires 266, 313

postmodernism 209, 214, 346

poverty 6, 15, 68, 71, 74

power 4

   approaches to community work 141–2

   critical research and 213

   knowledge and 201

   medical model of health 47–8

   qualitative research and 284

Powys Sure Start Programme 347–8

practice

   evaluation and changing 348–50

   qualitative research and 277

presenteeism 91

prevalence rates 246–7

prevention 9

   Tannahill model of health promotion 153–5

Prevention and Health: Everybody's Business 14, 70

prevention paradox 310

priority setting 317–18

private sector 123

problem definition 305, 306–7

   see also needs assessment

process evaluation 332, 333–4, 336

professional groups 112–18

programme planning 132

promoters of public health 101–28

   agencies 102–12

   informal public health workers 119–23

   people involved 101–2

   professional groups 112–18

   role of the media 118–19

Promoting Better Health 71

proposals for interventions 321

prostate cancer 25–6

psychiatric morbidity 248

psychological empowerment 207

psycho-social explanations 73–4, 88

public, conceptualising 10

public consultation 10

public health

   ethical issues in promoting 24–30

medicine and 48–9

origins of modern multidisciplinary public health 7–22

rationale for promoting 1–7

values 22–4

Public Health Act 1848 11

Public Health Departments 111, 247

public health genetics 78

Public Health Observatories (PHOs) 109, 217

public health practitioners 20

public health specialists 20, 115

public health workforce 20

values 22–3

Public Service Agreements (PSAs) 107–8

public service workers 117, 122

purposive sampling 264

qualitative research 48, 224–6, 268, 273–96, 337

aims in public health 274, 275–6

choosing between approaches 278–83

collecting data 286–8

combining qualitative and quantitative methods 268, 280–3, 316–17, 338–9

competing methodologies 278–80

contribution to public health 274–8

data analysis 288–91

early planning 283–6

evaluating 291–4

process 283–91

quality of life 261–2

quantitative research 48, 224–6, 231–71, 273

combining quantitative and qualitative methods 268, 280–3, 316–17, 338–9

demography 231, 231–9

epidemiology 48, 131–2, 231, 239–59

health surveys 231, 259–68, 273, 282, 337

quasi-experimental design 258, 337

questionnaires 264–6, 313

questions

communication and 149

formulating in information search 218–19

health surveys 264–6

radical humanist approach 157

radical structuralist approach 157

radical theories of community change 141–2

random sampling 264

randomised controlled trials (RCTs) 256–8, 336

rapid appraisal 315

reactive interventions 302–3, 304

realist approach 283

reasoned action, theory of 134–5

reflexivity 289–91

refugee children 181

Regional Assemblies 109–10

Regional Development Agencies (RDAs) 109

regional organisations 105–10

Registrar General 232

registration systems 235–9

relativist approach 283

relevance 142, 223

reliability 226, 263, 291

replicability 263

Report of the Chief Medical Officer's Project to Strengthen the Public Health Function 20

representativeness 263

research 199–229

biomedical research 205, 209–11

bodies of knowledge 200–1

children as social researchers 173–4

knowledge base of 201–4

lay research 205–9

process see research process

and promoting public health 204–15
    social science research 205, 211–15
research ethics committees 257, 284
research process 215–27
    criteria for assessing findings 226–7
    information search 217–23
    questions about data and sources 223–4
    research design 224–6
research proposals 321
researcher participation, degree of 287
resource, health as a 46
resource allocation 3
responsibilities 3–5
responsive interventions 302–3, 304
rhetoric 58
rights 2–3
    health as a right 3
    and responsibilities 3–5
risk 134
    children's understanding of health and 175
    clustering of health risk 171
    of health problems and obesity 357–60
role models 121, 135, 144
Royal College of Midwives (RCM) Campaign
for Normal Birth 50

salutogenesis 49–50
sampling 263–4
sampling frames 264
sanitation phase 11–12
Saving Lives: Our Healthier Nation 73, 110
schools
    promoting positive mental health 180–2
    sex education 186–7
Schoolwatch 180–1
scientific method 209–11, 240
Scotland 60, 108–9, 116, 177, 188

bullying and refugee children 181
    Healthy Respect initiative 188
    media campaigns against obesity 381–2
    STDs 247
Scottish Health Education Group 15
Scottish Parliament 108, 109
screening 25–6, 45, 57–8
seamless care 117
self-advocacy 206
self-help strategies 206
sense of coherence 49–50
settings approach 87, 138–9
sex 72, 76–81
    gender, health and 79–80
sex and relationships education (SRE)
186–9
sexual health promotion 182–9
sexuality, regulation of 184–5
Shaping the Future of Public Health 115–16
sickness 41–3
sickness absence 90–1
significant others 121, 135
Simon, John 11
Skills for Health 20–1
SMART objectives 318, 341
smoking 82, 256
    ban on 122
    bodies of knowledge and 200–1
    children and young people 172
    link with lung cancer 240, 256
    prevalence 83, 84
    rights and 4–5
    women and 88, 138
Snow, John 240
snowball sampling 264
social action 141
social capital 85–7, 119, 212

social care, holism and 56–7
social care workers 116–17
social causation of health and illness 51, 203
social class 167, 232–3
social construction of health 51, 203–4
social desirability 267
social exclusion 72, 87–8
Social Exclusion Unit 88, 88–9, 308, 309
social isolation 6
social justice 2–3
social marketing 147–8, 381–2
social model of health 50–6, 67, 205
    compared with holistic approaches 56
    criticisms of 54–6
social networks 72, 85–8
social planning 139
social science
    knowledge 201–2, 203–4
    research 205, 211–15
    understandings of obesity 364–7
social selection 71
social work, basic values of 29
socialist theories of community change 141–2
societal change approach 151–2
socio-environmental approach 72, 92–5, 130–1
solution generation 305, 307, 317–19
Speakeasy project 188
specialist community public health nurse 22
Stages of Change Model 135–6
stakeholders 319–20
standardisation 262–3, 267
Standardised Mortality Ratios (SMR) 243–5
Stepping Out programme 280–1
stereotypes 185, 310
stigma 365
stratified random sampling 264

street culture 276, 280, 285, 293
street-level bureaucrats 122
structural adjustment programmes (SAPs) 7, 105
Sudan 6
suicide rates 237–8
summative evaluation 332, 333–4, 336
Sundsvall Statement on Supportive Environments for Health 94
supermarkets 380
Sure Start 46, 138, 142
    Children's Centres 118, 178
    injury prevention 178
    programme evaluation 347–8, 349–50
Surrey County Council 183–4
surveillance medicine 17–18, 57–8
surveys see health surveys
sustainability 94
synonyms 220
systematic information search 222
systems thinking 138–9

teenage pregnancy 183
    Coventry special services project 308–9, 310, 312–13, 317, 320, 321–2, 337–8, 340–1, 343, 349
Teenage Pregnancy Partnership Board (TPPB) 312, 320
teleworking 282
Tescopoly Alliance 380
thematic analysis 288–9
theory 129–61
    behaviour change in individuals 132–8
    communication theories 143–50
    community change theories 138–43
    defining theory 131–2
    models of health promotion 151–7
    understanding theory 129–32

use in planning 303–8
time 251–2
Tower Hamlets 6
trade unions 123
traditional approach to health promotion 157
transport 384
Transtheoretical Model 135–6
Travelling Tutor scheme 46
Treasury 107–8
triangulation 226, 282, 334
Tripartite Group 20–1
trust in healthcare staff 114–15
trustworthiness of research 291–3
Turkey education project 104

unintentional injury prevention 177–80
United Kingdom Public Health Association (UKPHA) 107
United Kingdom Voluntary Register for Public Health Specialists (UKVRPS) 21, 115
United Nations 250
    Agenda 21 94, 111
    Convention on the Rights of the Child (UNCRC) 182
    Earth Summit 1992 94
    International Covenant on Economic, Social and Cultural Rights 1-2
    Universal Declaration of Human Rights 1
United States (USA) 251
Universal Declaration of Human Rights 1
upstream determinants of health 52–3, 72
urban spaces 384
user groups 206
user involvement 10, 120–1, 142, 177
utilitarianism 25–6, 210

validity 226, 263, 291
values 22–4

ethics 24–30
    and evaluation 345–8
VERB campaign 381
voluntary sector 119–23
voluntary visiting movement 12

waist circumference 361
Waist Watch Action 361, 362
Wales 108, 379
    Schoolwatch 180–1
    SMRs for cities 243
Wanless Reports 20, 107, 297
wealth 74–5
weight loss programmes 370
wellbeing, health as 44–5
Wellbeing in Wales 44, 110–11
Welsh Assembly 106, 108
wider public health workforce 20
women
    and autonomy 27
    and family health 121
    feminist perspectives on obesity 364
    and smoking 88, 138
    Stepping Out and young women 280–1
work/life balance 91–2
'Work–Life Balance Campaign' 92
working and living conditions 72, 88–92
World Bank 7, 104, 105, 217
World Health Organization (WHO) 18, 103, 138, 217
    Bangkok Charter 18–19, 123
    definition of health 2, 44, 45
    Diet, Nutrition and the Prevention of Chronic Diseases 376–7
    Framework Convention on Tobacco Control 103
    Global School Health Initiative 180
    Health for All 2, 16

Health 21 2
Healthy Cities Programme 53–4
infant feeding guidelines 166
obesity 360, 361, 363
Ottawa Charter 16–18, 19, 28, 46, 70, 103, 179
sexual health 182
Sundsvall Statement 94

World Trade Organization (WTO) 103, 104

X-perience projects 183–4

Young Carers' Initiative 173
young people *see* children and young people
Your Region, Your Choice 110
youth street culture 276, 280, 285, 293